COMPREHENSIVE GUIDE
TO INTERPERSONAL
PSYCHOTHERAPY

COMPREHENSIVE GUIDE TO INTERPERSONAL PSYCHOTHERAPY

MYRNA M. WEISSMAN, PH.D.,
JOHN C. MARKOWITZ, M.D., AND
GERALD L. KLERMAN, M.D.

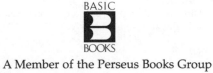

BASIC
BOOKS

A Member of the Perseus Books Group

Published by Basic Books,
A Member of the Perseus Books Group

Library of Congress Cataloging-in-Publication Data
Weissman, Myrna M.
   Comprehensive guide to interpersonal psychotherapy / Myrna Weissman, John C. Markowitz, and Gerald L. Klerman.
      p.   cm.
   Includes bibliograpical references and index.
   ISBN 0-465-09566-6
   1. Psychotherapy and patient.   2. Psychotherapy.   I. Markowitz, John C., 1954–   II. Klerman, Gerald L., 1928–   III. Title.
   [DNLM: 1. Depressive Disorder—therapy.   2. Interpersonal Relations.   3. Mental Disorders—therapy.   4. Psychotherapy—methods.   WM 171 W652c 1999]
   RC480.8.W445   1999
   616.89'14—dc21   99-046469

00 01 02 03 / 10 9 8 7 6 5 4 3

To Gerald L. Klerman
Loving and wise
A mind of crystal clarity

Gerald L. Klerman was ahead of his time. Mentor of Dr. Weissman (his wife) and Dr. Markowitz, he was convinced that interpersonal relationships importantly influenced the course and recurrence of illness, and that psychotherapy could potentially stabilize interpersonal relations. Gerry was the force behind the original ideas in the first Interpersonal Psychotherapy (IPT) manual (Klerman et al., 1984) and many of its adaptations. Yet his vision could not have anticipated the great interest in IPT that has developed since then.

Gerry died in April 1992. Even years after his death, his influence on IPT is pervasive. Out of respect for his contribution to the therapy, we are proud to name him a posthumous author of this book.

Contents

Preface   xi

Overview of IPT   1

PART I:
CONDUCTING INTERPERSONAL
PSYCHOTHERAPY OF DEPRESSION

1   An Outline of IPT   19

2   The Initial Phase   27

3   Grief (Complicated Bereavement)   61

4   Interpersonal Role Disputes   75

5   Role Transitions   89

6   Interpersonal Deficits   103

7   Termination of Treatment   117

8   Specific Techniques   123

9   Common Problems   139

10   Efficacy Data for Acute Treatment of Major Depression   163

PART II:
ADAPTATION OF IPT FOR MOOD DISORDERS

Introduction   173

11   Maintenance IPT for Recurrent Major Depression (IPT-M)   175

12   IPT for Dysthymic Disorder (IPT-D)   185

13   IPT for Depressed Adolescents (IPT-A)   195

14   IPT for Late-Life Depression   213

15   Conjoint Treatment for Depressed Patients with
     Marital Disputes (IPT-CM)   223

16   Bipolar Disorder   267

17   Primary-Care and Mentally Ill Patients   279

18   IPT for Depressed HIV-Positive Patients (IPT-HIV)   289

19   Depressed Ante- and Postpartum Patients   299

PART III:
ADAPTATION OF IPT FOR NON-MOOD DISORDERS

20   Substance Use Disorders   311

21   Eating Disorders: Bulimia and Anorexia Nervosa   317

22   Anxiety Disorders   329

23   Applications in Progress   341

PART IV:
IPT RESOURCES

24   IPT in New Formats: Group, Telephone, Patient Guide;
     Translation and Use in Other Languages and Cultures   361

25   Training and Treatment Manuals   375

PART V:
THE FUTURE OF IPT

The Future of IPT   395

Appendix: An Integrative Case Example   403
Literature References   435
Index   453

Preface

Interpersonal Psychotherapy (IPT) was first developed as a time-limited research treatment for depression by the late Gerald L. Klerman, M.D., Myrna Weissman, Ph.D., and colleagues. Since its efficacy has been demonstrated in numerous controlled clinical trials, IPT has been modified to treat different types of mood and non-mood disorders. These research advances, together with the ascendancy of managed care and its concern to reduce mental health costs, have accelerated clinical interest in IPT techniques and applications.

The idea underlying IPT is simple: psychiatric syndromes such as depression, however multidetermined their causes, usually occur in a social and interpersonal context. A marriage breaks up; a friendship dissolves; children leave home; a job is lost; a loved one dies; a person moves, is promoted, or retires. In IPT, patients learn (1) to understand the relationship between the onset and fluctuation in their symptoms and what is currently going on in their life—their current interpersonal problems—and (2) to find ways of dealing with the interpersonal problems, and thereby with the depressive symptoms.

IPT was first described in *Interpersonal Psychotherapy of Depression* by Gerald L. Klerman, Myrna M. Weissman, Bruce J. Rounsaville, and Eve S. Chevron (Basic Books, 1984). Since then, it has become a growth industry. Accordingly, what began as a modest revision of that book has matured into a comprehensive guide. It opens with an overview and outline of IPT's theoretical framework and strategies, which were designed specifically for the treatment of major depression in outpatients. This core application is then elaborated more fully than in the 1984 manual, with added case material. The clinical scripts assume the general clinical competence of the psychotherapist and must be used judiciously. Cases have been disguised or consolidated to preserve patient confidentiality.

Part I of the book describes the heart of the approach and is required reading for anyone wanting to learn IPT. The subsequent chapters present adaptations or new uses of this basic method. Parts II and III introduce adaptations of the core approach, in various stages of development, for treating mood disorders in different age groups, settings, and special populations, and for non-mood disorders. The rest of the book covers a wide range of resources for the spectrum of professionals who practice IPT: new therapeutic formats, treatment manuals, international references, history, and training procedures.

As this work has evolved over our professional lives, there are many people who contributed to it, including Bruce Rounsaville and Eve Chevron, who participated in writing the 1984 book, and the many IPT therapists and researchers who kept supplying us with their ongoing work. We are also grateful to the universities that supported us as scientists—Harvard and Cornell University Medical Schools, Yale University, and the Columbia University College of Physicians and Surgeons—and to the New York State Psychiatric Institute. We thank the government and private agencies that provided funds to carry out different studies: the National Institute of Mental Health; the National Institute of Drug Abuse; the Anne Lederer Pollack Foundation; the National Alliance for Research on Schizophrenia and Depression (NARSAD); the John D. and Catherine T. MacArthur Foundation; the Nancy Pritzker Foundation; and the fund established in The New York Community Trust by DeWitt-Wallace. We are especially grateful for the support received before we were established investigators and during periods when psychotherapy research was unfashionable.

Myrna M. Weissman, Ph.D.
John C. Markowitz, M.D.
New York, NY 1999

Overview of IPT

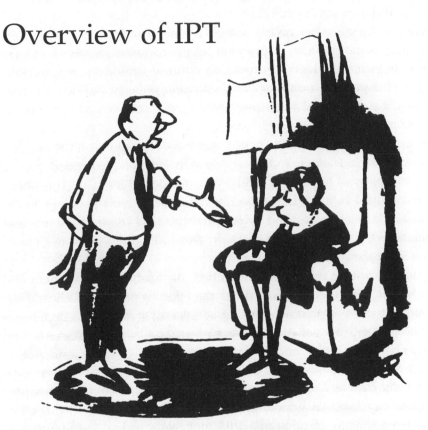

"I *do* like you. *You* don't like you!"
Drawing by Weber; © 1965
The New Yorker Magazine, Inc.

We begin with a description of major depression, as this was the starting point for IPT. The cartoon from *The New Yorker* illustrates many of the clinical features of depression. It is apparent that the woman is depressed. How do we know? Nonverbal and behavioral features convey her depressed state. She has a downcast gaze and a flattening of the nasolabial folds, depressive facial changes first described by Darwin. She sits slumped in her chair, a sign of "slowing down," or psychomotor retardation. She looks dowdy, reflecting the scant attention that depressed individuals pay to their dress and grooming. (On the other hand, she is not so paralyzed by her mood that she appears disheveled.)

That the depressed person is a woman is more than fortuitous: epidemiologic studies indicate that depression occurs more frequently in women than in men across diverse cultures. In addition, this woman is middle-aged, and depression occurs increasingly after puberty, peaking between the ages of eighteen and forty-four and declining somewhat in later years. This is probably not her first episode.

We also see that, although it is the woman who is depressed, the problem is a family affair. The man in the cartoon is irritated and frustrated. He has an air of futility as he says, "I *do* like you. *You* don't like you!" This observation captures an important aspect of the clinical phenomenology of depression: the fallen self-esteem, self-deprecation, and sense of helplessness, hopelessness, and worthlessness. Depressed individuals often negatively misinterpret the attitudes of others.

While the wife is depressed and sullen, the husband is impatient and even hostile. This precisely illustrates the effect of protracted clinical depression on interpersonal relationships. In the early stages of a depressive episode, patients may elicit sympathy, nurturance, and reassurance from family members, friends, and acquaintances. But if the depression is not resolved by what we may call "psychotherapy of everyday life," the response of those in the immediate environment tends to shift from support and encouragement to increasing irritation and frustration. At this point the patient is likely to be accused of "not really trying," of wanting to "make everybody miserable," or of "doing it to us on purpose." These pseudopsychological insights are usually expressed in a pejorative way, reflecting the frustration of those around the depressed person. This is a blaming of the patient for her illness rather than a scientific understanding of the complexities of the illness.

Let's reconstruct what might have happened to this couple. Over a number of months, the woman has slowly become depressed, perhaps after her children have left home and the "nest is empty." As part of the psychotherapy of everyday life, the husband has tried to reassure her and to provide optimism about the future. He has said, "I love you as much as when we first met," or "You are as beautiful as ever." These reassurances have evidently been of little avail. The wife continues to feel discouraged and worthless—depressed.

Thus far most clinicians and theorists would almost completely agree. However, depending upon theoretical orientation and training, a psychotherapist might conceptualize and intervene in this case in various ways. A strictly biological psychiatrist might interpret this picture as reflecting not psychological difficulty but altered neurotransmitter levels. The biological psychiatrist would invoke the medical model, label the patient as having a major depression, and might recommend treatment with an antidepressant medication. If that failed after six to eight weeks at adequate dosage, alternative medications might be considered or, if the depression were completely unresponsive to medication and the patient became more symptomatic, electroconvulsive therapy.

A psychoanalyst might interpret the patient's current situation as a reactivation of unresolved childhood difficulties and ambivalent identifications with the mother. Feelings of helplessness and hopelessness might be viewed as the response to inadequate mothering, most likely during the oral phase of psychosexual development. With the coming of menopause and the departure of the children, the patient experiences a loss of gratification from identification with the maternal role and regresses to early, oral, narcissistic stages of fixation. Perhaps psychoanalysis would be directed at uncovering childhood antecedents, particularly in the mothering relationship at the preoedipal phase, and working through the unresolved ambivalence toward the lost image of the idealized mother.

A practitioner of cognitive behavioral therapy (CBT) might note that the depression is producing distorted thoughts and perceptions of the patient's current situation. The patient believes these mood-congruent, irrational negative thoughts ("I'm worthless"; "Nothing ever goes right for me"; "Things are awful now, and will never get any better") and thus allows them to negatively influence her actions. If she can learn through homework to examine, test, and challenge the irrational thoughts, she may start to extinguish them and live her life again (Beck et al., 1979).

A family therapist might see this as a problem between husband and wife in the family system. Couples therapy would be recommended with the aim of improving communication between them and helping both partners to express their mutual frustrations and hostilities, in the hope that a new relationship would emerge.

A radical feminist therapist might say that the patient is not depressed but rather *oppressed*. Rather than seeing herself as ill, she should be encouraged to see her psychological state as reflective of the social position of women in a society dominated by male chauvinism. If she feels worthless and helpless, this is not a neurotic distortion of reality but rather a true perception of the low status of women. Without the childbearing role, she has no legitimate place in society. Lacking marketable skills, she is in fact worthless, and her feelings of helplessness reflect her inability to alter the power relationship between herself and her husband. Rather than needing medications or psychotherapy, she needs to become politically active and assertive, and perhaps independently employed outside the home.

These varied responses to the same clinical picture show the current diversity of psychiatry. There is no single, dominant school of American psychiatry, and no consensus on how best to regard the causes, prevention, and treatment of mental illnesses. Given this situation, how should the mental health professional proceed?

The authors believe that progress requires a pluralistic, undoctrinaire, and empirical approach that builds upon clinical experience and research evidence. Taking a pluralistic approach, we acknowledge the existence of multiple theoretical and clinical points of view; indeed, our work has been nurtured by them. We are convinced, however, that all theories and schools require evidence from testing, and that the most powerful evidence comes from carefully designed, well controlled investigative trials.

Treatment selection should consider a wide range of options—rather than simply the therapist's personal preference—and weigh the evidence for the likely efficacy of each: that is, treatment should be considered in the light of differential therapeutics (Frances, Clarkin, and Perry, 1984). Hundreds of different psychotherapies have been described, yet only a few have been tested and demonstrated to treat particular disorders. IPT and CBT are both proven approaches to treating major depression, as is antidepressant medication. We would have hoped that, in the interval between editions of this book, more therapists would have moved to such an outlook, but it remains unclear that this is the case. Too much therapy probably continues to be prescribed by therapists with a single approach to all comers.

Although many of its principles derive from the broader school of interpersonal psychotherapy, IPT is a psychological treatment originally designed specifically for the needs of depressed patients. It has since been modified for other disorders. IPT is a focused, time-limited psychotherapy that emphasizes the link between mood and the current interpersonal relations of the depressed patient while recognizing the roles of genetic, biochemical, developmental, and personality factors in the causation of and vulnerability to depression. IPT is not a causal explanation for depression, but a pragmatic treatment for it. We are convinced from clinical experience and research evidence that clinical depression occurs in an interpersonal context, and that acute psychotherapeutic interventions directed at this interpersonal context can facilitate the patient's recovery from an acute episode and possibly provide some preventive benefit against relapse and recurrence.

The first step in using IPT for depression successfully is to recognize just what depression is—making the distinction between normal and clinical depression, and observing the social, biological, and medical antecedents of clinical depression diagnosed through the use of a medical model. The original IPT book (Klerman et al., 1984) described in detail the then-current scientific understanding of depression and the empirical basis of treating it in an interpersonal context; the importance of attachment, bonding, stress, and interpersonal disputes in the development of depression; as well as the theoretical basis for IPT of depression, deriving from the interpersonal school of psychotherapy.

MAJOR DEPRESSION:
CURRENT UNDERSTANDING

The term *mood disorder* refers to a group of clinical conditions whose common feature is the patient's disturbed mood, which is either elated (in bipolar disorder) or depressed. This distinction does not imply a common etiology. Mood disorders are probably biologically heterogeneous, comparable in that sense to many medical presentations, such as jaundice. The major differentiation within mood disorders is between bipolar and "unipolar" depressive disorders; and, within the latter, between major depression and dysthymic disorder. IPT was originally developed to treat major depression. The characteristics of the other disorders are described with each adaptation.

The essential feature of major depression is either a dysphoric mood or loss of interest or pleasure in all or almost all usual activities and pastimes. The disturbance is prominent, persistent, and associated with other symptoms including appetite disturbance, change in weight, sleep disturbance, psychomotor agitation or retardation, decreased energy, feelings of worthlessness or guilt, difficulty in concentrating or thinking, indecisiveness, and thoughts of death or suicide, or suicide attempts. Major depression is only diagnosed in the absence of current or past manic symptoms (see Table 2–1 for DSM-IV criteria.) Although it is generally agreed that major depression is a heterogeneous disorder, there is no consensus on the utility of and little empirical basis for most of the subtypes in clinical use, such as endogenous, melancholic, and seasonal depression.

There is now considerable information about the rates of major depression from epidemiologic studies conducted in the 1980s across quite diverse cultures (Weissman et al., 1996). Studies conducted in the mainland United States, Canada, Puerto Rico, France, West Germany, Italy, Lebanon, Korea, and New Zealand all show convincingly that rates of depression are higher in women than in men, with an average twofold difference. Although rates of depression vary by country, its predominance in women is consistent across cultures. This finding has been replicated in studies conducted in the United States in the 1990s (Kessler et al., 1994).

These studies also show that the gender disparity in rates of the first onset of depression begins early, around thirteen to fifteen years of age, and persists throughout life. There is a peak in first onsets during the childbearing years and a decrease after age forty-five (Cross National Collaborative Group, 1992). There is no evidence for an increase in onset during the menopausal years. Longitudinal research suggests that depressed women have longer episodes of depression than men and a lower rate of spontaneous remission. The reasons for the sex differences in rates of depression are unclear (Wolk and Weissman, 1995). The epidemiological data support the importance of treating depression in the childbearing years, as the impact on offspring is enormous (Weissman and Olfson, 1995). There has been interest in adapting IPT for the treatment of depression during pregnancy and the postpartum period (see Chapter 19). Studies have also found an earlier age of onset of depression in more recent generations since World War II. Although women have had higher rates of depression than men in all countries, studies in the United States have suggested that, in recent decades, rates are increasing more rapidly in men.

Major depression is increasingly recognized as a worldwide source of morbidity, impairment, and health expenditures. The World Bank estimated that depression accounts for almost 30 percent of disability from neuropsychiatric disorders among women worldwide, but for only 12 percent among men (World Bank, 1993). The World Health Organization estimates that depression is currently the fourth leading cause of disability, surpassed only by respiratory infections, diarrheal diseases, and perinatal complications of women (Murray and Lopez, 1996). By the year 2020, depression is expected to be the second leading cause of disability.

Major advances in the treatment of depression have led to decreased hospitalization, reduced duration of episodes, and strategies to prevent relapse and recurrence. Most treatment for mood disorders is now ambulatory. Tricyclic antidepressants have been available for four decades, and the serotonin reuptake inhibitors for one. Their therapeutic value for both acute and maintenance treatment of depression is indisputable. There is excellent evidence that depressive symptoms can be reduced in two to four weeks of pharmacological treatment. Soon after antidepressant medications were introduced, however, investigators found that a high percentage of patients relapsed following short-term treatment. Continuation strategies then became common in clinical practice and were the subject of several research studies. The goals of continuation treatment are to sustain the remission brought about by acute treatment, to prevent relapse, and to facilitate social and vocational functioning. Beyond six to twelve months, treatment is considered maintenance or prophylaxis (see Chapter 11).

THEORETICAL AND EMPIRICAL SOURCES

We will briefly summarize the theoretical and empirical foundations of IPT. Among the founders of the interpersonal school were Adolf Meyer of Johns Hopkins University and his associate Harry Stack Sullivan. Meyer's psychobiological approach to understanding psychiatric disorders placed great emphasis on the patient's current psychosocial and interpersonal experiences, in distinction to the psychoanalytic focus on the past and the intrapsychic (Meyer, 1957). Sullivan, who linked clinical psychiatry to anthropology, sociology, and social psychology, viewed psychiatry as the scientific study of people and the processes that go on among them, rather than the exclusive study of the mind or of society. Sullivan popularized the term "interpersonal" as a balance to the then-dominant intrapsychic approach (Sullivan, 1953). In the interpersonal approach, the unit of observation and therapeutic intervention is the primary social group, the immediate face-to-face involvement of the patient with one or more significant others.

The IPT emphasis on interpersonal and social factors in the understanding and treatment of depression also draws on the work of many other clinicians, especially Fromm-Reichmann (1960), Cohen et al. (1954), and Arieti and Bemporad (1978). Becker (1974) and Chodoff (1970) also emphasized the social roots of depression and the need to attend to the interpersonal aspects of the disorder. Frank (1973) applied an interpersonal conceptualization to psychotherapy, stressing mastery of current interpersonal situations as an important component.

The interpersonal approach is specifically applied to understanding clinical depression, which we consider to have three component processes:

1. *Symptom function*: the development of depressive affect and the neurovegetative signs and symptoms (sleep and appetite disturbance, low energy, diurnal mood variation, etc.). These are presumed to have both biological and psychological precipitants.
2. *Social and interpersonal relations:* interactions in social roles with other persons derived from learning based on childhood experiences, concurrent social reinforcement, and personal mastery and competence.
3. *Personality and character problems:* enduring traits such as inhibited expression of anger or guilt, poor psychological communication with significant others, and difficulty with self-esteem. These traits determine a person's reactions to interpersonal experience. Personality patterns form part of the person's predisposition to depressive symptom episodes.

IPT intervenes in the first two of these three processes, symptom function and social and interpersonal relations. Because of its relatively brief duration and low level of psychotherapeutic intensity, there is little expectation that this treatment will have marked impact upon enduring aspects of personality structure, although personality functioning is assessed. On the other hand, many IPT patients gain new social skills that may help compensate for personality difficulties. Moreover, mood disorder and especially chronic mood disorder—dysthymic disorder—may mimic personality disorder. Thus personality disorder should not be prejudged in depressed patients: it is perilous to diagnose an Axis II disorder in the presence of an Axis I condition.

In our experience, most psychotherapies for depressed patients have paid insufficient attention to techniques directed at symptom reduction and amelioration of the patient's current social adjustment and interpersonal relations. IPT therapists do not attempt personality reconstruction. They rely upon well-established techniques such as reassurance, clarification of emotional states, improvement of interpersonal communication, and testing of perceptions and performance through interpersonal contact. Role-playing can provide important preparation for the patient making the life changes that will resolve the depressive episode.

Most of these techniques are conventionally grouped under the rubric of "supportive" psychotherapy. In our view, the term is a misnomer. Supportive psychotherapy has often been used as a loose, pejorative term to describe almost any psychotherapy that is not insight-oriented. Most formally "supportive" psychotherapies try to help patients adjust to their interpersonal relationships by building on existing defenses. They often aim to help patients accommodate to existing reality rather than try to help them change it.

IPT, on the other hand, intervenes with symptom formation, social adjustment and interpersonal relations, working predominantly on current problems and at conscious and preconscious levels. Although the IPT therapist may recognize unconscious factors, they are not directly addressed. The emphasis is on current disputes, frustrations, anxieties, and wishes as defined in the interpersonal context. IPT aims to help patients *change*, rather than simply to understand and accept their current life situation. The influence of early childhood experience is recognized as significant but not emphasized in the therapy. Rather, the work focuses on the "here and now." Overall treatment goals are to encourage mastery of current social roles and adaptation to interpersonal situations.

A key feature of IPT is that it approaches depression as a clinical disorder. Justifications for this are not only the widespread prevalence of depression but also the therapeutic importance of providing patients with a diagnostic label and legitimizing their assumption of the "sick role." This approach, which places IPT within the broad definition of the medical model, differs from that of many psychotherapists. In some of the psychotherapeutic community, although perhaps less so than in 1984, there remains an antidiagnostic bias and a tendency to depreciate symptoms.

IPT was based not only on theory but on empirical research on the psychosocial aspects of depression. There is evidence to support each of the three key interpersonal problem areas: that people become depressed in the contexts of complicated bereavement (Walker et al., 1977; Maddison and Walker, 1967; Maddison, 1968), marital disputes (Paykel et al., 1969; Pearlin and Lieberman, 1977), and the life changes encompassed by interpersonal role transitions (Overholser and Adams, 1997), particularly in the absence of social supports. Social supports—having intimate relationships, or even having a confidant to talk to—protect against depression (Henderson, 1977,

1979, 1981; Brown, Harris, and Copeland, 1977; Miller and Ingham, 1976; Prigerson et al., 1993). Early life events such as the death of a parent (Brown and Harris, 1978; Tennant, Bebbington, and Hurry, 1980), having a depressed parent (Weissman et al., 1997; Weiner et al., 1977), or poor parenting (Parker, 1979) can predispose to depression later in life, particularly when followed by later life stressors. Not only can life events trigger depression, but indeed the reverse clearly occurs as well. Once depressed, people have difficulty in communicating effectively (Coyne, 1976; Merikangas et al., 1979) as well as in generally handling their social roles, leading to strained relationships and adverse life events (Weissman and Paykel, 1974).

IPT COMPARED WITH OTHER PSYCHOTHERAPIES

IPT is not the only psychotherapeutic approach to treating depression. Several psychotherapies have been designed specifically for depressive disorders. Roth and Fonagy (1996) describe those psychotherapies with empirical support for treating depression. Both cognitive and behavioral approaches are similar to IPT in that they were developed specifically for depression, have been tested, and have been shown to be efficacious in randomized clinical trials. See Chapter 9 for a case illustration comparing IPT and different psychotherapies (see also Hamilton et al., in press).

Like Frank (1973), we believe that the procedures and techniques of many schools of psychotherapy share common ground. Important common elements include attempts to help patients gain a sense of mastery, combat social isolation, restore a sense of social belonging, and find meaning in their lives. A major difference among the therapies is their conceptualization of the causes of the patient's problems as lying in the remote past, the immediate past, or the present. IPT also differs from other approaches in particular techniques and in its overall strategies (Markowitz, Svartberg, and Swartz, 1998). Some of the differences *make* a difference: for example, IPT may be preferable to CBT for certain depressed patients, and vice versa (Sotsky et al., 1991).

CHARACTERISTICS OF IPT

Time-limited, not long-term

Considerable research has demonstrated the usefulness of short-term, time-limited psychotherapy in meeting the needs of most patients (Howard et al.,

1986). Long-term treatment is considered necessary to treat personality disorders, particularly maladaptive interpersonal and cognitive patterns, as well as some other chronic conditions. For immediate problems and for many Axis I disorders, however, short-term treatment is efficacious. Long-term treatment has the potential disadvantage of promoting dependence and reinforcing avoidant behavior. Short-term, time-limited treatment may well avoid these adverse effects.

Focused, not open-ended

In common with other brief psychotherapies, IPT addresses one or two problem areas in the patient's current interpersonal functioning. Patient and therapist agree on this focus after initial evaluation sessions.

Current, not past interpersonal relationships

The IPT therapist focuses the sessions on the patient's present social context, the patient's situation immediately before and since the onset of the depressive episode. Past depressive episodes, early family relationships, previous significant relationships and friendship patterns are assessed to enhance understanding of the patient's patterns of interpersonal relationships. In most cases, however, after a brief review of the patient's past relationships and interactions, the therapist focuses primarily on current social functioning.

Interpersonal, not intrapsychic

In exploring current interpersonal problems with the patient, the IPT therapist may recognize intrapsychic defense mechanisms such as denial, isolation, projection, undoing, or repression. Yet the therapist does not attempt to see the current situation as a manifestation of an internal conflict. Rather, the patient's behavior is explored in terms of interpersonal relations. An example of the interpersonal focus is the handling of dreams. Although the therapist does not request them, the patient may report dreams. If so, the therapist may work on the dream by focusing on the manifest content and associated affects, relating these to current interpersonal problems.

Interpersonal, not cognitive/behavioral

IPT tries to change the way the patient feels, thinks, and acts in problematic interpersonal relationships. Behaviors such as lack of assertiveness, guilt, lack of social skills, emphasis on unpleasant events, and negative cognitions are not focused on for their own sake, but in relationship to significant persons in the patient's life and to the way these behaviors or cognitions influence interpersonal relationships.

Like CBT, IPT is concerned with patients' distorted thinking about themselves and others, and about the options open to them. The IPT therapist may work with a patient on distorted thinking by calling attention to discrepancies between what the patient is saying and doing, or between the patient's standards and those of society. In general, however, IPT focuses directly on affects, or feelings, whereas CBT focuses on "hot" cognitions— thoughts with strong associated affects. Unlike CBT, IPT makes no attempt to uncover distorted thoughts systematically, by giving homework or other assignments, nor does it attempt to help the patient develop alternative thought patterns through prescribed practice. Rather, as evidence arises during the course of therapy, the therapist calls attention to distorted thinking in relation to significant others. The goal is to change the relationship pattern rather than associated depressive cognitions, which are acknowledged as depressive symptoms.

Personality is recognized, but not a focus

The patient's personality is often the focus of psychotherapies, but since IPT does not expect to alter personality, this therapy recognizes but does not focus on the patient's personality characteristics. The ability to "read" a patient's personality can help the therapist to understand the patient's relationship patterns and to build the therapeutic alliance. The IPT therapist is circumspect, however, about making Axis II diagnoses in the presence of a depressive episode (Markowitz, 1998). An exception to this general approach is the adaptation of IPT for borderline personality disorder (Chapter 23), but even here the personality disorder is not confronted directly. IPT does not assume that individuals who become depressed have unique personality traits. Whether they do or not is an empirical question that requires testing, and thus far research has yielded no conclusive answers (Hirschfeld and Cross, 1983).

Personality is, however, considered an important aspect of patients treated in IPT, as it is in all therapies. In IPT personality is believed to affect several aspects of treatment.

1. *Personality may predict psychotherapy outcome.* Patients with personality disorders may be less able to effectively use short-term psychotherapy than those with mild or absent personality pathology.

(This, too, is an empirically testable question.) One adaptation of IPT targets borderline personality disorder (see Chapter 23).

2. *Personality may alter the patient-therapist relationship.*

3. *Personality may be a determinant of the patient's recurrent interpersonal problems.* Although IPT therapists may make no attempt to explore antecedents of personality functioning or to change personality, they may help patients to recognize maladaptive personality features. For instance, to a patient with mild paranoid tendencies the therapist may point out a disposition to be "touchy" with certain people under certain conditions, and explore the interpersonal consequences. In trials of IPT, personality has so far not been found to be an important determinant of short-term outcome (Zuckerman et al., 1980; Markowitz et al., 1998).

4. *Although IPT does not target personality disorder as a treatment (excepting borderline personality disorder), it has been shown to build social skills.* Without fundamentally altering personality structure, IPT can thus significantly improve overall functioning even in the presence of a personality disorder. Learning to be more assertive or confrontative can make a huge difference in social functioning and quality of life.

5. *By relieving depressive symptoms, IPT may erase what appeared to have been a personality disorder,* or at least tone down maladaptive personality traits.

THE ROLE OF THE IPT THERAPIST

The therapist is a patient advocate, not neutral

The IPT therapist is nonjudgmental, communicating warmth and unconditional positive regard. In essence, the therapist is a benign and helpful ally. Confrontation is gentle and timely, and the therapist is careful to foster the patient's positive expectations of the therapeutic relationship. This, of course, does not mean that the therapist accepts all aspects of the patient; rather, the therapist conveys the message that the patient's problems can be resolved and do not necessarily represent permanent features of the patient's personality. (Many aspects that the patient may attribute to personality may in fact be symptoms of depression.)

In keeping with this stance, the therapist is optimistic and supportive, using reassurance and direct advice when they seem useful, usually during the initial sessions when the patient is feeling most symptomatic and helpless (see Chapter 8 for techniques). By avoiding a withdrawn, neutral role, the therapist minimizes the possibility that the patient will regress in the therapeutic relationship.

The therapeutic relationship is not a manifestation of transference

This is a corollary of the role of patient advocate, and of the medical model of treatment. Since the therapist offers an alliance, the patient's expectations of assistance and understanding are accepted as realistic, and the relationship between patient and therapist is also realistic. In general, the relationship is not seen as a fantasied reenactment of the patient's (or the therapist's) previous relationships with others. The therapist is sensitive to the patient's pattern of relating. For example, the therapist may try to avoid intellectualized argument with an obsessional patient by focusing instead on feelings and emotional issues.

Positive transference is left untouched, and attempts to interrupt or specifically explore patient-therapist interactions are made only when the patient's feelings about the therapist are disrupting progress. This stance is expected to reduce the likelihood of the patient developing angry or hostile feelings toward the therapist. When the patient's feelings about the therapist or therapy do seem to interfere with progress, as evidenced by problems such as lateness or missed sessions (see Chapter 9), then the patient's feelings about the therapist may be explored. We have rarely found this necessary. The overall strategy in this situation is to relate the patient's reactions to the treatment to his or her ways of handling interpersonal problems outside of treatment, and to help the patient learn alternative ways of handling these reactions both in and out of therapy.

Although IPT therapists offer assistance to patients, it is limited to helping them learn new ways of thinking about themselves in social roles and of solving interpersonal problems. The therapist keeps direct advice and reassurance to a minimum in order to foster the patient's own sense of competence. The time frame and emphasis on the patient's actions outside the office also tend to limit dependency.

The therapeutic relationship is not a friendship

Although the therapist is the patient's advocate, there are limitations to this relationship. On the one hand, the therapist can be selectively self-revealing and free in interactions with the patient. When relevant to the issues at hand, therapists may express personal opinions or give brief examples of problems from their own lives. If the patient asks a personal question, the therapist may feel free to answer. It may, however, be important to explore the patient's reason for asking, to determine whether it seems related to countertherapeutic attitudes or represent avoidance of self-revelation.

On the other hand, the therapist's openness to the patient does not include participation in activities unrelated to the tasks and goals of therapy. Thus the therapist would not become involved with the patient socially or in a business relationship.

The therapist is active, not passive

In structuring the therapeutic hour and focusing sessions, the IPT therapist takes a moderate position between the extremes of being highly active and merely reactive to the patient's productions. In keeping with the goals of IPT, the therapist is somewhat active in helping the patient focus on bringing about improvement in current interpersonal problem areas. In the initial session(s), the therapist actively elicits the history of the depressive condition, the history of the patient's significant interpersonal relationships, especially current ones, and helps the patient set treatment goals.

In intermediate sessions, the therapist actively guides the patient to cover material that is relevant to the treatment goals. If the patient does not bring in material, the therapist may elicit an update or more detailed information in one of the agreed-upon problem areas. If the patient is still unable to discuss the material, it may be advisable to ask whether some issue is difficult to discuss. It is a general rule that if a pressing issue is not discussed, other issues cannot be fruitfully explored.

Although the therapist is active, the ultimate responsibility for change lies with the patient. Even if therapists could solve patients' problems, the goal of the therapy is to help patients learn to solve their own problems and pursue their own goals. Thus therapists limit their interventions relative to patients' behavior both inside and outside the therapy session. In sessions patients are told that they will have the opportunity to discuss their concerns and problems as they see them, because the therapist cannot intuit what is important to the patient. The therapist gives the patient opportunities to discuss concerns, events, or thoughts about either the therapy or significant others that the patient would like to discuss. If the patient brings up material, the session may then be focused through a systematic exploration of the topic the patient chooses.

Outside of therapy, patients change their behavior at their own pace. Except in rare circumstances, the therapist does not directly intervene on behalf of a patient. The therapist does not usually make direct, specific suggestions, albeit specific suggestions for activities between sessions may be made in dealing with interpersonal deficits. Such patients may be encouraged to undertake social activities and report back to the therapist. Similarly, patients with unresolved grief may be encouraged to look over or bring in picture albums of the deceased. The therapist also does not assign formal homework, although the solving of the focal interpersonal problem area during the time-limited treatment provides implicit homework. The emphasis in IPT sessions is on planning and preparation for the patient to make interpersonal changes in their life outside the therapist's office.

PART ONE
CONDUCTING INTERPERSONAL
PSYCHOTHERAPY OF DEPRESSION

CHAPTER 1

An Outline
of IPT

We have conceptualized IPT at three levels: strategies, techniques, and therapeutic stance. IPT resembles many other therapies for the latter two, but it is distinct at the level of strategies.

The strategies of IPT occur in three phases of treatment. The first phase, usually the first 1–3 sessions, includes **diagnostic evaluation** and **psychiatric history** and sets the **framework** for the treatment. The therapist reviews symptoms, diagnoses the patient as depressed by standard criteria (American Psychiatric Association, 1994), and gives the patient the **sick role** (Parsons, 1951). The sick role may excuse the patient from overwhelming social obligations, but requires the patient to work in treatment to recover full function. During the initial session(s), the psychiatric history includes the **interpersonal inventory**, a review of the patient's current social functioning and current close relationships, their patterns and mutual expectations. Changes in relationships proximal to the onset of symptoms are elucidated: for example, the death of a loved one, children leaving home, worsening marital strife, or isolation from a confidant. This review provides a framework for understanding the social and interpersonal context of the onset and maintenance of depressive symptoms and defines the focus of treatment.

The therapist assesses the **need for medication** as part of treatment selection based on symptom severity, past history and response to treatment, and patient preference, and then **educates the patient about depression** by explicitly discussing the diagnosis, including the constellation of symptoms that define the diagnosis and what the patient might expect from treatment. The therapist then offers an **interpersonal formulation** (Markowitz and Swartz, 1997), linking the depressive syndrome to the patient's interpersonal situation within the framework of one of four interpersonal problem areas: **(1) grief; (2) interpersonal role disputes; (3) role transitions;** or **(4) interpersonal deficits.**

The depression is diagnosed within a medical model and explained to the patient. Having identified the major interpersonal problem area associated with the onset of the depression, the therapist makes an explicit treatment contract with the patient to work on this problem area. When this focus is agreed upon, the intermediate phase begins.

In the middle phase, the therapist pursues strategies defined in the manual (Klerman et al., 1984; see Chapters 3–6 below), which are specific to the chosen interpersonal problem area. For **grief,** defined as complicated bereavement following the death of a loved one, the therapist facilitates mourning and gradually helps the patient to find new activities and relationships to compensate for the loss. **Interpersonal role disputes** are conflicts with a significant other: a spouse, other family member, coworker, or close friend. The therapist helps the patient to explore the relationship, the nature of the dispute, and options to resolve it. Failing this, they may conclude that the relationship has reached an impasse or to end the relationship and replace it. **Role transition** includes any change in life status: for example, the beginning or end of a relationship or career, a move, promotion, retirement, graduation, diagnosis of medical illness. The patient is helped to deal with the change by recognizing positive and negative aspects of the new role they are assuming, and assets and liabilities of the old role this replaces. **Interpersonal deficits,** the residual fourth IPT problem area, defines the patient as significantly lacking in social skills, resulting in problems in initiating or sustaining relationships.

The principle of these four interpersonal problem areas derives from extant psychosocial research on depression (Klerman et al., 1984). Thus, every depressed patient qualifies for at least one of the four problem areas. The problem area may change during the course of treatment. The patient may have several related problem areas and may work on more than one, or may select the most salient or mutable. Adaptations of IPT to particular populations or disorders have in a few instances added new problem areas (e.g., depressed adolescents, Chapter 13) or focused on a particular area (e.g., dysthymic disorder, Chapter 12).

IPT sessions address present **"here and now"** problems rather than child-hood or developmental issues. Sessions open with the question: **"How have things been since we last met?"** This focuses the patient on recent interpersonal events and recent mood, which the therapist attempts to link. Patients who describe problem areas will be asked about recent mood and other depressive symptoms; alternatively, if the patient focuses on symptoms, the therapist asks about recent life events and inter-actions. Therapists take an active, non-neutral, supportive, and hopeful stance.

The final phase of IPT, typically the last few weeks of treatment, encour-ages the patient to recognize and **consolidate therapeutic gains** and to de-velop ways of identifying and countering depressive symptoms should they arise in the future.

The original description of IPT can be found in Klerman et al. (1984). The first compilation of adaptations of IPT appeared in Klerman and Weiss-man (1993), the modification for depressed adolescents in Mufson et al. (1993), for dysthymic patients in Markowitz (1998), and the patient book is Weissman (1995). The most recent review of efficacy studies is Weissman and Markowitz (1994). Efficacy studies of psychotherapy as an antidepres-sant and a general treatment have been reviewed in several publications: Klerman et al. (1994); Jarrett and Rush (1994); Weissman, Jarrett, and Rush (1987); and Conte et al. (1986).

The outline that follows will be useful to understand the structure of IPT, including its techniques and stance. The detailed discussions and case illus-trations in subsequent chapters in this section follow this outline. Most of the adaptations of IPT to particular depressed populations or other disor-ders follow the same format but have changed the initial sessions on "Deal-ing with Depression" to accommodate the special age group, time period, delivery method, and/or target diagnosis under treatment. These adapta-tions are discussed in Parts II–IV. Case examples and therapist scripts to il-lustrate the strategies can be found throughout the book. These scripts are intended as therapist guides only.

Outline of Interpersonal Psychotherapy for Major Depression

I. The Initial Sessions
    A. Dealing with the Depression
        1. Review depressive symptoms.
        2. Give the syndrome a name.
        3. Explain depression as a medical illness; and explain the treatment.
        4. Give the patient the "sick role."
        5. Evaluate the need for medication.
    B. Relate Depression to Interpersonal Context
        1. Review current and past interpersonal relationships as they relate to current depressive symptoms. Determine with the patient the
            a. nature of interaction with significant persons;
            b. expectations of the patient and significant persons from one another, and whether these were fulfilled;
            c. satisfying and unsatisfying aspects of the relationships;
            d. changes the patient wants in the relationships.
    C. Identification of Major Problem Areas
        1. Determine the problem area related to current depression and set the treatment goals.
        2. Determine which relationship or aspect of a relationship is related to the depression and what might change in it.
    D. Explain the IPT Concepts and Contract
        1. Outline your understanding of the problem.
        2. Agree on treatment goals, determining which problem area will be the focus.
        3. Describe procedures of IPT: "here and now" focus, need for patient to discuss important concerns; review of current interpersonal relations; discussion of practical aspects of treatment—length, frequency, times, fees, policy for missed appointments.
II. Intermediate Sessions—The Problem Areas
    A. Grief
        1. Goals
            a. Facilitate the mourning process.
            b. Help the patient reestablish interest and relationships to substitute for what has been lost.

2. Strategies
   a. Review depressive symptoms.
   b. Relate symptom onset to death of significant other.
   c. Reconstruct the patient's relationship with the deceased.
   d. Describe the sequence and consequences of events just prior to, during, and after the death.
   e. Explore associated feelings (negative as well as positive).
   f. Consider possible ways of becoming involved with others.

B. Interpersonal Role Disputes
   1. Goals
      a. Identify dispute.
      b. Choose plan of action.
      c. Modify expectations or faulty communication to bring about a satisfactory resolution.
   2. Strategies
      a. Review depressive symptoms.
      b. Relate symptom onset to overt or covert dispute with significant other with whom patient is currently involved.
      c. Determine stage of dispute:
         i. renegotiation (calm down participants to facilitate resolution);
         ii. impasse (increase disharmony in order to reopen negotiation);
         iii. dissolution (assist mourning).
      d. Understand how nonreciprocal role expectations relate to dispute:
         i. What are the issues in the dispute?
         ii. What are differences in expectations and values?
         iii. What are the options?
         iv. What is the likelihood of finding alternatives?
         v. What resources are available to bring about change in the relationship?
      e. Are there parallels in other relationships?
         i. What is the patient gaining?
         ii. What unspoken assumptions lie behind the patient's behavior?
      f. How is the dispute perpetuated?

C. Role Transitions
   1. Goals

a. Mourning and acceptance of the loss of the old role.
b. Help the patient to regard the new role as more positive.
c. Restore self-esteem by developing a sense of mastery regarding demands of new role.

2. Strategies
a. Review depressive symptoms.
b. Relate depressive symptoms to difficulty in coping with some recent life change.
c. Review positive and negative aspects of old and new roles.
d. Explore feelings about what is lost.
e. Explore feelings about the change itself.
f. Explore opportunities in new role.
g. Realistically evaluate what is lost.
h. Encourage appropriate release of affect.
i. Encourage development of social support system and of new skills called for in new role.

D. Interpersonal Deficits
1. Goals
a. Reduce the patient's social isolation.
b. Encourage formation of new relationships.

2. Strategies
a. Review depressive symptoms.
b. Relate depressive symptoms to problems of social isolation or unfulfillment.
c. Review past significant relationships including their negative and positive aspects.
d. Explore repetitive patterns in relationships.
e. Discuss patient's positive and negative feelings about therapist and seek parallels in other relationships.

III. Termination
A. Explicit discussion of termination.
B. Acknowledgment that termination is a time of grieving.
C. Moves toward patient recognition of independent competence.
D. Dealing with nonresponse.
E. Continuation/maintenance treatment.

IV. Specific Techniques
A. Exploratory.

B. Encouragement of Affect.

C. Clarification.

D. Communication Analysis.

E. Use of Therapeutic Relationship.

F. Behavior Change Techniques.

G. Adjunctive Techniques.

V. Therapist Role

A. Patient advocate, not neutral.

B. Active, not passive.

C. Therapeutic relationship is not interpreted as transference.

D. Therapeutic relationship is not a friendship.

CHAPTER 2

The Initial Phase

IPT has a dual focus: to reduce depressive symptoms and to deal with the social and interpersonal problems associated with the onset of the symptoms. The initial sessions are devoted to defining the depressive disorder and its interpersonal context, identifying the interpersonal problem areas, establishing the treatment contract, and dealing with the depressive symptoms. During the initial sessions, both the depression and the interpersonal problems are diagnosed and assessed. In these sessions, the therapist should accomplish four tasks:

1. Diagnose the depression;
2. Complete an interpersonal inventory and relate the depression to the interpersonal context;
3. Identify the major interpersonal problem areas;
4. Explain the IPT approach and make a treatment contract.

When these tasks have been accomplished, the intermediate phase begins.

THE INITIAL SESSIONS: DEALING WITH THE DEPRESSION

The first session begins with the patient's description of what has led to seeking treatment (the chief complaint), the recent history of the depressive condition, a review of the depressive symptoms, and an evaluation of the need for medication. A physical examination with a comprehensive medical workup should be required for all patients. If there has been no examination within the past year, the patient may be asked to have one. People over fifty, or who have a history of medical problems, should have had one even more recently.

The history of the depressive state should include a review of past episodes, of particular interpersonal precipitants and/or consequences of the depressions, and the ways in which previous depressive episodes were resolved. The patient's type and severity of depressive symptomatology are assessed in light of a possible need for concurrent pharmacotherapy. Suicidal intent must be carefully assessed.

Educating the patient about depression, including reassurance and guidance in managing symptoms, should be part of the first two sessions. This is important in establishing the patient's commitment to the treatment and in creating a sense that the problems are being "worked on" right away.

REVIEW OF SYMPTOMS

A detailed review of the patient's symptoms—of their presence, duration, and severity—should be undertaken in the initial session. This review of symptoms has three purposes:

1. It allows the psychotherapist to confirm the diagnosis.
2. It reassures the patient that the symptoms fit a pattern that is anticipated by the psychotherapist and is understood as a clinical syndrome. Thus the patient understands that seemingly inexplicable, aberrant, and unrelated symptoms and behaviors are part of a pattern, time-limited, and, although uncomfortable, treatable.
3. It sets the symptoms in a specific time frame and in the interpersonal context that will be the focus of the psychotherapy.

As part of this review, a detailed account of the patient's suicidal feelings, thoughts, and behaviors, past and present, should be obtained (see Chapter 9 for a discussion of suicidal patients). Guidelines for this review are the DSM-IV or ICD–10 criteria for depression (see Tables 2.1 and 2.2). To meet criteria for a DSM-IV Major Depressive Episode, a patient must have had at least five of nine symptoms most of the day, nearly every day, for a period

TABLE 2.1 DSM-IV Diagnostic Criteria for Major Depressive Episode (296.xx)

A. Five (or more) of the following symptoms have been present nearly every day during the same two-week period and represent a change from previous functioning: at least one of the symptoms is either (1) depressed mood or (2) loss of interest or pleasure.

   (1) depressed mood most of the day
   (2) markedly diminished interest or pleasure in (almost) all activities most of the day
   (3) significant weight loss, when not dieting, or weight gain (e.g., more than 5 percent of body weight in a month); or decrease or increase in appetite
   (4) insomnia or hypersomnia
   (5) psychomotor agitation or retardation (observable by others)
   (6) fatigue or loss of energy
   (7) feelings of worthlessness or inappropriate guilt
   (8) diminished ability to think or concentrate, or indecisiveness
   (9) recurrent thoughts of death (not just fear of dying), recurrent suicidal ideation, a specific suicide plan, or suicide attempt

B. The symptoms do not meet criteria for a mixed mood episode.
C. The symptoms cause clinically significant distress, or impairment in social, occupational, or other important areas of functioning.
D. The symptoms are not due to the direct physiological effects of a substance (e.g., drug abuse, medication) or general medical condition.
E. The symptoms are not better accounted for by bereavement, i.e., after the loss of a loved one, the symptoms persist for more than two months or are characterized by marked functional impairment, morbid preoccupation with worthlessness, suicidal ideation, psychotic symptoms, or psychomotor retardation.

(Adapted from DSM-IV)

of at least two weeks. The Hamilton Rating Scale for Depression (Hamilton, 1960) or the Beck Depression Inventory (Beck, 1978) can be useful guides to the systematic review of symptoms, their severity, and their change during the course of treatment. Any systematic assessment scale that includes the full depressive range of symptoms can be used, however.

The review of symptoms should cover many of the following areas:

1. Depressed Mood. Mood is assessed through such questions as:
    • How have you been feeling over the past two weeks, including today?
    • Can you describe what your mood has been?
    • Have you felt blue, down in the dumps, depressed, or sad?

TABLE 2.2   ICD—10 Symptoms for a Depressive Episode

The individual usually suffers from depressed mood, loss of interest and enjoyment, and reduced energy leading to increased fatiguability and diminished activity. Marked tiredness after only slight effort is common. Other common symptoms are:

(a)   reduced concentration and attention;
(b)   reduced self-esteem and self-confidence;
(c)   ideas of guilt and unworthiness (even in a mild type of episode);
(d)   bleak and pessimistic ideas of the future;
(e)   ideas or acts of self-harm or suicide;
(f)   disturbed sleep;
(g)   diminished appetite.

The lowered mood varies little from day to day, and is often unresponsive to circumstances. Differentiation between mild, moderate, and severe depressive episodes rests upon a complicated clinical judgment that involves the number, type, and severity of symptoms and social dysfunction present.

(Adapted from ICD—10)

- Have you wanted to cry? Does crying help? Have you felt that you would like to cry, but that you were beyond tears?
- Have you had these feelings most of the day, nearly every day, for the past two weeks? How long have you felt this way?

2.   Diminished Interest or Pleasure in Activities.
- Have you lost interest or pleasure in most of the activities you usually enjoy?
- Is there anything you can still enjoy? (How long does the pleasure last?)
- Has your lost of interest or pleasure been for most of the day, nearly every day?

3.   Change in Weight or Appetite.
- Has your appetite changed during this period?
- Have you been eating much more or less than usual?
- Do you have to push yourself to eat? Nearly every day?
- Has your weight changed in the last weeks or month?
- If so, how much weight have you lost (or gained)?

- Have you been dieting or trying to lose weight?
- Have your clothes been fitting you differently?

Assess the patient's maximum weight loss (or gain) since the start of the illness.

4. Insomnia or Hypersomnia.
    - Have you had trouble sleeping over the last two weeks?
    - (Early insomnia:) Have you had trouble falling asleep most nights?
    - Have you been taking sleeping pills?
    - How long does it take you to fall asleep?
    - What goes through your mind as you lie there?
    - (Middle insomnia:) When you fall asleep, do you sleep soundly?
    - Are you restless, or do you keep waking?
    - How many times a night do you wake up?
    - Do you get out of bed? Is that just to go to the bathroom?
    - (Late insomnia:) Do you wake up early in the morning?
    - If you awaken early in the morning, can you fall back asleep?
    - Do you get up earlier than you would normally get up?
    - (Hypersomnia:) Have you found that you've been sleeping too much lately?
    - How much time are you spending in bed?
    - How much more than normal is that? Do you take naps during the day?

5. Psychomotor Agitation or Retardation.
    - Has it been very hard for you to sit still lately?
    - Have you been so worked up and restless that other people have noticed?
    - Or have you felt slowed down? So slowed down that it's been hard to do anything, or even to think clearly?

These questions will help assess functioning during the past weeks. But the therapist should principally assess psychomotor agitation or retardation on the basis of observation in the interview, not simply on subjective complaints of restlessness or slowing down. Agitation is defined as restlessness associated with anxiety. It should be differentiated from anxiety, since it refers to observable phenomena of motor restlessness that are experienced as distressing. Note, for retardation, slowness of thought and speech, impaired ability to concentrate, decreased motor activity, or apathy and stupor.

6. Fatigue or Loss of Energy.
   - Have you found you've been getting tired easily?
   - Have you felt tired nearly every day?
   - Has your energy level been low?
   - Have you been spending a lot of time lying in bed?
   - Do your limbs feel heavy, like there are weights on them?
   - Are there parts of your body that feel particularly tired?

7. Feelings of Worthlessness or Inappropriate Guilt.
   - Do you feel lately that you're a bad or worthless person?
   - Have you been blaming yourself for things you've done, or not done?
   - Have you been down on yourself, critical of yourself?
   - Do you feel that you have let friends, family, or other people down?
   - Have you been feeling guilty about things?
   - Have you felt that you are to blame for your feelings?

8. Diminished Ability to Think, Concentrate, or Make Decisions.
   - Has it been hard for you to think straight or to concentrate lately?
   - How has that shown itself? Has it interfered with your work?
   - Has it been hard for you to make decisions?

9. Recurrent Thoughts of Death or Suicide.
   - Has death been on your mind a lot lately?
   - Have you felt so bad that life has not felt worth living?
   - Have you wished you were dead?
   - Have you thought about taking your life?
   - Do you have any plans for killing yourself? If so, what are they?
   - Have you made an attempt on your life?

Other symptoms, while not themselves diagnostic criteria, often help to define the depressive syndrome's effects on social, physical, emotional, and cognitive functioning:

10. Work and Activities.
   - Tell me about your work, housework, hobbies, interests, and so-cial life. Are you handling these any differently than usual?
   - Has the way you've been feeling interfered with your functioning at work or at home?

11. Psychic Anxiety.
   - Have you been feeling nervous, anxious, or frightened? Have you felt tense or found it hard to relax? Have you been worrying about little things?
   - Have you been feeling irritable, snapping at people?
   - Have you had a feeling, or dread, as though something terrible were about to happen?
   - Have you tended to become fearful in particular situations: being alone at home, going out alone, being in crowds, traveling?

12. Somatic Anxiety.
   - Have you suffered from: trembling, shakiness, excessive sweat-ing, feelings of suffocation or choking, attacks of shortness of breath, dizziness, faintness, headaches, pain in the back of the neck, butterflies or tightness in the stomach? Have you had pal-pitations or knots in your stomach?
   - How often? How badly?

This group of problems encompasses a number of somatic complaints common in anxious patients, including gastrointestinal problems such as flatulence and indigestion; cardiovascular problems such as palpitations; headaches; respiratory complaints; and genitourinary complaints.

13. Gastrointestinal Symptoms.
   - How has your appetite been? Have you had a heavy feeling in your stomach?
   - What is your pattern of bowel movements? Is this different now from your usual pattern?

14. General Somatic Symptoms.
   - Do you have any aches and pains? Feelings of heaviness?

This group of symptoms, related to fatigue, includes heaviness in limbs, back, or head; diffuse headache; loss of energy and fatiguability. Consider changes in intensity and frequency. In depression these are characteristically vague and ill defined, and it is extremely difficult to get a satisfactory description of them from the patient.

15. Sexual Symptoms.
- I want to ask you a few questions about your sex life. Have you lost interest in sex/your spouse/your partner recently? Have you had less sexual drive than usual? Difficulty in becoming aroused? Sexual relations less often? Difficulty in obtaining an erection [men] or reaching a climax?

16. Attitudes Toward Bodily Complaints.
- Have you been worrying a lot about your physical health?
- Thinking a lot about aches, pains, and bodily functions?
- Have you been worrying that there's something physically wrong with you?

This category refers to the patient's concern with bodily complaints, whether or not they have a realistic basis. The hypochondriacal patient is concerned with and keeps coming back to bodily symptoms rather than psychological complaints.

17. Insight.
- What would you say is the nature of your trouble?
- Do you regard yourself as being emotionally or psychologically ill?
- What caused what you're going through?

It is important to distinguish between a patient who has no insight and one who is reluctant to admit having "mental problems." Insight refers to the patient's awareness of a psychological disturbance and its depressive component. Degree of self-awareness, as well as understanding of psychodynamics and psychological causation, must always be considered in relation to the patient's thinking and background knowledge.

Everybody has a set of ideas and beliefs about illness, bodily or mental, and most people have their own classification and diagnostic systems. The patient's ideas should be elicited without disagreement or challenge. Some patients will see their experience in religious terms: "God is punishing me for being so selfish." Others will blame someone—a mother for not being loving enough, or a spouse for being cruel and insensitive.

18. Diurnal Variation.
    - Is there a characteristic pattern to your mood? Do you usually feel worst at one time of the day?
    - At what time of day do you feel best? Morning? Afternoon? Evening? At what time of day do you feel worst?

These queries are designed to discover consistent fluctuations of mood and other symptomatology in the first and second half of the day. As a rule, a patient will feel better during one or the other: most depressed people feel worst in the morning. Occasionally a patient feels better in the afternoon, or worse both morning and evening.

19. Depersonalization (and Derealization).
    - Have you been feeling as though you're in a movie or a dream?
    - Have you had the feeling at all that everything is unreal, that you are unreal, or that the world is distant, remote, strange, or changed? I don't mean just the feeling that you could not really imagine this illness would happen to you.
    - Have you felt as though you're outside yourself, watching yourself from a distance?

20. Paranoid Symptoms.
    - Has it been hard for you to trust other people?
    - Are you suspicious of other people? Do you think people are talking about you or laughing behind your back?

If a patient answers yes, probe for elaborations. Look for ideas of persecution that do not have a depressive element, that is, are not associated with guilt and a feeling that the persecution is deserved. If paranoid ideas do have such an element, this may be part of guilt or other depressive delusions.

21. Obsessional and Compulsive Symptoms.
    - Do you find that unpleasant, frightening, or ridiculous thoughts or words come into your head and won't go away, keep coming

back even when you try to get rid of them? Are you afraid you might commit some terrible act without wanting to?

- Do you find you have to keep checking or repeating things you have already done? Do you have to do things in a special way, a special order, or a certain number of times? Do you go through little rituals over and over, even in a superstitious sort of way, that help you feel better?

22. Depressed Feelings.
   - Have you been feeling helpless?
   - Hopeless?
   - Worthless?

RELATED DIAGNOSES

A comprehensive diagnostic workup for depression should consider potential alternative explanations for symptoms as well as comorbid diagnoses. Several standardized comprehensive diagnostic assessments are available that cover the major Axis I diagnoses. These can also be used to diagnose depression. They include the Schedule for Affective Disorders (SADS; Endicott and Spitzer, 1978), the Structured Clinical Interview for DSM-IV (SCID; First et al., 1995), and the Composite International Diagnostic Interview (CIDI; Wittchen et al., 1994). The latter two clinical interviews are based on American Psychiatric Association diagnostic criteria (American Psychiatric Association, 1994). The CIDI has been used primarily in clinical epidemiologic research, but has the advantage of generating both DSM and ICD diagnoses. For a comprehensive discussion of different diagnostic assessments in psychiatry, see the Handbook of Psychiatric Measures (American Psychiatric Press, to be published 1999).

The choice of instruments is less important in a clinical setting than the principle of making systematic inquiry about alternative and comorbid diagnoses to the depressive disorder. Standard DSM-IV or ICD–10 criteria (American Psychiatric Association, 1994) should be used in making a diagnosis. Treatment should be based on differential therapeutics (Frances et al., 1984)—that is, treatment should be determined by the diagnosis and needs of the patient, rather than based on therapeutic ideology. This may include IPT. For an excellent presentation of treatment guidelines for depression, see the Agency for Health Care Policy and Research (AHCPR) Depression Guideline Panel (1993).

In planning treatment, it is important to know whether the patient has bipolar disorder (manic depressive illness); nonpsychiatric medical illnesses and medications that might mimic the symptoms of depression; and bereavement (i.e., normal grieving in the wake of the loss of a loved one). In some instances, the standard model of IPT for depression has been adapted to particular disorders (see Parts II–III).

Bipolar Symptoms.
- Have you ever had periods in your life when you were feeling the opposite of depressed? Like you were walking on air? Feeling so good, or hyper, that other people thought you were not your normal self?
- Did your thoughts race? Did you talk faster than usual?
- Did you need less sleep?
- Did you spend a lot of money or do things impulsively that you later regretted?
- Did you think you had special powers?

(See Chapter 16 on IPT for bipolar disorder.)

General Medical Causes of Depression.
- Have you ever been diagnosed with a significant medical illness? Have you ever had problems with your thyroid gland?
- Have you been taking any medications (that might have contributed to your feeling depressed)?

Bereavement.
- Did someone you love die within the last year? If so, how did you handle that loss?
- Did you attend the funeral? Were you able to grieve?

(See Chapter 3 for bereavement-related depression.)

Since comorbidity is common for depression and can adversely affect the course of treatment, it is useful to assess other disorders, particularly anxiety disorders and substance abuse. The following questions may be useful as a screen for generalized anxiety or panic disorder.

Anxiety.
- Have you been feeling anxious or frightened?
- Do you find it hard to relax?

- Do you worry about little things?
- Have you had sudden, unexpected attacks of panic?
- Are you fearful when staying home alone or going out alone?
- Have you suffered from trembling, shakiness, sweating, feelings of suffocation or choking? Butterflies or tightness in your stomach or chest?

(See Chapter 22 for IPT adaptations for social phobia and panic disorder.)

Substance Abuse.

- How much alcohol have you been drinking lately? (How many drinks a night?)
- Other drugs? (Which ones? How often? How much?)
- Have you felt that you ought to cut down on your drinking or drug use?
- Have other people been worried about or complained about your drinking or drug use?
- Has your alcohol or drug use interfered with work, or with social or family life?
- Has there ever been a time when you drank or used drugs when it was dangerous to do so? (E.g., Have you driven or worked while intoxicated?)

If the answer is yes to any of the above for alcohol:

- Describe what kind of alcoholic drinks you have, and how many you drink in a typical day.
- If yes to drugs: Describe what drugs you are using, the route by which you take them, and how much you use in a typical day.

IPT has not been tested as a treatment for alcohol-dependent patients. Its efficacy for patients with serious drug dependence has not been demonstrated (see Chapter 20). A trial is under way at Cornell University assessing IPT administered in conjunction with Alcoholics Anonymous meetings as a treatment for dysthymic patients with secondary alcohol abuse (Markowitz, unpublished). Patients with a serious drug or alcohol problem should be referred to a drug rehabilitation program. Subsequently they might possibly receive IPT for comorbid conditions if these persist after the drug abuse or dependence remits.

GIVING THE SYMPTOMS A NAME

If, after the review of symptoms, the patient does indeed have a Major Depressive Episode (see DSM-IV and ICD–10 criteria, Tables 2.1 and 2.2), it is important to say so explicitly, to tell the patient that these multiple symptoms have a single clear name. (See Parts II-III for adaptations of IPT for other disorders and special treatment populations.) The patient should be told that the syndrome of depression has been diagnosed, and that the sleep and appetite problems, the headaches, the hopeless outlook, the lack of interest, the fatigue, are all part of the depression. If the results of the physical examination show no specific somatic causes for these symptoms, the therapist can confidently reassure the patient that they are due to depression. Patients need to know that they do not have a serious organic illness (although depression is a medical illness), that they are not "going crazy," that the sleep problems or difficulty in concentration are not due to senility.

The diagnosis might be conveyed to the patient in words like these:

> Your symptoms [state them specifically: headaches, sleep problems, fatigue, etc.] indicate that you have a major depression (not some other physical illness). Depression isn't just a bad mood: it's a combination of emotional, physical, cognitive, and interpersonal symptoms. The symptoms you describe are all part of being depressed. Your appetite and sleep are disturbed. You've lost interest in your usual activities. You're more irritated with your children and not getting along with your spouse. You can't imagine taking the job you were interested in before. You don't have energy and zest. This is all part of the clinical picture of depression. Your thoughts about death, your tiredness and feeling of futility, your questions about where your life is going, your lack of energy are part of the constellation of depression. The symptoms you describe are common for depressed persons. You are in the throes of a depression. And luckily, even though you may feel hopeless, depression is very treatable.

EXPLAINING DEPRESSION
AND ITS TREATMENT

After the specific diagnosis, the patient should be given some general information about depression and told what to expect:

Depression is a common disorder. It affects about 4 to 5 percent of the adult population at any one time. *It's an illness, and it's not your fault.* Even though you are suffering now and feel hopeless, depressions do respond to treatment. The outlook for your recovery is excellent. A variety of treatments are available, and you do not need to feel hopeless if the first approach doesn't work. Most people with depressions recover promptly with treatment. You will feel better and should return to your normal functioning when the symptoms disappear. Psychotherapy is one of the standard treatments of depression. It has been shown to be effective in a number of research studies. Psychotherapy should help you understand the problems that led to the depression and how to handle these problems in the future.

While you are depressed, you may not feel like being sociable or doing the things you usually do. You may need to explain this to your family members. You are going to be actively engaged in treatment, however, and you will be working hard toward recovery. The expectation is that, as you recover, you will resume your normal activities, and should be back to normal if not even better than that. In fact, there is every reason to hope that you will be better than before, although it may be hard to believe this when you're feeling depressed.

The underlying message of these explanations is that depression is a medical illness, not the patient's fault, and does not reflect a failure, character flaw, sign of weakness, or punishment for past sins. The patient does not have full control over the illness, but can take actions that will help bring about a remission. The prognosis is excellent. Moreover, in IPT the patient may not only treat symptoms but also solve a difficult interpersonal problem.

The diagnosis of major depression should not be given if there are extenuating factors that suggest other, confounding diagnoses such as bipolar disorder or substance abuse, or if the patient is taking medications or has a general medical condition that might explain the depressive syndrome. Other comorbid diagnoses, such as panic disorder, are not contraindications to IPT, but the presence of comorbid diagnoses should be discussed explicitly with the patient.

Thus, key themes to address include:

Depression is a common illness, not a unique character flaw of the patient.

Depression is an illness, not something the patient wanted, willed, or deserved. "The depression is not your fault."

Although the patient feels hopeless, depression is treatable. The chance of reaching remission and of recovering with treatment is excellent.

When the depressive episode remits, the patient should return to his or her usual self.

DETERMINING THE NEED FOR MEDICATION

Antidepressant medications have clear benefit for mood syndromes. Research has shown that depressed patients tend to respond to treatment with either medication or to IPT (e.g., Elkin et al., 1989). Thus, either treatment may suffice in many cases. In other instances, however, pharmacotherapy should be considered either as sole treatment or in conjunction with psychotherapy. Some patients are too depressed to participate in psychotherapy, although initial treatment with pharmacotherapy may later allow them to do so. Others are extremely unpsychological and/or may prefer medication to a talking therapy. A prior history of medication response should be taken seriously in considering treatment options, as should relative medical contraindications to pharmacotherapy.

Patients with recurrent depressive episodes, and/or with severe sleep and appetite disturbances, agitation, or lack of reactivity, are good candidates for antidepressant medications in addition to psychotherapy. Patients whose depression has melancholic features (see Table 2.3) may not respond as rapidly to psychotherapy alone as to psychotherapy and antidepressant medication combined (AHCPR guidelines, 1993).

The presence of life stress as a precipitating factor in the depression does not preclude the effective use of medication, either in place of or in addition to psychotherapy. In fact, the majority of patients identify a stress associated with the onset of depression. Nor does an acute depression superimposed on dysthymic disorder (Keller and Shapiro, 1982) preclude the use of antidepressant medication (Kocsis et al., 1988; Markowitz, 1994) in addition to psychotherapy (Rounsaville et al., 1980). Key clinical features to identify in evaluating the need for medication are the severity and recurrent pattern of

TABLE 2.3   DSM-IV Melancholic Features Specifier

A.   Either of the following, occurring during the most severe period of the current episode:

    1.   Loss of pleasure in all, or almost all, activities
    2.   Lack of reactivity to usually pleasurable stimuli (does not feel much better, even temporarily, when something good happens)

B.   Three or more of the following:

    1.   Distinct quality of depressed mood (i.e., the depressed mood is experienced as distinctly different from the kind of feeling experienced after the death of a loved one)
    2.   Depression regularly worse in the morning
    3.   Early morning awakening (at least 2 hours before usual time of awakening)
    4.   Marked psychomotor retardation or agitation
    5.   Significant anorexia or weight loss
    6.   Excessive or inappropriate guilt

(Source: DSM-IV, 1994)

the symptoms and the presence of specific ones: agitation, retardation, loss of interest or reactivity, and suicidality.

Psychotic symptoms such as depressive delusions and hallucinations require either electroconvulsive therapy (ECT) or pharmacotherapy with both antipsychotic and antidepressant medication. IPT alone has not been found useful in patients with psychotic depression, although it might be helpful in combination with pharmacotherapy.

Suicide is a tragic outcome of a depressive episode. Because depression generally responds more quickly to pharmacotherapy than to psychotherapy, antidepressant medication is an important option for suicidally depressed patients. On the other hand, medications such as the tricyclic antidepressants can actually be used as agents of suicide, and so should be dispensed cautiously to suicidal patients. Serotonin reuptake inhibitors have a far better safety profile and overdoses are much less likely to be fatal. Because IPT clinical trials, like those of other antidepressant treatments, have generally excluded acutely suicidal patients, there are few research data on the relative efficacy of antidepressant therapies for suicidal patients. Nonetheless, IPT may be helpful in combination with medication for suicidal patients (Markowitz and Weissman, 1999). The medical model of IPT makes it easily compatible with antidepressant pharmacotherapy.

Economic pressures have pressed mental health care in the 1990s to opt for relatively low-contact treatments: antidepressant medication accordingly has increasingly taken precedence over psychotherapy for depression. Yet research has demonstrated that IPT treats major depression in nonpsychotic outpatients essentially as well as pharmacotherapy, if not quite as rapidly. Patients should understand the array of available treatments for depression, and their risks, benefits, likely course, and potential combination. Although patients feel hopeless, depression paradoxically is extremely treatable. The more patients know about the options for treating depression, the less pessimistic they are likely to feel, and the more they may be able to view their symptoms as a recognizable and treatable illness.

In summary, severity of depressive symptoms and high suicide risk should raise the question of medication treatment and, when appropriate, psychiatric hospitalization. More severely and more chronically depressed patients may also be good candidates for combined treatment with IPT and medication, which can work better in synergy than either does alone (DiMascio et al., 1979). Because IPT and pharmacotherapy both employ a medical model of illness, they are easily combined as treatments.

Giving the Patient the "Sick Role"

The symptom review, the diagnosis, and the description of what the patient may expect, including the type and course of treatment, all serve deliberately to give the patient the "sick role." This role allows patients to receive in a compensatory, but time-limited, way the care that has not been adequately received—or felt to be received—from others.

The idea of the sick role was first presented by Talcot Parsons (1951). A professor of sociology at Harvard Medical School and one of the founders of the field of medical sociology, he noted that illness is not merely a "condition" but also a social role. The essential criteria of a social role concern the attitude both of the incumbent and of others with whom he or she interacts, in relation to a set of social norms defining appropriate behavior for persons in that role.

Parsons described four functions of the sick role:

1. The sick person is considered exempt from certain normal social obligations. This exemption must be socially defined and validated.

2. The person is exempt from certain types of responsibilities.
3. The sick person is considered in a state that is socially defined as undesirable, to be gotten out of as expeditiously as possible. The person is considered "in need of help."
4. Taking the role of patient carries obligations of its own, especially affirming that one is ill and cooperating with the helper in the process of getting well.

The review of symptoms allows the psychotherapist to determine whether the patient is entitled to the sick role. If the answer is yes, then this information is conveyed explicitly to the patient and, at times, to the family. This legitimizes the sick role and defines the patient as in need of help. It also temporarily exempts the patient from certain social obligations and from responsibility for the state of depression.

Describing the recovery process is essential, because it limits the sick role and informs the patient of the obligation to cooperate in getting well and relinquishing the sick role as soon as possible. A key element of this role is helping the patient to relinquish it and recover. The recovery phase should begin almost as soon as the patient is engaged in treatment.

The psychotherapist might give the patient the sick role by saying something like:

When you are depressed, you may not feel like entertaining or being sociable. You might explain this to your family. However, you should also explain that you are going to be actively engaged in treatment with me now, and over the next months we will be working hard toward recovery. The expectation is that you will be able to assume your normal life gradually and at the end of two months should be quite active. In fact, your interpersonal functioning is the focus of this treatment. As time goes on and we begin to understand and cope with the problems around your becoming depressed, we have every reason to hope that you will feel even better than before.

It is often helpful to provide a more obviously physical analogy of illness:

If you had a broken leg, you wouldn't expect—and no one would expect you—to run in a marathon. If you had appendicitis, you'd go to the hospital and you wouldn't blame yourself for missing work. Depression is another medical illness that has not only emotional symptoms—such as your mood—but also physical and cognitive symptoms: low energy, sleep and appetite difficulties, trouble concentrating and making decisions.

The central concept is that depression is a disorder of which they are not fully in control but from which, with treatment, they will recover without serious residual damage. Patients often take a moral view of their illness: that depression is failure, a sign of weakness, a just punishment for past misconduct, or even a deliberate act. They should be reassured that this negative view is part of the depressive affect.

An important aspect of the sick role is that it shifts blame from the patient (self-blame) onto the illness. Because depressed patients tend to be overly self-critical and to blame themselves unduly, the IPT therapist generally tends to balance the patient's outlook by helping the patient to shift blame from him- or herself onto the depressive illness and the interpersonal situation in which the patient presents. The sick role may be seen as one facet of the tendency of IPT to mitigate self-blame and to provide support for positive actions.

Many therapists learning IPT worry that giving the sick role will invite depressed patients to regress. In fact, if anything, it frees the patient from ruminative self-criticism that might interfere with activity. Although the IPT therapist does temporarily excuse the patient from activities that are too stressful, the therapist is always at the same time pressing the patient to socialize and participate in all activities that are feasible—it is precisely on these activities that IPT centers. The time limit of IPT also works against regression. Because the patient knows that the clock is ticking, and that treatment depends upon addressing an interpersonal problem within the limited time frame, the patient is pressed into activity, not passivity. Depressed patients also often feel too guilty to really relax: excused from one activity, they can be induced to undertake another. Thus, the absolution from self-blame that IPT provides through the sick role does not undercut the active nature of the therapy.

RELATING DEPRESSION TO THE INTERPERSONAL CONTEXT IN THE INITIAL SESSIONS

The Interpersonal Inventory

Having completed the review of depressive symptoms, the therapist should direct the patient's attention to the onset of symptoms and to the reason(s) for seeking treatment. What has been going on in the patient's social and interpersonal life that might be associated with the onset of symptoms? The review of key persons and issues often follows easily. If not, it is useful to begin an inventory of current and past relationships in order to understand the patient's important current social interactions.

Many depressed patients begin treatment with a clear formulation of the "cause" of their depression: "My husband left me," "I can't get along with my children." Other patients focus on their symptoms as a mysterious problem that "came out of the blue."

Even for patients who clearly understand the context of their depressive episode, a careful inventory of their relationships and life situation is helpful to get the full picture.

The systematic review of current and past interpersonal relationships involves an exploration of the patient's important relationships with others, beginning with the present. In this inventory, information should be gathered about each person who is important in the patient's life:

1. Interactions with the patient, including frequency of contact, activities shared, and so on;
2. the expectations of each party in the relationship, including some assessment of whether these expectations were or are fulfilled;
3. a review of the satisfactory and unsatisfactory aspects of the relationship, with detailed examples of both kinds of interactions;
4. the ways the patient would like to change the relationship, whether through changing his or her own behavior or bringing about changes in the other person.

Although the inventory is concentrated in the first two sessions, it may be expanded less systematically as treatment progresses.

IDENTIFICATION OF MAJOR PROBLEM AREAS

The primary interest in this review lies in determining which interpersonal issues are most central to the patient's current depression. The therapist should obtain enough information to define the primary problem area. Discussion of the problem area proceeds naturally in tandem with dealing with the depression itself, and it also helps move the patient away from sole concern with the present overwhelming symptoms. Since the discussion of the depression focuses on a discrete onset period, this is usually the best transition to a discussion of the interpersonal problems associated with the onset.

With the phrase, **"Let's try to review what has been going on in your life,"** the psychotherapist begins asking the patient about recent changes in life circumstances, mood, and social functioning. These questions are intended as guides for patients who do not fully respond to the initial questions:

- When did your symptoms first begin?
- Think about what was going on in your life at the time:
- Did something upsetting happen?
- Did someone close to you die? (Was it the anniversary of a death? Were you thinking about someone who died?)
- Did you or someone else get sick?
- Were you having problems at home with your partner? With your family? With friends? With children?
- Were you having problems at work?
- Were you put in a situation where you had to meet new people?
- Were chronic problems getting worse?
- What else had been happening in your life about the time you started feeling bad?
- Had anything changed in your life? At your work? At home? With your family? Your friends? Your social life? Your activities? Your health?

Determine how life circumstances relate to the onset of symptoms.

- When you learned of your husband's affair, was that around the time you started to feel sad and hopeless?

The therapist uses the problem areas to formulate a treatment strategy with the patient. Indeed, the problem area that emerges from the interpersonal inventory becomes the focus of the IPT therapist's formulation to the patient, and of the treatment that follows (Markowitz and Swartz, 1997). If IPT is short-term, as is the case in acute treatment, it usually concentrates on one or two of the four problem areas that depressed patients commonly encounter. (In long-term treatment, the problem areas may change over time; see Chapter 11.) This classification of problem areas conceptualizes interpersonal problems according to a system that focuses on potential areas of change in treatment. The classifications are not exhaustive and do not represent in-depth formulations, nor do they attempt to explain the dynamics of the depressive disorder. Instead, this classification system is intended to help the therapist outline realistic goals and follow appropriate treatment strategies.

The four interpersonal problem areas are:

1. **Grief** (complicated bereavement);
2. **Interpersonal role disputes** with spouse, lover, children, other family members, friends, coworkers.
3. **Role transitions**: e.g., a new job, leaving one's family, going away to school, relocation in a new home or area, divorce, economic or other family changes;
4. **Interpersonal deficits**—loneliness and social isolation.

These areas are not mutually exclusive. Patients may come for treatment with a combination of problems in several areas, or there may be no clear-cut, significant difficulties in any one area. (In the latter instance, interpersonal deficits becomes the focus.) For each person, the psychotherapist assesses individual needs and what the patient considers the factors that have contributed to the depression. For patients with wide-ranging problems, the therapist may be guided in the choice of focus by the precipitating events of the current depressive episode. Some adaptations of IPT have added additional problem areas (See Parts II-III).

Occasionally the patient and the psychotherapist disagree about the appropriate focus. Patients are sometimes unwilling or unable to recognize the degree to which a particular problem is distressing them. For example, patients with marital role disputes may be reluctant to complain of problems because they feel threatened by the possibility of endangering the marital relationship. A stormy marriage may have been tolerable until the children left home. Patients with pathological grief reactions may be unaware consciously of the source of annual episodes of depression. When the therapist and the patient do not agree about the desirable focus of treatment, the therapist can take one of three tacks:

1. delay setting treatment goals;
2. set very general goals in the hope of being able to focus more specifically as therapy progresses; or

3. accept the patient's priorities in the hope that after those issues are looked into, the focus can shift to more central matters.

The third approach worked well for a woman patient who came in with the complaint, "My children are driving me crazy." Several sessions later, however, after the therapist remarked that she never mentioned her husband, the patient brought up her more pressing distress at her husband's extramarital affair.

The specific stress area is usually determined by focusing on one or two areas that seem most troubling: threat of loss of job, problems with children, marital friction, relocation. The purpose is to identify and clarify the most recent stresses the patient is trying to cope with, which may be related to the depression, and to determine the problem areas that will be the focus of the remaining sessions. To target more than one or two interpersonal problem areas risks diffusing the focus of treatment, confusing the therapy for both therapist and patient. The simplicity of IPT in focusing on a single (or at most two) key interpersonal problems makes it easy for even significantly depressed patients to grasp and accept.

It is important to listen, to let patients describe the problems in their own terms and unburden themselves. But patients should not be allowed to dominate the interaction with irrelevant preoccupations. A systematic outline in which all salient historical points are listed can be useful in finding the best focus for a brief treatment.

These points do not have to be applied in mechanical order, but all the areas should be adequately covered. They should include the history of present symptoms; the history of current life circumstances; the history of current close interpersonal relationships; and the history of recent changes in all three.

A complementary patient book, *Mastering Depression: A Patient's Guide to Interpersonal Psychotherapy* (Weissman, 1995) contains an explanation of these procedures and patient worksheets with questions to complete prior to sessions. Some patients and therapists may find it useful in focusing and clarifying the treatment.

The psychotherapeutic task is to help patients identify the key persons with whom they are having difficulties, what the difficulties are, and whether there are ways the patient can make the relationships more satisfactory. The problems should be stated explicitly to the patient in formulations that show their derivation from what the patient has been describing.

It should also be made explicit that the purpose of the next visits is to help with the problems.

The therapist might say:

> It seems from what you have been telling me that you have been having difficulty [state the current problem or problems clearly—having trouble in your marriage, arguing with your spouse, afraid of losing your job, uncomfortable in your new apartment, lonely in the city, missing your old friends, etc.]. These problems can certainly be related to your depression. I'd like to meet with you over the next few weeks, as we have been doing, for about an hour each time, to see if we can figure out how you can better cope with the situation. As you solve this interpersonal situation—which we call [complicated bereavement; a role transition; etc.]—your depression should improve.

IPT is a relatively jargon-free therapy, but it is helpful to label grief (complicated bereavement), role disputes, and role transitions as such. For interpersonal deficits, the therapist might say, **"your difficulty in making [or keeping] relationships."** This identifies the interpersonal situation, like the mood disorder, as a commonly recognized problem rather than the patient's idiosyncrasy or personal weakness. It is also useful to elaborate the generic role transition with a more personalized metaphor or encapsulated summary, using the patient's own words if possible:

> We'll work on helping you solve your role dispute; or, as you called it, your boxing match with your husband.

Patient reactions to this type of exploration of the interpersonal nature of depression can be of at least three types:

1. Patients may insist that they have an undetected physical illness. (The recommended physical examination should rule this out.)
2. They may remain focused on the somatic symptoms of the depression—the sleep disturbance, the fatigue—and question or deny that these have any connection to life stress.
3. They may acknowledge to varying degrees some current life stress.

The first response is the least frequent and the most difficult to deal with. Obviously, the third response is the easiest to handle. In any case, a patient who responds in either the first or the second way—that is, with denial—should not be pushed or lectured. If the attitude persists, it may be necessary to postpone further sessions and offer the opportunity for a further physical examination, or perhaps a second opinion from another physician. At this point the therapist should go gently, reassuring the patient, not getting into an argument, not trying to change the patient's mind. It is more useful to follow the patient's lead, never denying the reality of the symptoms and the real discomfort they cause. When patients continue to deny current problems, always leave the door open for the next visit; tell them you'd like to help explore again what is going on in their life and see how they are getting on:

> I can understand that these [state patient's symptoms—headaches, sleep problems, etc.] are uncomfortable. I'd like to try to understand over the next few weeks what may be causing them. Let's see how you are doing next week.

In some cases it may be appropriate to negotiate with patients about their perceptions:

> We both agree that you have problems with [state symptoms—sleep, energy], but we have different ideas about what is producing them. Together let's see how things go for you and what we can find out over the next few weeks.

Psychoeducation is an important aspect of IPT. In our experience, many patients who initially misunderstand their depressive symptoms are relieved to have them reformulated as a treatable medical illness.

If after several sessions patient and therapist remain unable to agree on problem areas and/or treatment goals, IPT treatment may not be possible. The lack of an agreed-upon therapy contract may lead the patient to express dissatisfaction through silence, missed appointments, or termination. (The handling of such problems is discussed in Chapter 9.)

EXPLAINING IPT CONCEPTS AND THE TREATMENT CONTRACT

Even when taking the symptom history described above, it is important that the therapist ask questions in a way that conveys the message that depression is not a disease mysteriously visited upon the patient, but is related to interpersonal functioning.

EXPLAINING THE PROBLEM

Many depressed patients are aware that problems with others play an important part in their condition, but they often see their problems as entirely individual, related only to their personal failures or inadequacies, or to their early childhood experiences. They may have social relationships that are overtly untroubled, or they may be so socially isolated that they cannot see that interpersonal deficits increase their vulnerability to depression. These patients may need some such explanation as this:

> People play a large part in most of our lives, even if you tend to think that you face life alone. Although the causes of depression are unknown, its onset is frequently associated with problems in personal relationships, including dealings with your spouse, children, family, or colleagues. Problems in relating to others or the loss of loved ones may bring on depression in some people, while for others the symptoms of depression prevent them from dealing with other people as successfully as they usually do.
>
> In this treatment we will try to understand the relationship between your mood changes and your interpersonal problems. We'll try to discover *what you want and need from others* and *help you learn how to get it*. We will try to figure out what alternatives you have (there may be more than you've considered), which options are feasible and worth pursuing, and how you can use them to achieve what you want.

After this general explanation, the psychotherapist should give the patient an outline of the psychotherapist's initial understanding of the problems the patient is currently having in social relationships. To demonstrate the vital nature of interpersonal issues, patients may be asked what changes would make them feel better. The reply will usually involve improved interpersonal relationships, even if it does not do so obviously. Wanting more money, for example, can be seen as a step toward developing more satisfying relationships with others: more money is expected to bring more respect from others, less bickering, and so on.

The psychotherapist should then give the patient an explanation of the techniques of IPT. The "here and now" emphasis on current social functioning should be made clear:

> We'll be discussing your life as it is right now.

The patient should know that the general strategy of treatment is to review in detail current relationships (and relevant past ones) with the purpose of clarifying the problem areas and working toward resolving them.

> We'll be reviewing your relationships with important people in your life.

The patient's part in the process will be to decide, with the psychotherapist, on the focus of treatment and to bring in new material that pertains to the work at hand. Patients should know that they are largely responsible for choosing topics to discuss.

Whenever necessary, however, the therapist will refocus the discussion on the problem area after that has been agreed on.

> I'll expect you to be willing to discuss these relationships and your feelings honestly with me. If either you or I feel the direction of the session is not going to be useful, we should let the other know.

In addition, the patient should understand that it will not be enough simply to discuss solutions: to make real life changes, and to help alleviate the symptoms of depression, the patient will have to *do* things in his or her life between therapy sessions. Understanding motivation without making real life change is neither the primary focus nor an adequate outcome of IPT.

> If you can make the changes you want in your life situation, you're very likely to feel better.

SETTING THE
TREATMENT CONTRACT

The setting of two to three treatment goals takes place. Although improvement of interpersonal relationships is the goal of IPT, symptom reduction (eating better, sleeping better) is also an important component. As people work on their problems in therapy, they usually experience a relief of symptoms. Goals set should be attainable within the course of treatment, so that the emphasis is on progress toward solving a problem rather than lifetime solutions. For each problem area, the patient may be asked to define what would be the best possible outcome, the most expectable outcome, and the worst possible outcome. Being clear about hoped-for outcomes at the start may help patients see small increments of progress in the therapy.

Since treatment goals are set jointly by psychotherapist and patient, the therapist can use this process to provide evaluative feedback to the patient. This may include assessments of the psychotherapist's general understanding of the patient's particular interpersonal problem area and of the severity of the patient's difficulties. Many patients, experiencing psychiatric symptoms for the first time, may have an unrealistic sense of the severity of their problems. For example:

CASE EXAMPLE

A twenty-seven-year-old man came for treatment with a depression of moderate severity following his third loss of a job in the past several years. Reacting to his depressive symptoms, he was frightened that he was "going downhill" permanently. In the course of the initial interview, it became clear that the loss of the most recent job had been in part precipitated by the patient. As with previous jobs, when he began to get involved in the work, he also began to feel that coworkers and employers were "taking advantage" of him. He reacted to this with withdrawal, work slowdown, and absenteeism, behavior that always led to his quitting or being fired.

In setting up the treatment contract, the psychotherapist explained to him that he was suffering from a depressive condition of moderate severity, that there was a good prognosis for improvement, and that it did not portend more severe impairment or hospitalization. The therapist went on to relate the depression to the dispute at work. The therapist said that there seemed to be some regularity in the patient's problems at work, since the feeling of being exploited developed in each situation, and that one goal of treatment might be to figure out how this came about and help the patient find more satisfactory work in the future.

At this point, the practical aspects of treatment (length of sessions, frequency, termination date, appointment times, fee, missed sessions policy, and so on) should be agreed upon, and by the end of the first session an explicit treatment contract should be stated. The contract should emphasize:

1. The social or interpersonal context of the intervention:

We shall try to understand what current stresses and relationships in your life may be contributing to your depression.

2. The expected duration and frequency of treatment, and its time-limited nature. The precise duration and frequency will vary with the treatment setting. The key principle, however, is that a time structure is specified at the outset. For example:

   I'd like to meet with you once a week for twelve to sixteen more times for fifty minutes each time, to try to understand with you the stresses in your life and how they relate to your depression.

Maintenance treatment, for patients who are not acutely depressed but are in treatment to prevent recurrence, may meet less frequently but over a longer time frame. Other adaptations, including a group format or the use of telephone sessions (see Chapter 24), should also be explicitly discussed at this point.

3. A formulation of the (initial) problem area:

   From what you tell me, your depression began with recent transitions from college to graduate school. I'd like to discuss with you the areas you seem to describe as related to your depression. One is the transition you've had to make from being a college student to being a graduate student, and where this leads in terms of career directions as you would like to think about them, and how your life has changed recently with this transition. The second issue centers on how you develop and maintain intimacy with someone, whether a man or a woman. When I say intimacy, I mean a close and confiding relationship with someone you trust and feel understands you. Do these sound like the issues we should discuss?

4. Confidentiality:

   Everything that we discuss will be kept confidential. I will not discuss what happens in our sessions with anyone else unless you request a release of medical information; even then I would try to limit disclosure to what was medically essential. [If sessions are being taped:] We are recording these sessions for the purpose of supervision [or treatment adherence monitoring], but only my supervisor [or treatment raters] will have access to the recordings, which will be kept locked and anonymously coded.

The therapist needs the patient's explicit agreement to work on the interpersonal problem area in order to proceed. With the patient's assent on this formulation and focus, the intermediate phase of IPT begins.

TEACHING PATIENTS
THEIR ROLE IN IPT

In the first several sessions, while taking the history and helping the patient to delineate treatment goals, the psychotherapist is comparatively more directive and active than will usually be necessary in later sessions. It is important to convey to patients that they will be responsible for choosing the topics in the remaining sessions and that the psychotherapist will be less active. To prepare patients for their role in the exploration that therapy involves, a statement such as the following may be given:

Now that we have some sense of where we are going, here's how we'll proceed. Your task will be to talk about the things that affect you emotionally. We have already identified specific areas where there is room for change, and we have agreed upon certain goals. However, as we work together, other important issues may emerge—and you should feel free to raise them. I will be interested in what happened and in your feelings about these events. It will be your responsibility to select the topics that are most important to you. There is no "right" or "wrong" thing to talk about, as long as it is something that you have strong feelings about. This includes feelings about me, our relationship, or the therapy.

Patient and psychotherapist have specific roles in IPT. As a prototype for other relations, the reciprocal role expectations should be explicitly stated. This is a negotiation of the treatment contract, and the experience of negotiation can provide an example for the patient of dealing with interpersonal relations in the "here and now."

BEGINNING THE
INTERMEDIATE SESSIONS

The intermediate sessions, described in detail in Chapters 3 through 6, begin after the treatment contract is set and the initial problem areas to be worked on have been defined. (Defining the problem areas may take several sessions, and the areas may change during the course of treatment.) The psychotherapist's strategy during these sessions is based on the assessment of the problem areas.

The intermediate sessions focus on one or possibly two problem areas in each session. The therapist has three interrelated tasks:

1. helping the patient discuss topics pertinent to the problem area;
2. attending to the patient's affective state and to the therapeutic relationship, to maximize the patient's intimate self-disclosure; and
3. preventing the patient from sabotaging the treatment.

TOPICAL FOCUS

The patient is encouraged to take the initiative in choosing topics for discussion.

Each session begins, however, with the psychotherapist asking the question:

How have things been since we last met?

In keeping with the goal of exploring new material, this allows the patient to change the focus of treatment, when appropriate, and to bring up previously unrecognized or suppressed problems.

This initial question achieves several strategic goals. First, it focuses the patient on the recent past: the interval since the previous session. Second, it evokes one of two responses. Either the patient will answer by relating a mood ("I've been feeling terrible"; "I've had a couple of good days") or an event ("I had a fight with my wife"). The therapist then links the patient's response to its complement: that is, relates the patient's mood to recent events, or recent events to changes in the patient's mood. (See Table 2.4.) Therapist and patient explore important interpersonal events of the prior

TABLE 2.4   Key features of the Intermediate Phase of IPT

1. Opening question:

    How have things been since we last met?

2. Patient's response:

    Either a description of **mood** ("I felt sad") **or event** ("My children and I had a huge fight")

3. Therapist links mood to event (or event to mood)
4. Discussion and elaboration of emotionally charged event and its relationship to mood fluctuation
5. Therapist supports patient's successes
6. Therapist helps patient to understand setbacks:

    • **What did you want in that situation?**
    • **What options did you have to achieve what you wanted?**

7. Emotionally charged incident leads into the focal interpersonal problem area
8. Role playing:

    • **What could you have done? What can you do next time?**

9. Summary at end of session

week, noting the patient's successes (which may have improved mood) and setbacks (which may have worsened it). Usually the emotionally charged incident under discussion can be related to the interpersonal problem area that is the agreed-upon focus of the treatment. If things have gone wrong in these interactions, therapist and patient can work on strategies for handling such situations in the future.

If a patient is bringing in material that is relevant to treatment goals, this opening question may be sufficient to focus the session. But if a patient seems to be avoiding a subject of presumed concern, the therapist should give the patient time to see whether the material is truly irrelevant before trying to shift the focus to material more closely related to the goals of treatment. Relevance does not necessarily emerge at once. For example:

CASE EXAMPLE

A forty-three-year-old man with marital problems began one of his sessions with a lengthy discussion of his disgust with the slovenly, undisciplined ways of the residents of a poor neighborhood he drove through on his way to the session. This led, however, to a productive exploration of similar disgust with his wife's slovenly ways, and those of his mother earlier.

A patient's initial statements about the nature of the problem are often revised in the course of treatment. Either because of distrust of the psychotherapist or genuine misunderstanding of the problem, the patient may at first present relatively minor issues as important areas while deemphasizing major concerns. Alternatively, the psychotherapist may suspect that a problem area minimized by the patient is the most important one. In such cases it may be difficult to settle upon a treatment contract after only a few sessions. The focus of treatment may even change in intermediate sessions as issues are put into perspective. In general, though, the content of IPT sessions will follow directly from the interpersonal inventory and goal setting of initial sessions.

CASE EXAMPLE

A forty-five-year-old woman spent several sessions repeating her frustration at her teenager's messy rooms and noisy music, never mentioning her spouse. Finally, the therapist asked about the role of her husband in dealing with their child. The patient broke down in tears, revealing that she had recently learned that her husband was having an affair. She had suspected this for months, but had been too embarrassed to discuss it with the therapist, and so had initially denied difficulties with her husband.

With each problem area the sequence of movement in therapy is, first, a general exploration of the problem; second, a focus on patient's expectations and perceptions; third, an analysis of possible alternative ways to handle the problem area, and, finally, attempts at new behavior.

In exploratory phases of treatment, the patient is asked to review systematically the relationship with the person or persons with whom problems have arisen. In giving this history, including some explanation of mutual expectations and detailed descriptions of important interactions, the patient frequently reveals problem areas, such as poor communication or unrealistic expectations, that warrant more focused attention. Sometimes interpersonal difficulties do not result from maladaptive behavior by those involved but simply contradictory demands or expectations of each other. In such cases this situation should be made clear.

Upon discovering conflicting expectations, the patient is usually faced with a choice of either changing in some way or going on as at present while learning to accept limitations. At this point the psychotherapist's role is to guide the patient through a careful exploration of which options are open. If the patient chooses to attempt new behavior, the psychotherapist can then act as a collaborator in helping the patient assess his or her progress and develop new strategies of handling problems.

Chapters 3 through 6 focus on the particular social and interpersonal issues identified as focal problem areas.

CHAPTER 3

Grief
(Complicated Bereavement)

Grief is considered a problem area when the onset of the patient's symptoms are associated with a death, either present or past. Note that, for IPT, grief requires the actual death of a loved one; other losses are considered role transitions. Grief associated with the death of a loved one can be normal or abnormal. Efforts to modify IPT for normal bereavement are under way. The following section describes the use of IPT for episodes of depression associated with abnormal grief reactions, i.e., from failure to go through the various phases of the normal mourning process.

NORMAL GRIEF

The process of normal grief includes a full awareness of the reality of the death. The experience of normal grief after a beloved person dies has much in common with depression, but the conditions are not equivalent. In normal bereavement a person experiences symptoms such as sadness, disturbed sleep, agitation, and decreased ability to carry out day-to-day tasks. These symptoms tend to resolve without treatment in two to four months, as the bereaved person goes through a process of gradual weaning from remembered experiences with the loved one (Lindemann, 1944; Parkes and Weiss, 1983; Viederman, 1995) and begins to live with the reality of the loss. People who are experiencing normal grief do not generally seek psychiatric treatment, and normal grief is not a psychiatric disorder.

ABNORMAL GRIEF

An abnormal grief reaction may be diagnosed when grief is severe, protracted (compare DSM-IV criterion E in Table 2.1), and interferes with the resumption of functioning, or when the patient has been unable to grieve appropriately following the death of a loved one. The principal assumption behind the IPT strategy for dealing with abnormal grief is that inadequate grieving can lead to depression, either immediately following the loss or at some later time when the patient is somehow reminded of the loss.

Abnormal grief processes of two general kinds are commonly noted in depressed persons: delayed grief and distorted grief.

In *delayed grief reaction*, grief is postponed and experienced long after the loss. When this grieving occurs, it may not be recognized as a reaction to the original loss, but the symptoms are those of normal grieving. A delayed or unresolved grief reaction may be precipitated by a more recent, less important loss. In other cases, delayed reactions may be precipitated when the patient achieves the age of death of the unmourned loved one. Questioning the grieving person about earlier losses will show that this person is actually mourning the prior loss.

A *distorted grief reaction* may occur immediately following the loss, or years afterward. There may be no sadness or dysphoric mood; instead, apparently nonaffective symptoms may be present. These manifestations may lead to the involvement of different medical specialists before a psychotherapist deciphers the nature of such reactions. Other patients grieve interminably, unable to end their mourning and to return to their normal life role.

DIAGNOSIS OF
ABNORMAL GRIEF REACTIONS

It is often clear that the patient's depression began following a significant loss, but in other cases there may be only an indirect relationship between the current depression and a previous loss. In reviewing the patient's interpersonal relationships, it is important to obtain a history of relationships with significant others who have died. This history should include the circumstances of the death and the patient's behavioral and emotional reaction to it. Evidence that may suggest a pathological mourning process are found in Table 3.1.

Depressed patients suffering from complicated bereavement tend to have low self-esteem while often idealizing the lost other or their lost relation-

TABLE 3.1 Evidence of Abnormal Grief

Task	Therapist's Questions
1. Multiple Losses	What else was going on in your life around the time of the death? Has anyone else died or left? What has reminded you of it since? Has anyone died in similar fashion or when your circumstances were similar?
2. Inadequate grief in the bereavement period	How did you feel in the months following the death? Did you have trouble sleeping? Could you carry on as usual? Were you beyond tears?
3. Avoidance behavior about the death	Did you avoid going to the funeral? Visiting the grave?
4. Symptoms around a significant date	When did the person die? What was the date? Did you start having problems around the same time?
5. Fear of illness that caused the death	What did the person die of? What were the symptoms? Are you afraid of having the same illness?
6. History of preserving the environment as it was when the loved one died	What did you do with the possessions? The room? Were they left the same as when the person died?
7. Absence of family or other social supports during the bereavement period	Whom could you count on when the person died? Who helped you? Whom did you turn to? Whom could you confide in?

ship. Such a polarized, two-dimensional description should alert the clinician to the possibility of complicated bereavement. An aim of treatment is then to help the patient develop a clearer, more complex, and more realistic picture of the totality of his or her relationship with the lost person.

To diagnose abnormal grief, the psychotherapist might say,

> I notice that you didn't mention your mother when discussing your parents.
> . . . Has anyone you've been close to died recently? Could you tell me about the death? When did it happen? Where? Where were you, and how did you feel when you learned of the death? How were you during the next few weeks? Did you carry on as usual?

Some authors have distinguished between the complicated bereavement of depression and "complicated grief," meaning a nonaffective constellation of dysphoric symptoms, such as yearning, intrusive thoughts, and feeling numbed by the death, associated with enduring functional impairment (Prigerson et al., 1995). Although the terminology is potentially confusing, it should be clear that the complicated bereavement IPT addresses is the depressed state consequent to abnormal grief. Differential treatment effects of IPT on complicated grief and on bereavement-related depression have not been tested.

GOALS AND STRATEGIES
OF TREATMENT

The two goals of the treatment for depression that center on grief are:

1. to facilitate the delayed mourning process, and
2. to help the patient reestablish interests and relationships that can substitute for what has been lost.

The therapist's major tasks are to help patients assess the significance of the loss realistically and emancipate themselves from a crippling attachment to the dead person, thus becoming free to cultivate new interests and form satisfying new relationships. The therapist adopts and utilizes strategies and techniques that help the patient bring into focus memories of the lost person and emotions related to the patient's experiences with the lost person.

ELICITATION OF FEELINGS AND
NONJUDGMENTAL EXPLORATION

Abnormal grief reactions are often associated with lack of a supportive social network to help the bereaved person in the normal process of mourning. Consequently, the major psychotherapeutic strategy is to encourage the patient: (1) to think about the loss; (2) to discuss the sequence and consequences of events prior, during, and after the death; and (3) to explore associated feelings. Thus the psychotherapist substitutes for the missing social network.

- Tell me about ____. What was [the person] like?
- What did you do together? What was enjoyable? What did you dis-like? What didn't you get to do together that you had hoped you would do?
- How did [the person] die? When did you learn about the illness? Describe it.
- How did you learn about the death? How did you feel about all this?

REASSURANCE

Patients often express fear of bringing up something that has been "buried." They may be afraid of "cracking up," of not being able to stop crying, or of otherwise losing control. In such instances, the psychothera-pist may let the patient know that the fears expressed are not uncommon and that mourning in psychotherapy rarely leads to decompensation. There are a number of common themes in the mental life of persons experiencing the stress of bereavement.

Typical themes in the dysphoric thoughts of those who have experienced a stressful event such as a painful loss include: (1) fear of repetition of the event, even in thought; (2) shame at helplessness in being unable to post-pone or prevent the death; (3) rage at the person who died; (4) guilt or shame over aggressive impulses or destructive fantasies; (5) survivor guilt: the loved one has died and the person who survives is relieved to remain alive; (6) fear of identification or merging with the victim; and (7) sadness in relationship to the loss. It is helpful for the therapist to be alert to the ex-pression of these themes and to help the patient articulate them. In fact, it is frequently reassuring if the therapist can "anticipate" the patient's com-plaints by inquiring about thoughts and feelings along these lines (Horowitz, 1976).

It is quite normal to feel upset and confused when you talk about the loss. You will feel better again.

RECONSTRUCTION OF THE RELATIONSHIP

Patients with abnormal grief reactions frequently fixate on the death itself, thus avoiding the complexities of their relationship with the deceased. The therapist should lead a thorough factual and affective exploration of the patient's relationship to the dead person, both when the person was alive and in the present context. To facilitate this process and to help the patient review old memories, the therapist might encourage a review of old picture albums with friends or family, or to see old friends who knew the dead person in order to review past times together. The patient may not wish to acknowledge angry or hostile feelings toward the deceased, which may be due to feeling abandoned by the loved one. When the mourning process is blocked by strongly negative feelings toward the dead person, the therapist should encourage the patient to express these feelings, but the encouragement should not be through confrontation, which could provoke a shift of hostility from the deceased to the psychotherapist. If negative feelings emerge too rapidly, the patient may decide not to continue psychotherapy because of the guilt that is likely to accompany them. If, however, the psychotherapist reassures the patient that the negative feelings will be followed by positive and comforting feelings, as well as a positive attitude toward the deceased, the patient will be much better prepared to explore his or her ambivalence.

Tell me, how was your life with ____? How has it changed since ____ died?
Every relationship has its ups and downs—that's normal. What were yours?

CASE EXAMPLE

Stan, a forty-two-year-old gay man, came for treatment one year after the death of his longtime lover, Harry. As Harry's caregiver and companion, he had coped with the illness and death smoothly and courageously. Over the past year, he had been unable to work. His bills were in disarray, and he had had his electricity shut off several times. He had lost sixty-five pounds and was having trouble sleeping. He described the stable, loving ten-year relationship with Harry as one in which they had perfect synchrony on most major issues. He stated, "When Harry died, my life stopped."

The first five weeks of treatment were mostly consumed by a review of the details of their life together. Depressive symptoms persisted. Stan then mentioned the argument he and Harry had had about four years before the death. This dispute resulted in a five-month separation during which Harry was sexually promiscuous. It was probably at this time that he had contracted HIV infection. In one session, there emerged both the details of this dispute and Stan's anger at Harry for having exposed both of them to HIV. After this unburdening session, Stan became more active outside the home, his depressive symptoms diminished, and his picture of his partner became more balanced and less idealized.

DEVELOPMENT OF AWARENESS

The steps described above will help the patient formulate a new, healthier, and more balanced understanding of the memories of the person who has died. For instance, a patient may no longer consider a parent a villain but instead realize that the mother or father was a sick person, and thus be able to accept both the parent's behavior and his or her own reaction to it. To help achieve this new understanding, the therapist may try to elicit both affective and factual responses that will lead to more knowledge of the elements that contribute to the difficulty of mourning. A patient who feels a need to maintain a pathologically strong bond to the deceased can be comforted by answering such questions as:

What were the things you liked about _____? What were those you didn't like?

FACILITATING EXPRESSION OF AFFECT

Catharsis is an important aspect of treating grief. Encouraging the patient to look through belongings or pictures of the deceased may evoke painful grief feelings that the patient has avoided. When these feelings arise during IPT sessions, the therapist can often best encourage their expression through silent listening. In our experience, a mistake of beginning IPT therapists, who often feel the need to be "active," is that they feel anxious in the presence of such affect, and may interrupt the patient with questions. This conveys the wrong message: namely, that such feelings are dangerous or intolerable. The IPT therapist should be as active as necessary in priming the expression of grief but, once having succeeded, should quietly allow it to surface.

BEHAVIORAL CHANGE

Catharsis, although important, is not in itself sufficient to treat complicated bereavement. The necessary next step is to change interpersonal interactions. As patients lose their investment in maintaining continued, abnormal grieving, they may be more open to developing new relationships to fill the "empty space" left by the lost loved one. At this point, the therapist may be very active in leading the patient to consider various alternative ways (dating, church, organizations, work) to become more involved with others again.

What is your life like now? How have you tried to make up for the loss? Who are your friends? What activities might be enjoyable?

ABNORMAL GRIEF: THE CASE OF MARY

Mary, a married woman in her late fifties, was admitted to a local general hospital because of paralysis of her right leg from the hip down. Until the symptoms started to appear two months earlier, Mary had been very active in her community, dedicated to her church, and happily married. Until about a year before her admission, she and her husband had lived on the upper floor of a two-family house, with her mother living on the first floor. Mary defied the efforts of internists, neurologists, neurosurgeons, and orthopedic surgeons. Sophisticated laboratory procedures repeatedly confirmed a healthy person who should be up and walking.

Mary was clinically depressed. She spoke slowly, reported difficulty sleeping and early-morning awakenings with ruminations about past failings. She looked sad and she had lost ten pounds over the past six weeks. She had no previous history of depression. Careful evaluation revealed that about three months before admission, Mary's doctor, who had cared for her since she was a young girl, had died of a painful and unpleasant disease. She did not know precisely what the illness was, but said his death had greatly affected her. She mentioned only in passing that her mother had died about a year earlier, and said that this death had not caused her much difficulty.

In the third session, more information about the mother developed. Mary's mother had lived downstairs in the same house for the past few years. Mary had to wait on her mother, coming down several times a day, because the mother's right leg was paralyzed and she could not move. When Mary's mother died, it must have been a great relief, and it caused only a very mild grief reaction. About a year later, however, there was a reaction of intense guilt. Mary started to carry her mother's cane and progressively stopped walking downstairs and outside. It appears that the paralysis was Mary's way of coming to grips with the guilt caused by her feelings about her mother's death, and her grief at her doctor's death compounded the problem. Mary entered the hospital on the first anniversary of her mother's death.

The therapeutic stance with the patient was supportive and nondirective. Reconstruction of the patient's relationship with both deceased persons was the first step in the therapy. She was encouraged to describe in detail the circumstances around the death of her mother, including the physical care she had provided during the last few years, the details of their daily activities, and her reactions both during these years and at the time of the death. She was also encouraged to describe the circumstances and her reactions when she learned of her physician's illness and death, since she particularly turned to him for comfort.

No joint interpretation of the possible meaning of the paralysis could be attempted. In fact, when the therapist in one session referred to the relationship between the mother's paralysis and her use of the mother's cane, Mary nearly terminated treatment.

Initial Phase (Sessions 2–3)

In the first session, Mary described her guilt about not providing sufficient care for her mother. She felt that had she made her mother adhere to the special diet prescribed and massaged her good leg, her mother might be alive today. She also regretted her lack of compassion toward her family physician, who himself was ill although she hadn't known it, and whom she called repeatedly for help and advice about her mother.

By the second session, Mary had gradually begun to walk with the cane, and by the third week she could walk without it. She was discharged from the hospital but continued the weekly psychotherapy. Her sleep and appetite disturbance improved, although she was still slowed down.

Intermediate Phase (Sessions 4–9)

During the middle phase of treatment, more of Mary's anger at both her mother and her doctor became overt. She described her mother's unreasonable screaming at her to come downstairs and care for her, so that for the six months before the death Mary was virtually never out of the mother's apartment. Mary resented not being able to visit her grandchildren and having to give up church activities and all social life with her husband. Though he didn't complain overtly, her husband became more withdrawn and less emotionally available to her.

Further discussion revealed long-term bitterness between Mary and her mother, who had forced her to leave college and go to work because "college is wasted on a girl." In contrast, her brother had attended law school. She felt angry that she had to carry all the family burdens and he could visit once a week, bring flowers or candy, and be viewed as the "good son," while she, who was giving virtually all the physical care, could never please her mother.

During the terminal phase of the mother's illness, when Mary went to see her doctor because she felt so drained and fatigued, she was told that he couldn't see patients and was referred elsewhere. She felt abandoned and rejected by the doctor, whom she had used as a confidant since she was a girl.

TERMINATION PHASE (SESSIONS 10–12)

As therapy ended, Mary was asymptomatic and was not using the cane. She had resumed her church activities and was planning to move downstairs and rent the less convenient upstairs apartment. She and her brother had a good talk about the circumstances of her leaving college and she had been able to tell him her feelings about it. She described her satisfaction with her own children and grandchildren and the full life she and her husband had together.

Mary expressed some reluctance at termination, but she had found a new family doctor who would probably act as confidant in periods of stress. She left without ever having discussed the possible psychogenic origins of her paralysis, but she was completely without depressive symptoms at termination.

In some ways this case is not typical for IPT, since the therapeutic contract was not explicit. Nevertheless, the reexamination of the relationship and the opportunity to express the appropriate feelings directed toward the dead mother contributed to a more successful resolution of the grief.

"OVERGRIEVING"

Many patients with complicated bereavement have avoided grieving, seemingly having found the emotions of mourning too uncomfortable to tolerate. For these patients, the therapist encourages the expression of feelings. An alternative if perhaps rarer problem is the patient who has wholeheartedly accepted the mourner's role and has trouble giving it up. Such patients have become "professional mourners": grieving has taken over their lives, often for prolonged periods of time, and they seemingly "can't turn off the tap." Other aspects of their lives atrophy. Sophocles' Electra, who grieved from youth "till I'm past childbearing, till I am past marriage," is an example.[1]

"Overgrieving" patients frequently see mourning as an expected role and a duty. Some may feel unexpressed guilt about some aspect of their relationship with the lost loved one for which their grieving atones. The therapist's role in treating overgrieving patients is to help them find a graceful way to return to formerly satisfying activities or develop new ones without feeling that they are abandoning or betraying the mourned other. In doing so, the therapist must be careful not to echo the responses of others around the patient, who frequently have become irritated by the patient's behavior and say, "Enough, already!" They need not stop mourning, and will not forget their lost other; but mourning need not occupy every moment of their lives.

"OVERGRIEVING": THE CASE OF LESLIE

Leslie, a sixty-three-year-old widowed homemaker, was brought to treatment by her sons. Her husband had died seven years before of the complications of diabetes. Leslie had attended the funeral, where she made a dramatic display of her intense bereavement. Following the wake, however, she had retreated into her home, claiming ill health. She withdrew from her small circle of friends. She claimed she was too exhausted to walk, and during the years since had remained homebound, expecting her sons to bring her groceries and other necessities. She maintained her husband's room and belongings as he had left them, almost as a shrine. The local priest visited her and discussed her prolonged mourning, since she felt too prostrate to attend church. Her physician gave her Valium (diazepam) to "calm [her] nerves."

The sons were driven to distraction. Every attempt they had made to induce their mother to give up her withdrawal and constant obsequies was met with more tears and accusations of disloyalty to their father. When they brought Leslie for a psychiatric consultation, she came reluctantly. She was indifferently groomed, wore no makeup, and cried throughout the interview. She denied depression, but said that her husband had been her whole life and that since his passing she had nothing to live for. She denied active suicidal ideation. She reported chronic sleep disturbance, low energy, trouble making decisions and concentrating, intrusive ruminations about her husband and their marriage, and a variety of somatic and anxious symptoms. There was no evidence of psychosis.

The history revealed that Leslie had indeed depended on her husband in many respects: for income, for many of the errands she had now transferred to her grown sons, and for their social life, which mainly involved "his" friends. She described the marriage and her husband in transparently idyllic terms, but her asides and the sons' comments indicated that there had been numerous tensions. Among other things, Leslie apparently felt that her husband's illness had prevented him from giving her proper attention, and also that her demands for attention might have damaged his health. She also revealed that an argument they had had shortly before her husband's death, over getting his insulin from the pharmacy, was her fault and has hastened his death. Now she owed him her prayers, and in any case there was nothing to be done for her.

The therapist listened sympathetically, commented on what a terrible loss her husband's death had been for her, and diagnosed her problem as major depression. Validating mourning as appropriate following the death of a loved one, he said that her situation still needed "attention," and that it would make sense to talk things over to try to treat the depression. He emphasized that his goal was not to stop her from mourning. Still somewhat reluctant, Leslie agreed to a twelve-week treatment.

Early sessions focused on the marital relationship, initially emphasizing its positive aspects, but soon delving into its more painful issues as well. Leslie felt she had kept her husband from pursuing job opportunities by refusing to move, and that she had hurt him with her temper. He had been a quiet, submissive man, "although I never liked pushing him." The therapist gradually helped her to develop a more three-dimensional picture of the strengths and weaknesses of her husband and of their relationship. A discussion of the events surrounding his death also made clear that, as distressing as the death had been, Leslie was not to blame.

As these feelings came out, with Leslie bringing photograph albums to some of the sessions, the therapist also explored Leslie's social skills and interests. She did have some friends with whom she had played cards; some of her "husband's friends" were in fact also friends of hers; and she had once been a regular churchgoer. Therapist and patient discussed how pleasurable these activities had once been, and whether resuming them would betray her husband's memory. The therapist gently pressed Leslie to consider leaving her house to *honor* her husband's memory: to go to the grave site, to church, to see their grandchildren. Protesting, she nonetheless began to do so.

Within six weeks, Leslie's mourning had diminished in intensity, her depressive symptoms had faded, and she rarely cried in sessions. She had stopped taking the diazepam (with an appropriate taper). After initially expressing guilt about activities, she conceded she was enjoying herself more. She did recontact friends, who greeted her happily. And after exploring her options, she decided that one way to honor her husband was to join the local diabetic fund-raising organization. By the end of the twelve-week treatment, she was euthymic. She sent Christmas cards reporting her continuing good health and happiness—with sadness about her husband, "but not depression," she wrote—during the three subsequent years.

This case presented the danger that this apparently highly dependent woman would simply shift her dependence from her sons to the therapist. The limited time frame of the treatment, the uncovering of the patient's guilt, and the therapist's emphasis on redeveloping outside interpersonal personal relationships helped to reduce that risk.

NOTES

1. A related literary example that comes to mind is Miss Havisham in Charles Dickens's *Great Expectations*. Her life stops when she is jilted by her fiancé: the wedding table is left to rot, the clock is stopped at the tragic hour, and she wears a wedding dress that has turned to rags. Because grief in IPT requires a death, however, this problem would be termed a role transition rather than complicated bereavement.

CHAPTER 4

Interpersonal Role Disputes

An interpersonal dispute is a situation in which the patient and at least one significant other person have nonreciprocal expectations about their relationship. An example is the wife who expects the spouse to take care of her financially but must take an outside job to help meet their bills, whereas the spouse expects his wife to share financial responsibility. Another is the mother who expects her teenage daughter to confide in her fully the details of her friendships, as the mother had with her own mother, while the teenage girl feels that to grow up she must figure some things out on her own. In both examples, the parties have different expectations about the relationship. These expectations conflict—i.e., are nonreciprocal—and hence define a dispute.

The IPT therapist focuses on interpersonal disputes if they seem important in the onset and perpetuation of the depression. This usually occurs when the disputes are stalled or repetitious, leaving little hope for improvement. In such circumstances, depressed patients lose self-esteem, feeling they can no longer control the dispute, and feeling threatened by the loss of what the relationship provides, or incompetent to manage their own lives. Typical features that perpetuate role disputes are the patient's demoralized sense that nothing can be done (that the dispute has reached an *impasse*), poor habits of communication, or truly irreconcilable differences.

DIAGNOSIS OF INTERPERSONAL DISPUTES

For the therapist to choose role disputes as the focus of IPT, the patient must give evidence of current overt or covert disputes with a significant other.

Such disputes are usually revealed in the patient's initial complaints or in the course of the interpersonal inventory. In some IPT research, role disputes with a spouse have been the most common problem area. In practice, however, recognition of important interpersonal disputes in the lives of depressed patients may be difficult.

Depressed patients are typically preoccupied with their hopeless feelings and consider themselves solely responsible for their condition. When there is no clear precipitant to a depressive episode, and when the patient does not identify problems in current interpersonal relationships, it is important while eliciting the interpersonal inventory (as described in Chapter 2) to listen as much for what is omitted as for what is said. Insufficient or overidealized descriptions of current or recent important relationships may provide clues to difficulties that the patient is reluctant to recognize or explore. The therapist should question the patient carefully about how relationships have changed prior to or after the onset of depressive symptoms. An understanding of how interpersonal problems may have precipitated the depression or how they are involved in preventing recovery may suggest a strategy for therapy.

GOALS AND STRATEGIES OF TREATMENT

The general goals for treatment of interpersonal role disputes are to help the patient first identify the dispute, then make choices about a plan of action, and finally modify maladaptive communication patterns or reassess expectations, or both, for a satisfactory resolution of the interpersonal disputes. Improvements may take the form of a change in the expectations and behavior of the patient and/or the other person; changed and more accepting patient attitudes, with or without attempts to satisfy needs outside the relationship; or satisfactory dissolution of the relationship. The IPT therapist has no commitment to guide the patient to any particular resolution of difficulties and makes no attempt to preserve unworkable relationships.

Treating a patient with an interpersonal dispute often resembles a unilateral form of marital therapy. The therapist must decide whether it makes sense to bring in the other party, and if so, for how much of the treatment. In instances where the other member of the dispute is a work colleague or boss, or an unwilling spouse, the issue may be moot. An advantage of working with the patient alone on an interpersonal dispute is that the patient can take credit for all achievements that emerge, whereas in a conjoint therapy the therapist will invariably be credited.

The general IPT treatment strategy with interpersonal disputes is to help the patient understand how nonreciprocal role expectations relate to the dispute and begin steps that will bring about resolution of disputes and role negotiations. This movement from exploration to action may take place over the entire course of therapy, with early sessions devoted to exploration and communication analysis, and later sessions to decision analysis. In dealing with particular, circumscribed problems, however, exploration and decision making may occur in a single session.

In developing a treatment plan, the therapist first determines the stage of the role dispute:

1. *Impasse* implies that discussion between the patient and the significant other has stopped and that the low-level resentment typical of "cold marriages" exists.
   - Have the discussions between you and [the other person] stopped?
   - Do you use the "silent treatment" on each other?

2. *Renegotiation* implies that the patient and the significant other are openly aware of differences and are actively trying, even if unsuccessfully, to bring about changes.
   - Are you and [the other person] aware of the differences between you?
   - Are you trying to change things?
   - Do you often argue?

3. *Dissolution* implies that the relationship is irretrievably disrupted.
   - Are the differences between you so great that you're considering ending the relationship?

The therapist's tasks and expectations at these three stages differ. For example, intervening in an impasse situation may initially increase apparent disharmony as negotiations are reopened, while the task of treating a dispute at the stage of unsatisfactory renegotiation may be to calm down the participants to facilitate conflict resolution. In addressing either renegotiation or impasse, the therapist's treatment goal is often to help the patient learn new ways of communicating and self-assertion in order to facilitate a resolution of the dispute. The treatment of disputes at the stage of dissolution has much in common with the treatment of grief described in Chapter 3, in that the therapist tries to help the patient put the relationship in perspective and become free to form new attachments.

In exploring role disputes, the therapist seeks information on different levels. At a practical level, these questions are answered:

- What are the ostensible issues in the dispute?
- What are the differences in expectations and values between the patient and the significant other?
- What are the patient's wishes in the relationship?
- What are the patient's options: which have been explored, and which remain?
- What resources does the patient have to bring about change in the relationship?
- What does the other person want?
- How have they resolved disagreements in the past?
- What are the strengths and weaknesses, the high points and disappointments of the relationship?
- What changes are realistically possible?

To understand the importance of the particular dispute under discussion, the therapist looks for parallels in previous relationships. The parallels may be obvious—for example, when a patient has repeatedly gotten involved with alcoholic men. Others are more subtle, as when patients keep manipulating others into rejecting them. Useful questions are:

- Has this happened to you before?
- Do you have other similar relationships? The relationship you describe sounds like the one you had with ____.

When parallels are discovered, the key questions to explore are:

- What does the patient gain by the behavior?
- What are the central unspoken assumptions that lie behind it?

- What leads the patient into similar unpleasant situations?

It is important that the therapist not blame the already self-critical depressed patient for situations to which the depressive state itself may have contributed. The tone of these questions should always be curious and optimistic:

Let's figure out what went wrong here, so that we can decide how to help you make it better.

Attention to the interpersonal strategies of the disputants frequently reveals problems in communication patterns. For instance, repetitious, painful disputes are frequently perpetuated when the participants are afraid of confrontation and expression of negative feelings and try to ignore solvable problems by simply waiting for things to "blow over." It may be useful to ask the patient:

- Have you told ____ directly how you feel? (If so: What response did you get?)
- What do you think would happen if you did? (Could you try?)

The aim here is to help patients recognize their complex, mixed feelings of anger, fear, and sadness, and devise strategies for managing them, such as avoiding situations in which they arise, expressing wishes directly, and reducing impulsive behavior based on irrational suspicions. Depressed patients typically have difficulty in asserting their needs and in appropriately expressing anger in interpersonal situations.

When a patient has developed a sufficiently clear understanding of role disputes, including the part he or she plays in them, therapist and patient can proceed to a thorough consideration of the consequences of a number of alternatives before taking action.

A role dispute can be renegotiated successfully if the patient becomes able to express needs and wishes directly to the other person, and together they are able to work out a resolution that incorporates the needs of both. There will be some understanding of each other's needs and some compromise on both sides. Role playing is often a crucial preparation to help patients anticipate problems and rehearse the expression of their emotions and wishes in the dispute.

AN INTERPERSONAL ROLE DISPUTE:
THE CASE OF ALICE

Alice was twenty-eight years old and had been married for ten years when she began treatment. She worked with her husband in his business. Her chief complaints were a lack of interest in everything around her, increasing irritability, and marital problems. Her symptoms included sad mood, difficulty falling asleep, loss of appetite and interest, and a profound sense of her inadequacy as a woman. Her relationship with her husband had deteriorated markedly over the previous four months.

She believed he took her for granted and was interested in her only insofar as she fulfilled his needs as a sex partner and as an employee. Alice vacillated between self-blame and feelings of helplessness on the one hand, and angry accusations about her husband's inattentiveness and lack of concern for her wishes on the other. As she talked of first one area and then the other, she tended to lose track of what she was saying. She related her depression to her husband's all-consuming interest in his business and what she perceived as the resulting change in their relationship.

Although she dated the onset of her difficulties as four months before seeking treatment, she was unable to identify any specific event. Instead, she spoke about her growing dissatisfaction with what she perceived as her husband's selfish and controlling attitude and his lack of consideration for her feelings.

As Alice reviewed the history of their marriage, she expressed nostalgia for the "good old days" when they were poor but happy. She reported feeling increasingly left out since he purchased the business five years ago. Exploration of her interpersonal relationships revealed a paucity of social supports as well as lifelong feelings of loneliness associated with her inability to establish and/or maintain intimate relationships. She had been one of nine children in a somewhat fragmented family. Although they all lived in the same city, she had only minimal contact with them now. Alice had felt fairly close to her mother, but this relationship was somewhat strained by her belief that her mother had never approved of Alice's husband.

After gathering information about the current depression, the events surrounding the onset, and Alice's perception of its effect on her relationship with her husband, the therapist tried to explore what Alice hoped to get out of therapy—how she expected therapy to be helpful to her. She indicated that she wanted: (1) "someone to talk to," because she felt unable to discuss these issues with her husband; (2) to learn how to stand up to her husband; and (3) to get her husband to respect her, to relate to her as a wife and not as an irresponsible child or employee.

At the end of the first session, the therapist was still uncertain how to conceptualize the patient in terms of IPT problem areas. Although the social history made it clear that the patient had interpersonal role deficits, she had come for treatment with the specific problem of an interpersonal role dispute with her husband, and as the session developed, marital disputes in an impasse phase became the central focus.

INITIAL PHASE (SESSIONS 2–4)

In the early sessions, Alice focused on her ambivalence vis-à-vis her marriage and her dependence on her husband. She continued to express disappointment with what it meant to be a "married woman," and she described the gradual process by which she had become more and more dependent upon and controlled by her husband. She related to him as if he were a disapproving father; she was afraid of offending him, yet angry that she seemed unable to please him. She had a severely restricted view of the options available to her, thinking she must either deny her own wishes to please her husband or get out of the marriage. The interpersonal inventory revealed a pattern of withdrawal, denial, and/or indirect communication of her wishes. She seemed to expect others to "know" what she needed and felt rejected if her needs were not magically anticipated and met.

Much of the work in these sessions focused on sorting out with Alice her expectations in the marriage and how she thought things would have to change if she were to be more comfortable. Since she was committed to the marriage, goals were set in terms of working on improving communications with her husband and in developing some independent interests so she would be less dependent on him to fulfill all her needs.

Alice's communication problems with her husband were discussed first. She described a fight they had had the previous night. She acknowledged that her customary way of avoiding confrontation on the real issues was related to the couple's increasing estrangement. She said she could express her real wants only when she was angry, but the depth of her rage frightened her and made her feel guilty—and so she would withdraw into silence but continue to seethe. During these sessions she started to talk, albeit indirectly, about her suspicions that her husband was "fooling around" with a young woman who worked in the store with them. As if she couldn't trust her own judgment, she remarked, "Everybody says it's so but I just can't see it . . . I don't know." Later she said that her husband had had a series of girlfriends over the past few years, but she felt certain he wouldn't leave her. The fourth session ended with her assertion that she was going to try to begin to talk to him about what she expected of him without waiting until she blew up, but, typically, she put a damper on it by saying, "But you'll see . . . it won't work."

INTERMEDIATE PHASE (SESSIONS 5–8)

Alice began the fifth session by bringing a letter her husband had written to her the previous night. Many individuals communicate by letter since they find face-to-face discussion of difficult issues easier if they first communicate in writing. In the letter, he talked about his love for her, his sadness about their deteriorating marriage, and his frustration about his seeming inability to "turn things around." She expressed doubts about her husband's sincerity: "I just can't get myself to believe it—it seems he just wants to get me where he wants me, and then it just starts all over again." When the therapist suggested that it might be helpful to have him join them for one session, she became quite restless and said, "I don't want to talk about him any more. I just want to talk about my problems." Later, she agreed to ask him but felt that he wouldn't come.

When they both came for the conjoint session, the communication problems reported in previous sessions were played out in this hour. Alice remained silent for most of the hour, allowing her husband to do most of the talking. When she reluctantly began to talk about her complaints, she finally confronted her husband, Mark, about his involvement with the saleswoman, which he promptly denied. By the end of the hour they had begun to talk to each other more directly, rather than entirely through the therapist.

After the conjoint session, there was a marked change in Alice's appearance. Up to now she had looked rather shabby and sullen—usually dressed in black. She started wearing bright colors and her overall attitude had a bright, confident, "up" quality. She and Mark had gone out to dinner a couple of times, and had visited relatives whom they hadn't seen for a long time. Although she acknowledged feeling some satisfaction with this broadening of their activities, she nevertheless continued to express doubt about Mark's motives. She described several occasions on which she felt rebuffed when she had begun to express her wishes to him. What was most impressive, however, was her determination to "let him know what's on my mind whether he wants to hear it or not."

Alice also spoke about her fear that people (especially her family) might think that she had gotten "uppity" since she and her husband had become financially secure. She described her humble background and her own discomfort with Mark's new, "classy" ways. Whereas Mark enjoyed his success and the community respect it brought him, Alice felt somewhat embarrassed by it, because it seemed to represent yet another barrier separating her from her family and former friends. She was cut off from her roots, so to speak, yet ill at ease with her new status in the community.

During these middle sessions, much of the time was devoted to exploring the couple's efforts to reestablish some contact with each other and with their families. Toward the end of the eighth session, Alice acknowledged her anxiety about termination. The following week, Mark telephoned to cancel his wife's appointment because "Alice is sick and she didn't want to call you herself."

TERMINATION PHASE (SESSIONS 9–12)

At the next scheduled session, Alice once again started to talk about difficulties with her husband over his business. Both the content and the quality of her comments were reminiscent of the first sessions. The relatively introspective stance of the previous sessions had all but disappeared. Midway into the hour, however, Alice became quiet and somewhat thoughtful. She finally said, "I'm scared to show Mark my love, that's all it is." As the therapist began to discuss these feelings, she commented, almost casually, that her husband had been talking about getting a divorce. Despite her insistence that she really didn't take it seriously, it seemed to have a disorganizing effect on her functioning. Toward the end of the hour, she again raised the issue of termination and voiced her concern about not yet feeling strong enough to go it on her own.

In the following sessions, the therapist continued to explore with Alice her feelings about termination, but Alice had a tendency to avoid the issue or deny having any special feelings about it. The couple had been arguing more frequently. Part of the conflict seemed to focus on Mark's desire for a child and Alice's extreme ambivalence about being further tied down. She was also afraid Mark might leave her if she had a baby, and this was not completely irrational, since both Mark's and Alice's fathers had abandoned their families. Another part of her resistance to becoming pregnant was her feeling that this would represent just one more way she would be "giving in" to her husband. Despite the increase in arguments between them, she reported feeling less depressed than she had the previous week; "letting it out is better than keeping the stuff inside," she said. At the final session, Alice was somewhat agitated and attempts to explore her feelings about the termination were met with denial and thinly disguised anger.

Three days after this stormy termination session, however, Alice telephoned to "apologize" and to say she was in fact feeling better after all. She refused referral for further treatment: "I think I'd like to try it on my own."

While the course of IPT in this case did not fully resolve the dispute, the patient by the end of treatment was asymptomatic and had identified the key issues in the dispute. Whether or not she would resolve them on her own, or even with additional treatment, was left uncertain, but she was now at least in a better position to try.

AN INTERPERSONAL ROLE DISPUTE:
THE CASE OF SAL

Sal, a thirty-one-year-old married man, was unemployed at the time of the first interview but within a week found a job as a television repairman's assistant. His chief complaint was a history of decreased energy and motivation over the past several months. He reported having difficulty finishing projects on his house because he quickly became physically exhausted. He also slept less and had little interest in sex. "My feelings have left me," he said.

Initial Phase (Sessions 1–4)

Sal was the oldest male in a traditional Italian family. His mother was the emotional caretaker for the family and his father was a stern, "cold" man whom Sal could never get along with. He was critical, unavailable, and "browbeating." Sal described himself as an underachiever in school: he was not interested in schoolwork. He dropped out of high school in the eleventh grade and joined the Marines as a challenge to his father's assertion that he'd never make it. After his hitch was up he became a construction worker under the direction of his father, who was a foreman. Their work relationship was often stressed by disagreements.

Five years ago Sal had had a fall that injured his knee and leg; he could no longer do construction work, which he had found productive and lucrative. He then became more dependent on his wife, who quit her job to care for him while he was in a wheelchair. Sal said that if he had not had the fall, or if he had been able to go back to his old job after it, he would be a foreman by now. As a result of this physical handicap, he changed jobs and became a TV repairman, receiving vocational training through workmen's compensation.

He tended to minimize the effect of his injury on his self-esteem, and talked mainly about his marital difficulties. He often came to his appointments looking tired and disheveled, and did not spontaneously volunteer information. As a result, the therapist maintained an active profile by asking specific questions and taking a careful interpersonal inventory. The central theme that emerged was Sal's feeling of inadequacy and powerlessness in relation to life in general, but more specifically in relation to his father and his wife.

By the end of the initial sessions, it had become clear that Sal's depressive symptomatology was associated with marital disputes with his wife. These seemed largely related to an impasse in relation to his wife, his problems in expressing his wishes to her, and their increasing estrangement. Treatment centered on his understanding the impediments prohibiting him from constructively communicating with his wife.

INTERMEDIATE PHASE (SESSIONS 5–8)

When Sal began to explore his relationship with his wife in more detail, in Session 5, he started crying as he described his unhappiness in his marriage and his difficulty articulating his feelings because he felt "numb." He said that he had been "holding on" to many of his feelings, which was causing a break in the relationship with his wife. In the next session he again addressed family issues, and for the first time he began to see some similarities between himself and his father. He said he thought he was treating his wife in many of the same distancing ways that his father treated him.

Session 7 proved to be a turning point. He was more self-revealing, and he described the ways he and his wife had been very "emotional" and close with each other during the past week. They had talked more openly and had finally been able to make a joint decision to accept a lump sum of money from an insurance company for the leg disability rather than accept compensation in the form of disability payments. This decision, which would relieve the couple of a great deal of their financial burden, had been worrying them for more than a year.

In Session 8, Sal said he felt improvement in his overall attitude. He stated that as he tried to change, to share thoughts and feelings with his wife, she began to meet him halfway, which favorably surprised him. He and the therapist discussed possible ways in which he could further involve his wife in how he was feeling.

TERMINATION PHASE (SESSIONS 9–12)

During this phase, Sal was laid off. He explored some of the circumstances leading up to the layoff and the feelings of hurt and anger surrounding the event. He was puzzled that he did not go out and look for work immediately, but thought this was due in part to receiving the insurance settlement and in part to a need to assess his job situation and plan more carefully. He had made use of the layoff to seek his wife's opinion. He thought that in the past he would have picked a fight with his wife, indirectly thrusting his job worries onto her. He planned to start looking for work the following week, after he had a chance to consider his options.

In Session 5, Sal had said that before he began treatment he had withdrawn too much from his wife, and he was now risking more openness with her. He had been surprised to find that she had not responded negatively or "violently" when he expressed his feelings. He went on to say that he could not continue to prejudge his wife's responses, but he still felt he could not share too many intimate feelings with her for fear she would get upset. In discussing termination, he said that initially his major concern about involving himself in treatment was his fear of disclosing feelings that he did not want to reveal. He was afraid the therapist would "jump into my head" and force feelings out. Rather, he had been pleasantly surprised to experience therapy as enabling him to explore and find out about himself.

In Session 11, Sal initiated the session by stating that he had a great deal to say. He was happily thinking about going into work as a subcontractor in which he would be his own boss. He felt more confident and less lethargic at home, able to accomplish home chores more willingly; as a result, he experienced less pressure from his wife. He had been communicating more directly with her, saying so when he wanted to help her and not pushing her away without explanation. He acknowledged that the financial problems and the enforced idleness after his injury had been extremely demoralizing. And his feeling like a failure while he was working as a repairman had also contributed to the depression, because he was not producing up to his potential. In talking about terminating, Sal said he was still baffled that he hadn't been able to express as much to his wife as he had with the therapist.

In the last session, Sal expressed positive feelings toward the therapy and said he had experienced a sense of "reawakening" within himself. He felt relaxed in the treatment and wanted to create the same openness with his wife that he felt with the therapist.

AN INTERPERSONAL ROLE DISPUTE:
THE CASE OF LISA

Lisa, a twenty-eight-year-old artist, presented with the chief complaint: "This last year of my life has been hell." She reported having been depressed for much of the past year following the breakup of her relationship with her ex-fiancé.

INITIAL PHASE (SESSIONS 1–2)

Lisa reported that she had been engaged for nearly three years, during which time her fiancé, Roy, had insisted on having unprotected sexual intercourse. He began to lose weight over time, a fact to which she paid little attention until the day he told her that he was leaving her for a man, and that he had AIDS. She reported she felt "a little angry" upon hearing this, but almost immediately criticized herself for having negative thoughts about "a dying man." She then developed a major depression, including a hopeless mood, loss of sleep, appetite, and energy, and passive suicidal ideation. Her Hamilton Depression Rating Scale score was in the mid–twenties.

Although Roy left their apartment, taking many of their common belongings, they maintained a relationship thereafter in which he frequently called her to complain about physical aches and pains, interspersed with reports about his numerous (unprotected) sexual exploits. Lisa frequently brought him chicken soup. She continued to make deposits in their joint checking account, from which he made the withdrawals. She withdrew from her friendships, and refrained from telling her friends the details of the rupture or of Roy's behavior. She had tested HIV-negative, but was still within the time frame for possible seroconversion.

From the interpersonal inventory emerged other instances of Lisa's rather passively complying with the domineering and sometimes sadistic behavior of others, including her autocratic father. She was generally cheerful, supportive, unassertive, and quietly dissatisfied with but rarely overtly angry in her relationships. From a psychodynamic perspective, she might easily have been considered to have a masochistic personality disorder; alternatively, the diagnostic question arose of whether she had suffered from a mild form of dysthymia prior to this major depressive episode. The IPT therapist, while noting this behavioral pattern, emphasized to Lisa that she had a treatable major depression, and emphasized the connection to the role dispute: "It's hard not to believe that your depression is connected to your still-persisting relationship with Roy." Lisa agreed to a fourteen-session treatment.

INTERMEDIATE PHASE (SESSIONS 3–10)

Early sessions in this phase focused on Lisa's feelings about Roy and their relationship. The therapist tried to help her recognize the anger about which she continued to feel guilty. They discussed Roy's infidelity and his putting her at risk for HIV infection through unprotected sex while knowing he was positive. The therapist called these transgressions, breaking the explicit or implicit agreed-upon rules of common decency in relationships: "No one should behave that way; if they do, you have a right to feel angry." After a few sessions, Lisa conceded that perhaps she had some reason to feel angry, and began to express this in sessions. Role playing helped to prepare her to confront Roy, but as the weeks passed, the confrontation failed to occur. The therapist began to feel frustrated, but relied on the time limit and on gentle exhortation to push events forward. Lisa felt somewhat relieved at voicing her anger in sessions, but remained depressed.

Lisa came to Session 9 in high spirits, bustling through the door. She reported that she had accidentally bumped into Roy in a restaurant. She was initially unsure what to say, but when he made a provocative, critical remark, she "let him have it": she angrily told him that he had had no right to treat her that way, had put her life in danger, and owed her an apology. How dare he! Furthermore, she continued, she wanted her belongings back, and he had better march to the bank with her to close their joint checking account. And if he continued to have unprotected sex with others, she would tell their friends about his disgraceful behavior. He was apparently surprised, and sufficiently chastened that he ceased stalling and did close the bank account with her.

Buoyed by her success, Lisa immediately felt euthymic, and her other depressive symptoms resolved. Emboldened, she also called her father—whose behavior had not been a focus of the therapy—and told *him* off about his treatment of her, too. The therapist congratulated Lisa on her self-assertion, and pointed out the relationship between her taking control of these relationships and expressing her feelings, and the improvement of her depressive symptoms.

The following week, Lisa seemed a bit lost, unsure of what to do next, but she never again appeared depressed. In subsequent sessions, she moved from her apartment, which contained bad memories of her relationship, and found a new job at higher pay.

TERMINATION PHASE (SESSIONS 11–14)

In the final sessions, the therapist and Lisa reviewed her impressive gains, and the vulnerabilities that might have made her unhappy in relationships. Lisa reported that her friends had noticed her new attitude: she herself had realized that she deferred too much to others in relationships, and was handling them differently, more assertively. She was no longer depressed, and recognized the appropriateness of ending IPT, but asked about referral to a psychodynamic treatment "to figure out how I tick." The referral was made accordingly.

*   *   *

This last case demonstrates some differences between IPT and psychodynamic psychotherapy, which might well have focused on the patient's "characterological" masochism, confusing it with the primary problem of the mood disorder. The psychotherapy also focused on the current interpersonal crisis rather than, for example, on the patient's relationship with her father. IPT made no attempt to change character, but did help the patient to develop new social skills, to assert her feelings, and to express anger. When treatment ended with the major depressive episode resolved, referral to psychodynamic psychotherapy seemed reasonable for a different treatment indication.

CHAPTER 5

Role Transitions

Depression associated with role transitions occurs when a person has difficulty coping with life change. Almost everyone has multiple roles in the social system, and these roles become indelibly interwoven with the sense of self. The roles themselves, as well as the status attached to them, have an important influence on the individual's social behavior and patterns of interpersonal relationships. Impairment in social functioning frequently occurs in response to demands for rapid adaptation to new, strange roles, especially changes that are experienced by the individual as loss. Not all individuals undergoing role transitions experience the change as a loss. Those who are clinically depressed are more likely to experience role changes as loss. The loss may be immediately apparent, as in the case of divorce, or it may be more subtle, like the loss of leisure following the birth of a child. Retirement or some other change of social or professional role, especially one that brings diminished social status, is often another kind of subtle loss. Moving, changing jobs, leaving home, economic change, and changes in family roles due to illness, new responsibilities, or retirement are other examples of role transition.

The most frequently encountered role transitions occur with progression to another part of the human life cycle. Since these changes are expected as part of the timetable of biological growth and development or are dictated by social and cultural patterns, they are considered normative transitions. The transition to adolescence, childbirth, the end of childbearing potential, and the decline of physical capacity with aging are biologically normative.

Social transitions, which are heavily determined by social class and historical era, include entering college or leaving home for the first time, marriage, job promotion, and retirement. It is important to remark that most transitions are neither inherently good nor bad, and generally entail both advantages and disadvantages. Depressed individuals, of course, will focus on the negative aspects of the change and may fail to see its potential benefits.

People who feel they are failing in a new role, or who are not satisfied with the role or its status, may become depressed. These difficulties are often related to ideas about the new role that the patient is only partly aware of and that may be discovered through a systematic attempt in therapy to find out what the change means to the particular person. People who, paradoxically, become depressed after a sought-after promotion are commonly troubled by conflicts about responsibility and independence. They were actually more comfortable in the old, subordinate role, in a less demanding job with more direction from others.

Depression frequently results when a person recognizes the need to make a normative role transition but has difficulty with the changes required, or when a person correctly recognizes failure in a particular role but is unable to change the behavior or to change roles. In depressions associated with role transitions, the patient feels helpless to cope with the change in role. The transition may be experienced as threatening to one's self-esteem and sense of identity, or as a challenge one is unable to meet. Patients frequently view life as having been comfortable before the change, and describe a sense of chaos and lack of control over the transition.

In general, difficulties in coping with role transitions are associated with the following issues:

1. loss of familiar social supports and attachments;
2. management of accompanying emotions, such as anger or fear;
3. demands for a new repertoire of social skills; and
4. diminished self-esteem.

Depression is commonly associated with developmental role transitions. For example, depression in late adolescence or early adulthood (late teens and early twenties) typically involves difficulties in achieving a satisfactory sense of role identity or in forming intimate relationships outside the family.

Patients with these problems may remain overattached to their parents. Other role transition problems that are typical of young adult life include adapting to occupational or marital roles and to the role of parent.

In the middle adult years, depression may be related to failure to find satisfaction or success in one's chosen career, marriage difficulties, or a decrease in the parental role. In old age, depression may be related to a loss of role and status through retirement, decline in health, or loss of social supports through illness, relocation, or death of relatives and friends. Although the normal bereavement process may have ended, the loss of a childhood friend or close family member may have left a difficult gap to fill.

DIAGNOSIS OF ROLE TRANSITION PROBLEMS

To diagnose role transition as a problem area for IPT, the therapist requires evidence that the patient's depression and related clinical problems have followed life changes related to role transitions. In most instances, this relationship will be apparent to patients and their significant others, and the patient will readily identify the transition: for example, leaving school, seeking a first job, impending marriage, recent divorce, or retirement.

In exploring role transitions, such inquiries as these have proven helpful:

- Have there been changes in your life recently?
- Have you been separated or divorced?
- Have your children left home?
- Has someone moved in with you?
- Have you moved?
- Did you start or end school or a job?
- Were you promoted or demoted?
- Did you retire?
- Have you had financial problems? Health problems?
- Have you started living alone?

Tell me about the change [retirement, leaving home, the divorce, etc.]. How did your life change? What important people were left behind? Who took their place? How did you feel in the new role [as retiree, divorcée, student]?

What was life like before the change?

The therapist should look for age- and stage-appropriate life changes, such as graduations from school, moving in or out of a home or of a relationship, getting or losing a job, being promoted or demoted, having significant financial reversals, or developing a significant illness. Each of these events may be accompanied by changes in relationships with significant others.

PLANNING TREATMENT
FOR ROLE TRANSITION

Although the issues may vary according to the life phase the patient is in, certain elements common to all role transitions can help define the tasks and goals of IPT treatment for depression connected with these transitions. Problems in managing role transitions center on four tasks:

1. giving up the old role;
2. expressing guilt, anger, loss;
3. acquiring new skills;
4. developing new attachments and supports, and identifying positive aspects of the new role.

Table 5.1 outlines these tasks and offers suggestions for questions the therapist can ask to check the patient's progress with them.

EVALUATION OF OLD ROLE

This first task resembles the facilitation of grief described in Chapter 3. The psychotherapist helps the patient put the lost role in perspective by evaluating the activities and attachments that were given up. In general, patients who are having difficulty managing role transitions tend to idealize the benefits offered by the old role while minimizing its negative aspects. In reviewing the aspects of the role that has been lost, it is useful to help the patient acknowledge the difficulties of the old role, while also trying to discover and grieve the loss of its positive aspects. For example, one patient had great difficulty managing her separation from her husband because, to her, being married, regardless of the circumstances, was socially expected of women. She had suppressed the extent to which her marriage had been a

TABLE 5.1   Checking the Parent's Progress

Task	Therapist's Questions
1. Facilitate evaluation of role that has been lost.	Tell me about the old whatever has been left or lost or changed—the old house, the former job, living with parents, the former spouse, etc. What were the good things? The bad? What did you like? Not like?
2. Encourage expression of emotions.	How did it feel to give up or leave _____? Tell me the details of your leaving. How did you feel in the new situation? What was it like at first?
3. Develop social skills suitable for the new role.	What is required of you? How hard is this? How does it make you feel? What is going well? Badly?
4. Establish new interpersonal relations, attachments, and social supports.	Whom do you know? Who can help you? Are there people you want to get to know?
5 Identify any positive aspects of the new role.	What is your new life like? Are there any benefits? Potential benefits?

failure and a destructive element in her life because the role of divorcée was unacceptable.

ENCOURAGING EXPRESSION OF AFFECT

Even when a change is desired and sought, giving up the old role may be experienced as a loss, so that a mourning process occurs. The patient may have experienced the satisfaction of mastering the requisite social skills needed to perform in an old and familiar role, and may have derived great pleasure from rewards unique to that phase of life. Management of the old role also may have involved development of a satisfying system of social supports that were vital to maintenance of self-esteem.

To facilitate the transition, it is useful to elicit the feelings about the change, including grief, guilt—perhaps at not having entirely lived up to self-expectations—anger, and disappointment.

Developing New Social Skills

Most important transitions involve acquisition of new skills. The IPT psychotherapist is not a vocational counselor whose task is to determine the patient's aptitude for taking on different kinds of jobs. The therapist instead helps the patient to assess the meaning of the role expectations, and tries to discover the beliefs and emotions that are hindering the patient from making full use of potential coping skills.

The new role may require new skills, both to respond to new role demands and to form new relationships and attachments. The therapist may help the patient go through a realistic assessment of assets and skills for managing the transition, while carefully looking out for areas in which the patient may be over- or underestimating them. Such skills might include finding an apartment on one's own, learning to get around in a new community, finding a new job, learning to entertain. Frequently, difficulty in managing new demands is related to performance anxiety. To help with this, the therapist may engage the patient in a kind of rehearsal of difficult situations, asking the patient to imagine, for example, the worst thing that could happen, and role playing the situation.

Another important type of difficulty involves incorrect or stereotyped assumptions about the new role. These attitudes are often formed through observation of and identification with key individuals in the patient's past who provided undesirable models. To counter these attitudes, the therapist can frequently help the patient recognize examples of specific cases that contradict the stereotype. For example, one sixty-two-year-old woman had a great deal of difficulty getting involved with a senior citizens' group because this meant that she was "old." However, an evaluation of what she meant by "old"—which included isolation, lack of activities, and lack of interests—actually described her own socially isolated situation. In contrast, even the little contact she had with the senior citizens' group showed her that they were less "old," and more lively and involved, than she was.

Establishing Social Supports

Taking on a new role often means developing a new system of social supports, forming new types of relationships as well as familiar kinds of relationships with new people. In addition, the types of rewards offered by the new social role may be unfamiliar and less avidly desired than those offered by the old one. This sort of change may occur when a woman returns to the workforce after her children no longer need her as a full-time caregiver. Although she may have had previous work experience, the demands of the job may have changed markedly since then, or they may seem more difficult to manage after a lapse of some years. Often too, the kind of job the patient wants or finds available is entirely different from the earlier one. Many women feel apprehensive about entering what is still often perceived as the "man's world" of the workplace, and though they have less time to enjoy old friendships, they may hesitate to form comparable relationships with work associates.

To help the patient develop the needed social supports, the therapist might review the opportunities available in the new role for getting involved with others. Depressed patients are likely to have overlooked opportunities for forming supportive relationships and to have become socially isolated. Positive aspects of the new role, including new social supports and opportunities, are discussed.

ROLE TRANSITIONS: THE CASE OF ELLEN

Ellen was a twenty-seven-year-old part-time salesclerk and mother of a six-year-old son. She came for treatment three weeks after a suicide attempt with a combination of nonprescription medications. The precipitant had been the end of an extramarital affair. She had been chronically dissatisfied with her marriage of ten years to an alcoholic husband, who provided her with steady financial support but little affection. Moreover, when the husband drank, which occurred several times weekly, he became verbally abusive and sometimes physically assaultive. Ellen's extramarital affair, she said, "made me realize what I had been missing." The affair had lasted only a few months, and the lover had returned to another woman. Feeling abandoned and hopeless, Ellen made her impulsive suicide attempt immediately after getting the news. She was treated in an emergency room and sent home, where she developed severe depressive symptoms. When these persisted for three weeks, she sought professional help. This was her first depressive episode.

INITIAL PHASE (SESSIONS 1–3)

Ellen saw her depression as clearly related to her difficulty in ending the marriage and disrupting the attachment. She had left her husband several years before, but his behavior toward her improved while they were apart and she returned after two months. Old patterns had quickly been resumed, and Ellen had felt trapped again. She said that she hoped treatment would "help me to leave him." She felt she deserved better treatment than she received from her husband, but was unsure that she could actually make the break. She felt apathetic, anhedonic, and pessimistic that any positive changes could take place.

Ellen and a sister five years younger were raised by a domineering, passive/aggressive mother, her father having left the family for another woman when the patient was six years old. Her mother did not become involved with other men, and Ellen recalled feeling that the family seemed to her to be unattractive, outcast women who could not gain the attention of a supportive man. This view of herself and her family contrasted with her personal attractiveness and social abilities. In fact, she herself was a popular student, as well as a good one, throughout her high school years. Her mother's relationship with her was excessively close—overwhelming—and her marriage at the age of seventeen was seen as a means of leaving mother and home. However, this did not completely interrupt her mother's intrusiveness into her affairs. She still had qualms about contradicting her mother and felt that this was also something that she would like to work on in treatment.

By the second session, Ellen had asked her husband to leave the house and he had willingly agreed, expressing his own discontentment with the marriage. Ellen felt elated and reported an improvement in the depressive symptoms. She also described feeling surprisingly free of conflict about breaking up with her husband, in spite of her years of being unsure about doing so. She also described becoming more forthright and direct with her mother in discussions about such matters as when she would take a vacation. These two sessions were largely taken up with reviewing her relationships with her husband and mother. From this discussion, it emerged that she avoided taking responsibility for her decisions and got others, such as her mother or her husband, to make decisions for her. She distrusted her own judgment and was hesitant about thinking things through. Related to her discomfort with taking responsibility for herself was her conviction that losing her man (or getting him to leave) would mean being unattractive, unwomanly, and devalued, as she felt her mother and she were after the father left. Her pattern of relations with a man was to get involved and stay with the man at all costs, overlooking all faults. She also, however, expressed fears of being alone, having never lived on her own as the head of a household.

From the information gathered in the first three sessions, it was decided that the focus of therapy would be helping Ellen manage the role transitions involved in separating from her husband. It was anticipated that this would involve the following steps: (1) helping her identify new sources of emotional support to replace her husband and her husband's family, (2) exploration and correction of fears of being alone and her tendency to distrust her own judgments, (3) helping her develop a new repertoire of social skills, such as the discipline of her child, and (4) helping her recognize the distinction between her own value and having a man, any man. It was decided to treat her case as one of role transition rather than role dispute because of Ellen's conviction that the differences between her and her husband were irreconcilable, and her professed certainty that she wanted to end the marriage.

INTERMEDIATE PHASE (SESSIONS 4–10)

Ellen continued to feel good about the separation from her husband. In search of alternative sources of support, she had first turned to her extended family, including her in-laws and her mother, who had all urged her to reconcile with her husband, describing, for instance, how "pathetic" he seemed to be without her. Realizing that seeking help from these people had contributed to her previous reunion with her husband, she began to reestablish old relationships with women friends. Before the fifth session, the husband had come to ask her to take him back and she had refused. She noted that he was drinking at the time of the request. The psychotherapist then explored the possibility of a reconciliation, asking the circumstances under which she would find reconciliation acceptable. Ellen felt that there were no circumstances under which she would be willing to reestablish the marriage.

Four weeks after the separation, she began to date again. She found this a positive experience, though she felt strange, after ten years, at having to consider what she wanted and expected from the men she went out with. Just at this time, she began to have trouble with her son, who was beginning to act up at school and at home. She realized that she had tended to leave the disciplinary role to her husband and that she had been uncomfortable about discussing the separation with the child. Several sessions were spent discussing in detail how she related to her son, how to talk with him about the separation, and alternative approaches to discipline. The son's behavior improved at home and at school, and she began to feel closer to him.

From Session 5 on, Ellen's symptoms improved. She still had good and bad days, but the anhedonic, lethargic, hopeless feelings had passed. Ellen continued to date, and became interested in one man. In treatment she examined her initial attraction to her husband. He was "safe" because he had become dependent on her, and because he was so "pathetic" without her. She realized that she was attracted to men who were quickly and unconditionally interested in her because she felt so fearful of being rejected by men. As a result, she was not discriminating about the men she became involved with. She also began to discuss with the psychotherapist early signs she might use to help her detect similar nonproductive patterns in her future relationships with men.

TERMINATION PHASE (SESSIONS 11–13)

As the end of treatment approached, Ellen reported feelings of emptiness and boredom, and a sense that her life was going nowhere. She did not relate this to the end of treatment, but spoke principally of her reemerging sense of worthlessness in living without a man, even if this was recognized as not necessarily a permanent situation. More material about her adolescent feelings of self-condemnation and worthlessness without a father were discussed, and Ellen began to talk about such dismaying things as growing old and ugly. The therapist related these feelings to the termination and Ellen's fears of being on her own, and tried to contrast her fears with her actual level of competence and indicators of her attractiveness.

At this time the husband made another attempt to induce Ellen to take him back. Although tempted, she again reminded herself of the old patterns and decided that even though she felt lonely and unhappy now, she would be condemning herself to a more enduring unhappiness if she resumed the marriage. In the final session, she reviewed the changes in attitudes and behaviors that she had made during the treatment, including her improved relationship with her child, her growing circle of friends, both male and female, her dating, her greater ability to communicate her needs and disagreements to others, and her improved sense of independence and competence. On the basis of this, she concluded that she did not want to resume her old life, even if she had to put up with a certain amount of loneliness.

*   *   *

The patient's immediate depressive episode was precipitated by an extramarital affair that brought into focus the things that were missing in her marriage. Although she had long recognized her dissatisfaction with her husband, she had been able to ignore it until she experienced what an alternative relationship could be like. She came to treatment wanting to escape her destructive marriage but feeling unable to make the change on her own. The therapist helped the patient to evaluate the new demands, available social supports, and rewards associated with becoming a more independent single parent. The demands of separation from her husband included: (1) tolerating loneliness; (2) maintaining her self-esteem without being identified with a man; (3) parenting her child; and (4) making new friends and dating. In each case the therapist helped her examine the fears associated with the demands and determine that she in fact had the resources to meet them.

In the situation of her disciplining her son, the therapist not only evaluated

Ellen's attitudes about being a single parent but was active in teaching the patient ways to think about and talk with him, information that she had not obtained elsewhere. As for social supports, the therapist helped the patient identify new supports that were less conflicted than her relationships with her mother and in-laws. To help the patient enter the new role, the therapist helped her clarify her feelings about the role she wanted to leave—being married to her husband and highly involved with her mother. From this process, the patient decided that she was losing far more than she gained in these relationships, and this view helped to provide incentive for accepting the strain of making the transition she wanted. And in jointly considering the rewards of the new role, the therapist helped the patient recognize the relief and pride she felt in relying on herself.

ROLE TRANSITION: THE CASE OF ROGER[1]

Roger, a fifty-year-old separated businessman, presented with a three-month history of major depression. Although he denied any precipitants, it soon became apparent that he had recently been passed over for a job promotion. Having just turned fifty, he saw that he would never reach the pinnacle of the company in which he had worked for twenty-five years. His social supports were limited, as he had typically given precedence to work over his family and other relationships. His wife of twenty-seven years had asked him to move out the year before, and his two children were away in college. His circle of friends consisted of business colleagues with whom he competed and was ashamed to tell of his debacle. His symptoms included passive suicidal ideation, a hopeless feeling that his life was over and might as well be ended. Sleep disturbance and poor concentration impeded his ability to work. His Hamilton score was 23. A previous episode of depression, at age thirty, had concerned a lesser setback at work and had been successfully treated with antidepressant medication by his internist.

INITIAL PHASE (SESSIONS 1–3)

The therapist sought in constructing the interpersonal inventory to determine whether Roger was facing role disputes as well as the evident role transition. He maintained a coolly distant relationship with his wife, and a fonder distance from his children, whom he supported financially with only occasional disagreements. There appeared to be no major conflicts with his boss or coworkers: it was in fact difficult to determine from Roger the reasons for his not being promoted. The therapist also weighed the benefits of other treatment modalities. Roger had a history of antidepressant medication response; yet it seemed clear that, even if medication again relieved his symptoms, he would need psychotherapy to resolve this major life crisis.

The therapist offered him the formulation of a role transition, in part because Roger seemed far more focused on his career change than on any relationships. Having ruled out obvious role disputes as the central problem, the therapist told Roger that he had a major depression and linked it to a role transition: namely, the realization that he would never achieve the high title he had long coveted. The therapist acknowledged that this was painful, but insisted the situation was not hopeless: Roger had options that would be worth exploring. Although Roger proved a difficult, not particularly psychologically intuitive patient to work with, the therapist gradually built a supportive alliance.

INTERMEDIATE PHASE (SESSIONS 4–10)

Roger began to work in IPT while simultaneously taking a serotonin reuptake inhibitor. The IPT therapist began by helping him to mourn his lost dream of success: the office, the perks, the prestige he had anticipated, and his perceived humiliation in the eyes of his peers. The therapist allowed him to ventilate his feelings. At the same time, he pushed Roger to interact with the colleagues from whom he had withdrawn. With renewed contact, Roger recognized that his peers were not treating him with condescension; on the contrary, many seemed sympathetic and shared war stories of their own. At a meeting with his boss that had been rehearsed with role playing in IPT sessions, Roger assertively, but without anger or overreaction, asked for and received an explanation of his situation. Roger felt less humiliated upon learning that corporate circumstances, rather than some personal failing on his part, had largely obstructed his promotion. Following the meeting, he felt that he could continue to work with his boss.

In exploring his options, Roger also looked into alternative job opportunities, although none met his scrutiny. He felt "too much at home" where he was, felt his age worked against him in applying elsewhere. He gradually reconciled himself to remaining where he was. In the meantime, his therapist encouraged him to talk to friends and family. They were for the most part far more sympathetic than he had anticipated; he was relieved to find that they, too, did not see him as weak or a failure, but rather still as a high-powered executive. Roger eventually got an offer for a high-ranking position at another company, but in the meantime had come to terms with his own company and his superiors. Although he never got the promotion he craved, he was given a face-saving raise and decided to stay. His Hamilton score was within the normal range—5—by Session 9.

TERMINATION PHASE (WEEKS 11–14)

Roger remained euthymic as the end of treatment approached. He made provision to see the therapist for medication follow-up on an every-three-month schedule. He expressed some relief that the therapy was ending, that he had "pulled himself together" without endless treatment; at the same time, somewhat to his own surprise, he conceded a fondness for the therapist and the treatment process. Therapist and patient reviewed the interpersonal stress, the blow to his self-esteem as an executive, that had contributed to his getting depressed; and his need to maintain social supports, which he should not neglect for his work. They also reviewed all he had done to improve his status. Finally, they discussed the risk of recurrence in the wake of two prior depressive episodes, and the need for prophylactic treatment. Roger remained euthymic on medication during a three-year follow-up.

NOTES

1. Adapted from J. C. Markowitz and H. A. Swartz, Case formulation in interpersonal psychotherapy of depression, in *Handbook of Psychotherapy Case Formulation*, ed. T. D. Eels (New York, Guilford Press, 1997), 192–222.

CHAPTER 6

Interpersonal Deficits

Interpersonal deficits are chosen as the focus of treatment when a patient with major depression presents with a history of social impoverishment, inadequate or unsustaining interpersonal relationships. Patients with such deficits may never have established lasting or intimate relationships as adults, or have pervasive feelings of loneliness and social isolation not specifically related to recent transitions or interpersonal disputes. In general, patients with a history of interpersonal deficits tend to be more severely disturbed than those with other presenting problems. If patients describe both interpersonal deficits *and* one of the other interpersonal problem areas, it is preferable to focus on the latter.

Included are patients who:

1. are socially isolated, lacking relationships either with intimate friends or at work. They have chronic difficulty in developing close relationships.
2. have an adequate number and range of relationships, but find them unfulfilling and/or have difficulty in sustaining them. These people may have chronic low self-esteem, despite apparent popularity or success at work.
3. have lingering symptoms, untreated or inadequately treated in the past, that interfere with relationships.

It is important to rule out dysthymic disorder among patients with interpersonal deficits, as chronic depression often presents with social impover-

103

ishment, chronic low self-esteem, and seemingly "characterological" features. In our experience, indeed, depressed patients who present with interpersonal deficits—that is, lacking an acute precipitant like grief, role dispute, or role transition—often have an underlying chronic depression. The major depression they present with may represent a worsening from their chronic baseline, constituting "double depression" (Keller and Shapiro, 1982). The reason to distinguish dysthymic disorder among patients with interpersonal deficits is that the approach to such patients differs. An adaptation of IPT for dysthymic patients (IPT-D) is discussed in Chapter 12. Some of these patients also may have social phobia (see Chapter 22 for that adaptation of IPT). With these rule-outs, we suspect that interpersonal deficits, already a rare interpersonal problem diagnosis (Wolfson et al., 1997), will become still rarer.

DIAGNOSIS OF
INTERPERSONAL DEFICITS

Optimal social functioning includes close relationships with intimates or family members, less intense but satisfying relationships with friends and acquaintances, and adequate performance and relationships in some sort of work role. For patients with interpersonal deficits, it may be useful to focus on those who are socially isolated. The socially isolated group may lack relationships with either intimates or friends, or may not have a work role. They may have long-standing or temporary deficiencies in social skills.

GOALS AND STRATEGIES
OF TREATMENT

The goal of treatment of interpersonal deficits is to reduce the patient's social isolation. Because there are no current meaningful relationships, the focus of treatment is on past relationships, the relationship with the therapist, and beginning to form new relationships.

The three tasks involved in handling a problem of interpersonal deficits are:

1. review of past significant relationships, including negative and positive aspects;

2. exploration of repetitive or parallel problems in these relationships; and

3. discussion of the patient's negative and positive feelings about the therapist and parallels in other relationships.

The review of past significant relationships, particularly childhood relationships with family members, assumes greater importance with these patients. Depressed patients often forget or minimize positive experiences from their past. As each relationship is reviewed, it is important to determine both its best and its worst parts. Discussion of past relationships at their best may provide a model for helping the patient to develop satisfying new relationships. The therapist might ask:

- Do you have any close relationships? With whom?
- Tell me about your current friends, your close family. How often do you see them?
- What do you enjoy with them? What problems do you have with them?
- Do you find it hard to make friends?
- Is it hard for you to keep close relationships once you make them?
- Is getting close to people something you enjoy, or would like to do? What about it makes you uncomfortable?

The therapist may then continue reviewing relationships from most current to less recent:

- How can you find friends and activities now that you used to enjoy in the past?

CASE EXAMPLE

A positive relationship in the past was used to help Joe, a highly withdrawn twenty-eight-year-old man, find more satisfying current relationships. Although he had broken off contact with his parents in his late teens, Joe remembered with satisfaction the task-oriented work he and his father had done together. Since he was unable to enjoy the company of others in unstructured situations, he reduced his isolation by taking a volunteer job at a local hospital.

Detailed evaluation of failed relationships or of past interpersonal difficulties may alert the therapist about predictable problem areas in new relationships. The therapist should look for patterns in the kinds of situations that lead to difficulty for the patient and help the patient identify these situations, with the hope of avoiding them in the future or of working on gradual resolution of the difficulties. For example:

CASE EXAMPLE

A thirty-year-old woman had closed herself off from social contacts with others and had lost a job largely because of her extreme anxiety at interacting socially with more than two or three people at a time. She absented herself in an embarrassing manner on many occasions. She felt excluded, disliked, and anxious, and these feelings were related to her earlier family situation. When she was able to identify her problem, she found more acceptable employment in a small business in which she had frequent interactions with only one boss. She also reduced her isolation somewhat by entertaining friends at home one at a time.

Attention to the patient-therapist relationship is more important for socially isolated patients than for those with other types of problems. This relationship provides the therapist with the most direct data about the patient's style of relating to others. In addition, solving problems that arise in this relationship may provide a model for the patient to follow in developing intimacy in other relationships. Open discussion of the patient's distorted or unrealistic negative feelings about the therapist or the therapy is especially important. Typically, patients in this group prefer severing relationships to openly confronting others and resolving issues. For example:

CASE EXAMPLE

A twenty-four-year-old man was particularly silent at the beginning of the seventh session and began to discuss quitting. He stated that he did not think that he could be helped. When the therapist asked whether he had been upset about something the therapist had done or not done, he replied that the therapist was just rejecting him as others had done. When he was asked to explain what he meant, it turned out that he had completely misheard an encouraging statement the therapist had made. The patient was relieved at having discovered his mistake and also at having expressed his complaint. This interchange provided the basis for more extended discussion of the patient's generally inhibited communication with others.

For patients with interpersonal impoverishment, dealing with negative feelings toward the therapist not only provides a model of interpersonal learning but also acts as a safety valve to prevent the patient from terminating treatment prematurely because of some imagined slight. The therapist might say:

> Since we're going to focus on your getting more comfortable in relationships with other people, it will be really important during our meetings for you to tell me if I do anything that bothers you, makes you feel angry or uncomfortable. I won't be offended if you bring these things up: in fact, I want you to tell me if something I do bothers you, so that we can figure out what's going on and how you can handle it.

In helping the patient apply the learning that takes place in treatment to outside situations, the therapist may make extensive use of communication analysis and role playing. When the patient has tried, successfully or unsuccessfully, to increase his interactions with others, a detailed review of these attempts may reveal easily correctable deficits in the patient's communication skills. In helping the patient overcome his hesitation in approaching others, the therapist may invite the patient to role-play difficult situations:

> Let's pretend you are going into a room full of strangers at a party. What could you do to meet people? How do you begin conversations?

It should be emphasized that brief treatment of interpersonal deficits is difficult. Goal setting should therefore be limited to "starting" to work on these issues, not necessarily resolving them. Patients with interpersonal deficits are harder to treat in any modality, and they lack the interpersonal life situations and skills on which IPT focuses. If a patient presents with alternative interpersonal problem areas, interpersonal deficits should not be chosen as the focus. Nonetheless, patients with such deficits often can be successfully treated in IPT.

While grief, role dispute, and role transition are useful terms with which to explain an interpersonal focus to patients who have such foci, "interpersonal deficits" may sound pejorative. The formulation is better stated:

> Your depression seems related to your difficulty in making (or sustaining) relationships with other people. If we can help you to develop more comfort in

dealing with people over the next twelve weeks, your depression is likely to improve as well.

INTERPERSONAL DEFICITS:
THE CASE OF BOB

Bob was twenty-two years old, single, and was working as a cook while going
to a local college part-time. He lived with his mother. Bob came for treatment
at his employer's suggestion. He complained of depressed mood and irritability for the past one or two months. His symptoms included anorexia (with a
ten-pound weight loss over the previous month), sleep disturbance, crying
spells, decreased interest in his normal activities, lack of energy, anhedonia,
and irritability. He denied suicidal ideation. Two weeks before the evaluation,
he had had an argument with his mother and struck her. He denied ever having hit her before. He had had no previous psychiatric contact.

Bob dated the onset of symptoms to approximately a month before the
breakup of a three-year relationship with a woman, Jill. He said that Jill had
decided to end the relationship because of his "moodiness" and emotional unavailability. He had not seen or talked with Jill since the breakup.

Bob was born out of wedlock to a nineteen-year-old woman in a rural
Southern community. During the pregnancy, Bob's father was said to have run
off with another woman, settled in a nearby town, and had other children. Bob
was raised solely by his mother and had no further contact with his father.
When he was thirteen, he and his mother moved to New England. Bob experienced this as a very difficult transition: he felt out of place, embarrassed
about his Southern accent and his ineptitude at sports. He had few friends and
led a rather lonely existence. Over the next few years, he did poorly at school
and argued constantly with his mother about his behavior.

Soon after entering high school, he met Jill. She was a successful student
who attended a special community high school geared toward encouraging
academic achievement for students of ability but prior poor performance. She
persuaded Bob to transfer to this alternative school, and he soon took much
greater interest in his studies, developed himself as an athlete, and stopped his
self-destructive behavior. He became interested in a career in teaching, and after graduation he enrolled in college and began working part-time to pay for
his education.

Two years before he began treatment, Bob's mother, who had been working
as a keypunch operator, was hospitalized because of complications resulting
from diabetes mellitus; she subsequently became depressed. Because she had
no health insurance, there were substantial medical bills to pay. Shortly before
his mother's hospitalization, Bob had made plans to move out on his own,
partly because Jill wanted him to have his own apartment so the couple could

have some privacy. Concern about his mother's psychological state as well as her debts made him decide to continue living with her, and to work full-time, cutting back on his studies. At the time of the evaluation, Bob's mother had still not returned to work.

INITIAL PHASE (SESSIONS 1–4)

During the initial evaluation, Bob wore wrinkled, loose-fitting clothes. He sat slumped in his chair and spoke so softly that it was often difficult to hear him. He was severely depressed. After the appropriate medical workup, he was given a course of antidepressant medication. In addition, it was agreed that Bob would meet with his therapist twice a week until there was a significant improvement in his symptoms, at which time the meetings would be held once a week. During each of these early sessions, time was spent reviewing Bob's symptoms and discussing questions relating to the medication regimen. Beginning with the second session, Bob gradually appeared less depressed, talked more, and began taking more care with his appearance. The therapist was highly active in helping Bob manage day-to-day problems at work that had arisen because of his severe depression.

The therapist also began exploring Bob's relationship with Jill, his lack of social skills, and the events leading to the breakup. The relationship with Jill had been vital to him because she was his model for adapting to life in the Northeast and helped coach him in relating to other people. However, the relationship was much like that with an older sister. Bob was frightened of the intimacy and attachment Jill wanted and tended to withdraw when her demands increased. He couldn't sustain the attachment. He felt inferior to his girlfriend and unworthy of her interest. He felt guilty, too, since he perceived that his involvement with Jill meant being disloyal to his mother. In fact, the immediate precipitant of the breakup had been his refusal to move into an apartment with her.

Review of Bob's relationship with his mother showed how his perception of the mother's expectations was affected by his being a male only child of a woman who married neither his father nor anyone else. His mother treated him as very special but also as someone she could rely on to replace the need for a man in her life. His mother had told him that when he was born she had been urged to give him up for adoption but had chosen to keep him despite the humiliation and inconvenience this had caused. Although Bob's mother made him feel that he was essential to maintenance of her well-being because she needed his love and care, she also made him feel that he represented the residue of the totally irresponsible father who had left her pregnant with him. The bad father was frequently brought up as an example of what the boy might become. Hence Bob saw his desire for relationships with other women and his plans to leave home as indications that, like his father, he was a worthless man who wronged his mother.

Discussion of current relationships revealed that Bob felt close to no one but his mother at the time he began treatment. Relationships with men were avoided because he felt clumsy, inarticulate, and inadequate in comparison with them. Moreover, although he felt unmasculine and overidentified with strong women such as his mother and Jill—his only relationship with a woman that had been more than casual—he also felt contempt for many male friends because of their irresponsibility about drugs and women. Although he felt able to meet women, he could not sustain relationships. Bob's relationships at school and at work were relatively superficial. He worked hard to escape notice for either very good or very poor performance.

Because of the paucity of current interpersonal relationships and Bob's lack of social skills, the problem area was identified as interpersonal deficits and the strategy was as follows:

1. to focus on past significant relationships, to clarify perceptions of his mother's expectations of him, to identify positive experiences that could be models for new attachments, and to help him reexamine his view of his father, with a more realistic and balanced picture emerging. By reviewing these relationships, the therapist hoped to help the patient clarify how he used them as models in a way that prevented him from forming meaningful adult attachments; and
2. to focus on the patient-therapist relationship as a direct source of information about Bob's style of relating to others, in order to modify current interpersonal problems.

The immediate focus was on Bob's current living situation and his relationships with his mother, girlfriend, and peers.

INTERMEDIATE PHASE (SESSIONS 5–8)

By the end of the fifth session, Bob was virtually asymptomatic, and tolerating the medication well. His mood was brighter; his appearance had changed rather dramatically as he paid more attention to his clothes and grooming; and he felt an increased interest in activities. The fifth session occurred after a one-week break due to the therapist's planned vacation (which had been discussed with the patient at the beginning of treatment). Bob reported that he had gone out to a few sporting events by himself, and was spending time painting and writing, two activities he had avoided for the past few months. To the therapist's question about whether he was considering beginning to date again, he responded that he was frightened of involvement with a woman because he became emotionally attached quickly and then would, as he put it, "get detached quickly." He did not comment directly about the therapist's absence the previous week. Because he appeared to be doing well, the therapist recommended meeting once a week for the remainder of the treatment, and Bob agreed.

On the day of Session 6, a coworker of his called to say that he was out of town and would not be able to keep his appointment but would be there the following week. However, he did not appear for—nor call to cancel—his next scheduled appointment. When the therapist reached him at work the next day, he said he had forgotten about the appointment but would come for his next appointment the following week at the regular time. Thinking about the two successive missed appointments and reviewing Session 5, the therapist decided that Bob was probably quite angry about the therapist's vacation, and perhaps about the change from twice-a-week to once-a-week meetings.

Bob arrived the next week at the regular time. He explained that he had missed his session two weeks before because he had gone to another city to visit his two stepsisters, his father's other children. He had not mentioned the sisters before. Now he said that he had talked to them about his father and they had confirmed his view that the father was indeed an irresponsible man. Bob went on to say that he had missed the next session because he had met a woman he liked and had been with her on the afternoon his appointment was scheduled. He had realized he was missing the appointment but thought it more important for him to remain with the woman. The therapist asked for the details of the encounter: how it went, and what Bob felt.

The therapist questioned that Bob had never commented on his feelings about the therapist's vacation. After maintaining that he had not minded it, he acknowledged that he had really been furious with the therapist for leaving "just when we were getting started" and had even considered stopping treatment at that point. The therapist pointed out that Bob had in fact taken a vacation (to see his sisters) just as the therapist had, and he allowed that there might be a connection between the two events. The therapist then raised the question of why he had not said anything about his feelings earlier. This led to a productive discussion of his difficulty expressing angry feelings, and specifically his fear that if he were to express those feelings, things would inevitably get out of control and he would either be thrown out or have to leave in order to "save face." He was able to acknowledge his attachment to the therapy, and said he was surprised and grateful that the therapist didn't have a negative reaction to his anger. During this period, Bob also brought up recent efforts to make friends at work, describing his discomfort at approaching one of the coworkers. Role playing was undertaken in which Bob practiced what he might say.

TERMINATION PHASE (SESSIONS 9–11)

In the next session, Bob discussed his feelings about a man his mother had begun dating. He felt the man was irresponsible, as his father had been, and thought his mother was using poor judgment in spending time with him. Bob was considering talking either with her or with the man about his disapproval of the relationship. The therapist questioned the appropriateness of getting involved in his mother's social life, but Bob asserted that it was appropriate for him to "look out for" his mother. This led to a further discussion of his feelings of indebtedness to his mother because of her decision not to give him up as a child, and of his fear that he, like his father, had an irresponsible streak. He talked about how difficult it had been for his mother during his early adolescence, and his wish to "make it up to her." In response to this, the therapist suggested that Bob's mother's dating might be an indication that she too was getting ready for a separation, and explained that although Bob need not give up helping his mother, being more concerned with his own needs and relationships was appropriate at his age. He was encouraged to discuss directly with his mother what her wishes and expectations about separation were.

In the following session, he expressed more strongly than before his wish to be out on his own and his feeling that not having moved out sooner had contributed to the breakup with Jill. He talked of his wish to "see the world" while still young. He also discussed his wish to learn more about his father and described a poignant scene: when he was sixteen he had visited his Southern relatives and an aunt had spent a few hours telling him about his father's early life. Although he wanted to talk with his mother about his father, he had felt from a very early age that this would make his mother too uncomfortable, and had never done so. Mention of his father had been limited to brief angry episodes. Now he said he intended to talk with his mother about his father but was not ready to do it quite yet. The therapist helped him practice what he might say to his mother and he speculated on what he might expect to hear. Bob discussed his feeling that even to understand the negative side of his father would be preferable to the emptiness he felt when he thought about him.

At the beginning of the next session, Bob announced that he had decided to move out of his mother's apartment at the end of the coming summer. The decision had been made after a long conversation with his mother in which she had surprised him by agreeing that he needed independence. He acknowledged that he had liked the idea of his mother's dependence on him; he had seen it as his chance to make up to her all she had given him. He was disturbed that she had taken the discussion of his wish to move with such equanimity, and wondered whether his view of her as a rather fragile woman was accurate. Although he had talked to his mother about his father, she had been unwilling or unable to enlarge on the same stereotyped images she had always used. Bob was planning a trip to the South that summer to see his relatives and ask them about his father. He also planned at the end of the summer to take a vacation in the Caribbean, something he had wanted to do for a long time. He and his mother had discussed the fact that she would go back to work when she felt better. He had decided that he could move out and still help his mother financially, and that she was well enough now to go back to work.

As the end of therapy approached, Bob reported becoming more assertive in work and school relationships and showing more initiative in seeking out male and female friends. He felt surprised and relieved about his mother's cooperation in his plans to move out on his own and was already feeling more independent. Although he discussed continued feelings of sadness about the lost relationship with Jill, and expressed a desire to try to see her, he felt that he might want to become involved in a new relationship in which he felt he had more to give the woman. He had been off medication for several weeks and experienced no return of symptoms. At the end of the last session, he became tearful and thanked the therapist for his help.

Although Bob started treatment with a severe depression and had had significant and long-standing problems with interpersonal relationships, he was able to use several aspects of the brief treatment to make substantial gains. He had required pharmacotherapy because of the severity of his symptoms, and an active, supportive, structuring stance from the therapist to help him manage day-to-day functioning. With the symptomatic relief that followed this approach, he was able to make several important changes. First, in the interaction with the therapist around the therapist's vacation and his own missed sessions, he was able to acknowledge his desire to form a relationship with a supportive man. More important, he was given the opportunity to discover that angry feelings can be fruitfully discussed in a relationship and do not necessarily spell the end of it. Being able to discuss his anger with the therapist made him feel affirmed and valued and more able to continue the therapeutic work.

Review of Bob's current relationship with his mother revealed appropriate desires for independence, and over the course of subsequent sessions he was able to recognize that many of the feelings that kept him living with his mother—such as excessive guilt and fear of being identified with his father— were irrational. In addition, he was surprised to find that his mother supported his moving, having her own life to lead, including beginning to date a new man.

Finally, discussions of Bob's feelings about his father enabled him to recognize that he could be a man without being the same kind of man as his father.

He began trying to sort out the myths from the realities concerning his father by questioning relatives about him. This was an important process because he felt that he could not really know who he was without knowing who his father was. Although Bob ended treatment with much work to be done to develop a satisfactory adult life for himself, he felt stronger and more optimistic than he ever had.

The major goals of the early sessions had been to obtain essential background information, form a therapeutic alliance, and help the patient manage his symptoms and reduce his social isolation from his peers. The therapist maintained a warm and supportive stance but remained relatively unintrusive, sensing that Bob needed to "open up" at his own pace, lest he feel threatened. Because of the relative absence of here-and-now "live" relationships, emphasis was placed on an exploration of the patient's feelings about relationships in the past, particularly within the family, with the goal of helping him broaden his social contacts both within the extended family and among peers. Later sessions dealt with termination issues and served to consolidate his understanding of the origins of some of his interpersonal difficulties. He began to resume activities and his social isolation was reduced.

The case of Bob was an early example of IPT, and some aspects of the therapist have shifted over the years. In treating the same case today, an IPT therapist might be quicker to address the patient's difficulty in expressing angry feelings in social situations outside the therapeutic relationship, rather than focusing on the vacation issue within it. Such difficulty in appropriately expressing anger could be anticipated as a typical difficulty of depressed patients. As IPT proved itself in clinical trials, IPT therapists gained confidence in the interpersonal method, and moved away from more psychodynamic techniques. The following case illustrates some subtle shifts in treatment strategy that have developed over the years.

INTERPERSONAL DEFICITS: THE CASE OF MICHAEL

Michael, a forty-two-year-old data clerk, presented with a history of depression dating from age seventeen, accompanied, in fact, with dysthymic disorder. His depression had worsened, resulting in increasing lateness and worsening work performance that threatened the loss of his job. He lived with his parents and siblings, had unbalanced relationships with a few friends, and had barely dated.

INITIAL PHASE (SESSIONS 1–3)

The Hamilton Depression Rating Scale yielded a score of 21, apparently somewhat higher than his usual depressed state. The interpersonal inventory was notable for a paucity of relationships and his difficulty within these. Michael answered to his friends' needs while neglecting his own. He would run errands for his friends instead of taking care of his own affairs. He had enormous difficulty expressing his needs in relationships, and was afraid to go out to meet people because he could not believe anyone would find him interesting. He was a virgin who seemed overwhelmed by the idea of more than casual contact with women, and unsure how to negotiate even that level.

This case could well have been treated as dysthymic disorder, but the therapist instead used the interpersonal deficits model. She told Michael he was depressed, and that his depression seemed related to his difficulty in making and handling social relationships. She reassured Michael, however, that in the sixteen weeks of IPT he could learn new ways to handle social situations and thereby improve his depression. He was cautious and skeptical, but willing to try.

INTERMEDIATE PHASE (SESSIONS 4–12)

The interventions focused on helping Michael handle his interpersonal situations at work, home, and socially. Therapist and patient discussed the difficulty in functioning at work without energy, sleep, and motivation, and the need to make the most efficient use of the resources he had. After some weeks of encouragement, with role playing as preparation, Michael met with his boss and discussed ways to make his job more interesting. To his surprise, the boss was sympathetic and allowed him to make some changes in his routine that made the work far more enjoyable. Again with role-playing rehearsal, Michael also managed to tell his friends that he could no longer do their errands as he had to take care of his own work. This freed up needed time and energy to handle his job, and enabled him to do better work for himself.

Living in his parents' home with his siblings, Michael reported that his brother's loud stereo system bothered him greatly, but he felt unable to do anything about it. The therapist's questions elicited his wish to get his brother to lower the volume; she then asked how this option might be achieved. After some discussion, Michael acknowledged that he had some rights in the house, and that there was no harm in asking his brother to lower the volume, particularly late at night. It required some role playing to help him choose his words and tone of voice, but he then successfully delivered the message—again, with a successful outcome that surprised him.

More delicate was his relationship with a woman he had met once or twice for dates. She was perplexed by his behavior: when she spoke to him on the phone, he seemed willing to see her, but then he would sometimes not answer his door when she came over. In sessions, Michael revealed that he felt too panicked to see her at times, too afraid he would mishandle their fragile friendship. One simple solution was to suggest that he simply tell her when he did not want her to come over: an option that had not appeared obvious to him, and which represented an important assertion of his needs. His new-found ability to tell this woman when he did and did not want to see her allowed Michael to feel far more in control of his relationship and his mood, which was now euthymic. The relationship, while still unconsummated, appeared to grow stronger.

TERMINATION PHASE (SESSIONS 13–16)

The final sessions focused on the relationship between Michael's gains in self-assertion, the subsequent improvements these had made in his work and social life, and the relationship of these to his mood disorder. He said he felt better than he ever had before. He had some doubts and fears about the therapy ending, although he also acknowledged fears of dependence on the therapist should the therapy continue. Therapist and patient discussed depression as a potentially recurrent disorder, and that it was not the patient's fault. He remained euthymic at termination and on six-month follow-up.

This case demonstrates the use of the interpersonal-deficits model in a case of dysthymic disorder. In fact, many of the key elements are similar: the focus in such cases is on the patient's illness as a medical disorder rather than as a personality disorder, and generally requires the patient to develop social skills such as the appropriate expression of needs or anger. Sixteen weeks will not suffice to completely overhaul the life of such patients, but it can provide relief from depressive symptoms and the beginning of a new direction in social functioning. The most important aspect of the IPT approach in interpersonal deficits is that the therapist must avoid prejudging the patient as personality-disordered. It might have been possible to consider Michael avoidant, self-defeating, or even schizoid; yet these apparently chronic "personality" issues showed significant improvement in a short course of IPT, and more likely reflected the chronicity of his mood disorder.

CHAPTER 7

Termination of Treatment

IPT is explicitly defined as time-limited, not open-ended, treatment. Frequency and duration are defined at the outset in a contract the therapist makes with the patient. The duration and frequency of IPT can vary: e.g., for treatment of an acute depressive episode, weekly and sometimes twice-weekly sessions of forty-five to fifty minutes for twelve to sixteen weeks have been used. In maintenance treatment, two dosage schedules have been used: weekly sessions for six months in one study, and monthly sessions for three years, in two other trials. Other dosages are possible and are being tested. The dosages used to date have been primarily determined by research protocols, which may be preferable to the current determination of the length of many therapies by third-party payors and managed care. In any case, it is important to maintain the initial contract. The optimal duration of treatment may vary from patient to patient; nonetheless, in each case, a time frame should be specified at the outset of treatment in order to focus on goals. Changes in this contract should be explicitly renegotiated.

As in other time-limited therapies, termination should be specifically discussed at least two to four sessions before it occurs. At termination, the patient faces the task of giving up a relationship and establishing a sense of competence to deal with further problems without the psychotherapist's help. Failure to accomplish these tasks may lead to a return of depressive symptoms as the end of treatment approaches or shortly after its end. This symptomatic worsening may in turn bring on a renewed sense of hopelessness.

117

To facilitate the tasks of termination, the last three to four sessions should contain: (1) explicit discussion of the end of treatment; (2) acknowledgment of the end of treatment as a time of potential grieving; and (3) movement toward the patient's recognition of his or her independent competence.

Presumably the patient has been trying new ways of coping, so that he or she is likely by now to have regained a sense of self-esteem. Despite this, the patient may feel that the improvement has depended entirely upon the psychotherapist's help, and that when this help is gone regression will be unavoidable. It must be emphasized to the patient that the goal of the treatment is to help the patient deal successfully with life (work, love, friendship) on the outside. The therapist-patient relationship is meant to enhance the patient's health and competence on the outside and is not a substitute for "real world" relationships.

With at least three or four sessions to go, the therapist should raise the topic of the end of treatment and elicit reactions to it if the patient has not already volunteered such information. Many patients are unaware of having any feelings about the end of treatment. Others may hesitate to acknowledge that they have come to value the relationship with the therapist. If they find themselves already missing the relationship or experiencing a slight recurrence of symptoms as termination approaches, they may interpret their feelings as a relapse. To prevent this misunderstanding, such patients should be told that toward the end it is usual for patients to have feelings of apprehension, anger, or sadness about ending treatment, and that the appearance of these feelings does not portend a return of depression. In fact, such feelings usually present an opportunity for the therapist to help the patient distinguish between appropriate *sadness* at breaking up a successful team and the related but pathological symptom of *depressed mood*.

> I think we both feel sad, approaching the end of this, after working together so well. Is sad the same as depressed? Are you feeling guilty, or suicidal? Or is this an appropriate feeling of sadness when you experience a loss or disappointment in your life? Now that you're out of the depression, it's important to distinguish between depression and the helpful emotion of sadness, which tells you something about what's happening in your environment.

To aid the patient's perception of his or her own competence to cope with new problems, the therapist should systematically, throughout treatment but particularly in its final phase, call attention to the patient's independent successes, to the friends, family, church, and other supports that are available on the outside, and to the ways in which the patient has begun to handle his or her own difficulties. In the last visit, the therapist may bolster the patient's sense of being able to handle future problems by discussing areas of future difficulty and guiding the patient through an exploration of how various contingencies could be handled. Since the patient has in fact done most of the interpersonal work outside of the office setting, the therapist can make it clear that although therapeutic coaching may have helped, the patient deserves the real credit for undertaking social risks and developing social skills even while in the midst of a depressive episode. And frequently the list of the patient's accomplishments, even during the relatively brief time frame of the treatment, is impressive.

> I appreciate your wanting to give me the credit, and we have been working together as a good team. But who's the one who actually went out there and confronted your husband [asked for a raise, etc.]? I may have helped as a coach, but you're the one who really has made the changes in your life that have helped you get out of this depression.

Particularly important is the patient's future ability to judge when he or she needs to seek further help. Early warning signals of distress and situations of stress should be identified, and ways of coping—family, friends, and other resources—discussed. Relapse or recurrence of depression should be discussed as an aspect of a frequently recurrent illness, not the patient's fault.

The previously established work pattern of treatment need not be disrupted as termination approaches. Some patients continue to bring up new issues even at the end of treatment. More typically, as the final session approaches, the opening of new problem areas ceases, providing opportunities to review the course of treatment and the options that remain open. The patient should be given the opportunity to evaluate the treatment and to assess future needs. Many patients actually terminate IPT with surprising ease. They feel empowered by their gains, pleased with their relationship with the therapist, but also relieved not to need a lengthier treatment.

IPT is not a panacea, and not all patients respond to it. If the patient has made an effort to work in therapy and has failed to respond, it is important that the therapist counter the patient's guilt by pointing out—just as in a pharmacotherapy trial—that the patient has tried his or her best, and **it is**

the treatment that has failed. Using the important IPT concept of the need to explore one's options, the therapist should then encouragingly emphasize to the patient that depression is very treatable, and that although it is discouraging not to have a treatment succeed, there are fortunately many other effective alternatives. Hope remains.

Even patients who do not experience an improvement of mood symptoms, however, do not necessarily leave IPT without gains. In many cases, they have in fact altered the interpersonal problem area that was the focus of the treatment, and can feel some satisfaction in having changed an important aspect of their lives even in the face of depression. Recognition of such accomplishments can help to make clear the uncoupling of the promised link between interpersonal accomplishments and improvement of mood. The therapist can say:

> You did what you set out to do, and you've really taken important steps to resolve your [complicated bereavement, role dispute, role transition]. I told you that in IPT, solving the interpersonal problem area leads to an improvement in depressed symptoms, and that's usually the case. You did your part: it's the therapy that let you down, not the other way around.

DIFFICULTIES WITH TERMINATION

Because some remitted patients have discomfort with termination, a decision not to terminate as planned should not be based on the patient's discomfort. A patient who does not want to terminate should be told that further treatment is possible, but—unless symptom criteria suggest otherwise—there should be a waiting period of at least four to eight weeks, to see if it is really needed. Exceptions to this are made for patients who are still significantly symptomatic, having shown little or no improvement in the course of therapy. In such cases, alternative treatments, including use of medications not previously tried, a psychotherapy of a different type, or psychotherapy with a different therapist should be considered and, if necessary, begun at once.

To the patient who is free of serious symptoms but feels uncomfortable or hesitant about termination, the psychotherapist might say:

> Many patients have some uneasiness about ending these sessions if they have found them helpful. We have found that a treatment-free period is usually help-

ful. Let's see how you are doing over the next eight weeks before making any decisions about further treatment. You can, of course, call me if you need to and treatment will be arranged.

It may take a while to feel secure that the depression is really gone and that it won't come back—it's often the case that people early in remission feel that way. You should stay aware of the symptoms of depression and the life situations that might provoke depression for you, such as ____, which you should now be able to handle differently.

Some therapists have difficulty with termination as well. It is important that therapy not continue simply because of the therapist's discomfort with ending. Ending psychotherapy may be the difficulty with which long-term therapists have the most trouble, and can be one of their struggles in adapting to time-limited psychotherapy. Until you have the confidence to know that you *can* end treatment with many patients in twelve to sixteen weeks, it may be hard to do so. Research suggests that you often can. Attitudes can be infectious: if the therapist does not face termination with confidence, it will be hard for the newly remitted patient to feel confident about stopping. It is important that the therapist remind both parties that the goal of the treatment has been to treat the depressive episode, not to continue indefinitely.

INDICATIONS FOR LONG-TERM TREATMENT

For certain patients, longer-term treatment is indicated. Such patients may include those with long-standing personality problems, those who can initiate relationships but not sustain them, those with interpersonal deficits who lack the skills to initiate relationships and thus feel perpetually lonely, those with recurrent depression who require maintenance treatment to prevent relapse (see Chapter 11), and those who have not responded and are still acutely depressed.

In time-limited treatment, the initial time contract should be maintained. Patients who require longer-term treatment should be referred elsewhere or should make a new and different contract, involving a change in focus and techniques, with the same therapist.

CHAPTER 8

Specific Techniques

Many of the techniques used in IPT are common to psychodynamic psychotherapy and were long ago described by Bibring (1954) and by Menninger and Holzman (1971). On the other hand, IPT differs from psychodynamic psychotherapy in important respects (Markowitz, Svartberg, and Swartz, 1998). The IPT techniques are used as part of a strategy that differs from psychodynamic psychotherapy: to treat a depressive episode rather than principally to increase insight. Each technique is used in a specific sequence and with varying frequency, depending on the characteristics of the patient and the particular interpersonal problem the patient describes. These techniques, which will be familiar to clinicians who practice many forms of psychotherapy, are defined here to specify the range of options open to the therapist practicing IPT. Techniques are not the major element of IPT: it is the strategies, described in the previous chapters, that are distinctive.

Each patient needs a different combination of techniques. The techniques are listed here in order of increasing intrusiveness on the part of the therapist and, with the exception of the adjunctive techniques, in the order they are most often used as the therapeutic relationship develops.

Patients are encouraged to use the time-limited treatment as a time to discuss feelings about, as well as to take action to change, the interpersonal problem area. Patients are encouraged to be open about their feelings, painful and pleasant, and (to use a phrase from Christopher Fairburn's Oxford IPT group) to use the time in therapy to change things.

EXPLORATORY TECHNIQUES

Systematically gathering information about the patient's symptoms and presenting problems using exploratory techniques can be either direct or indirect.

Nondirective Exploration

The term *nondirective* means using general, open-ended questions or verbalizations. When eliciting information from patients, it is best to allow leeway in the style (choice of words, use of detail) of their responses to questions. To facilitate relatively free discussion of material, general, open-ended questions are best, especially in the first phases of a session. The therapist usually begins sessions with the focusing but still open-ended question: "How have things been since we last met?"

If material is being discussed in a productive way, nondirective techniques can be used to encourage the patient to continue talking. These techniques include:

- *Supportive acknowledgment*, a nondirective technique that includes such metacommunication as nodding, saying "Mm-hm," "I see," "Please continue," or other comments designed to encourage the patient to continue talking.
- *Extension of the topic discussed*, a nondirective technique in which the therapist directly encourages the patient to continue on an initiated subject, invites the patient to return to a subject presented earlier, or repeats key or charged words the patient has used.
- *Receptive silence*, a nondirective technique in which the therapist maintains an interested and attentive attitude that encourages the patient to continue talking.

Nondirective exploration is most useful in allowing the patient to bring up new material, to identify problem areas not touched on in initial sessions, or to update events that have occurred since the previous session. By refraining from structuring parts of a session, the therapist facilitates the patient's sense of responsibility in the treatment (since the patient can choose areas to concentrate on) and the patient's feelings of being understood and accepted by the therapist (the therapist accepts his or her choice of concerns as legitimate).

Guidelines for Using Nondirective Exploration

The optimal use of nondirective exploration is with the verbal patient who has a sense of his or her own problems and is usefully communicating to the therapist. It can also be useful when the therapist feels that the patient is struggling to relate something previously undisclosed or is usefully trying to shift the focus of the treatment. It is a mistake to use this technique when the patient is nonverbal or stuck and groping for direction, or when more active or specific techniques are called for, such as decision analysis or communication analysis.

DIRECT ELICITATION OF MATERIAL

This technique uses directive questioning or therapist-initiated inquiry into a new topic. Formal questionnaires such as a review of depressive symptoms would be included in this category of therapeutic techniques. Open-ended questions should precede more detailed inquiry; for example, in inquiring about a patient's spouse, the first question, "Tell me about your husband," would be followed by progressively specific questioning. Included in direct elicitation is the interpersonal inventory, a systematically detailed exploration of the patient's important relationships with significant others (see Chapter 2).

Guidelines for Using Direct Elicitation

Direct elicitation is best used to obtain a thorough evaluation of a particular problem area and to check the therapist's interpersonal hypotheses. Specific questions should be asked only with some purpose in mind—such as to help the patient see his or her role in a situation, or to develop a data base, or to elicit an avoided affect—and in some semblance of flow from where the discussion has moved. Too much skipping around and too many specific, close-ended questions should be avoided. It is a mistake to ask overly specific questions with nothing in particular in mind, questions that interrupt a patient who is already doing well in discussing an issue, or questions that inhibit expression of affect.

ENCOURAGEMENT OF AFFECT

Encouragement of affect denotes a number of therapeutic techniques that are intended to help the patient express, understand, and manage affect. The relatively free expression of affect in psychotherapy distinguishes it from other relationships, in which affective components are often highly constricted. The learning in therapy is an emotional learning, and dealing with affect is essential in bringing about changes. In developing new interpersonal strategies, the elicitation of affect about others may help patients decide on priorities and strive toward emotionally meaningful goals.

Depending on the nature of the affect and the patient, the IPT therapist may pursue three general strategies:

1. facilitating acknowledgment and acceptance of painful affects about events or issues that cannot or should not be changed;
2. helping the patient use his or her affective experiences in bringing about desired interpersonal changes; and
3. encouraging the development of new and unacknowledged desirable affects which, in turn, may facilitate growth and change.

ACCEPTANCE OF PAINFUL AFFECTS

Many patients have excessive guilt feelings related to strong hostile or sexual feelings about significant others. They may be only partly aware of such emotions. For example, an important aspect of distorted or delayed grief reactions is often unacceptable to the patient. When the patient gives evidence of painful, unacknowledged, or suppressed feelings of this sort, the therapist's job is to encourage the clear expression of the affect. One way to do this is to inquire into sensitive areas, perhaps by eliciting the details of a patient's interactions with significant others or extending discussions of topics to which the patient has shown an emotional response. A second way is to repeatedly inquire about feelings the patient is experiencing while discussing emotionally charged issues in treatment. As the feelings are expressed, it is important for the therapist to help the patient accept them. Direct reassurance, through statements like "Most people would feel like that" or "Of course you're angry," may be helpful. At other times, through simple silence the therapist conveys the tacit acceptance of the patient's feelings. For patients who are afraid that their hostile or sexual feelings will be acted upon, it is important to clarify the distinction between feelings and actions: the latter are not necessarily the consequence of the former.

Using Affects in
Interpersonal Relationships

Some schools of psychotherapy hold the belief that the best way to manage affects is to express them in a cathartic fashion, both in and out of the therapy. In IPT the expression of strong feelings in the therapeutic session is seen as an important starting point for much therapeutic work, but their expression outside the session is not a goal in and of itself. Since the goal is to help the patient act more effectively in interpersonal relationships, this may involve either expressing or suppressing affects, depending on the circumstances.

The IPT therapist may help the patient manage his or her affective experience in several ways. First, the patient and the significant other may negotiate to bring about changes that eliminate the circumstances that evoke painful feelings. For example, a patient who feels repeated disappointment and anger with a spouse's behavior may not feel this way if the behavior changes. Second, the patient may learn to avoid painful situations when appropriate. A third way of managing affect is to delay expressing it or acting on it until one has calmed down. This might include such strategies as planning with a spouse to postpone an argument until a time when both have achieved some distance on the matter to be discussed.

A fourth way of changing painful affects is to help patients revise their thinking about an affect-laden topic, so that the affect that arises in response to this thinking is also revised.

> Because you're depressed, you're likely to anticipate the worst. How likely is that to happen? (And even if it were to happen, perhaps there's a way to handle that worst-case situation.)

This cognitive strategy is particularly important in the management of anxiety. Depressed patients frequently have high levels of anxiety in relation to irrational thoughts and fears. By exposing the irrational thoughts and helping the patient to arrive at alternative ways of understanding a situation, the therapist may help to reduce anxiety. Anger can also be mitigated through revising the patient's understanding of the situation in which anger arose. Often this revised understanding involves a more mature acceptance of unchangeable circumstances.

HELPING THE PATIENT
GENERATE SUPPRESSED AFFECTS

Some patients are emotionally constricted or have a maladaptive lack of emotion in situations in which strong affects are normally felt. They may be so unassertive that they do not feel anger when their rights are violated by others. Some patients may feel anger but lack the courage to express it in assertive behavior. Others may not feel angry because it has never occurred to them that others should act differently toward them. With these patients, it may be useful to point out that they are being abused. Patients who have difficulty feeling and expressing other types of feelings—such as affection, gratitude, or caring—may be helped to discover irrational fears that led to the suppression of these emotions.

Guidelines for Using Encouragement of Affect

For extremely emotionally constricted individuals, this technique cannot be overused, particularly when the patient seems to be unaware of strong feelings such as sadness, anger, or love. The therapist should usually be listening for emotionally important statements and encouraging their expansion.

However, for patients who are troubled by intense, diffuse, and flooded affective experiences, the strategy may be to help suppress these overwhelming experiences. In addition, mere repetition of angry, hostile, or sad outbursts without an attempt to understand these feelings is probably counterproductive. In such cases, the therapist may interrupt an affective display by, for instance, inquiring about the patient's thoughts regarding the strong feelings. Alternatively, the therapist may explore with the patient various strategies for delaying action on impulsive feelings, to allow time to think over the consequences.

It is a mistake to fail to distinguish patients in whom affective responses should be encouraged from those who should not be encouraged. Other mistakes include missing cues from the patient about emotional issues, failure to use the technique when appropriate, and verbal or nonverbal disapproval of the patient's feelings.

CLARIFICATION

The therapist uses clarification to restructure and feed back the patient's material. The short-term purpose is to make the patient more aware of what has actually been communicated. In the longer term, this may facilitate the patient's discussion of previously suppressed material. Specific techniques for clarification include:

Asking patients to repeat or rephrase what they have said. This is particularly useful if the patient has made a misstatement, said something in a surprising or unusual way, or contradicted previous statements.

The therapist may rephrase what the patient has said and ask the patient if this is what was intended. The rephrasing should be done in a way that places the patient's statement in an interpersonal context. For instance, a patient discussing an incident in which his wife had come home late described his feelings by saying, "There was anger," to which the therapist replied, "You were angry with her?"

The therapist may call attention to the logical extension of a statement that the patient has made or point out the implicit assumptions in what was said.

Calling the patient's attention to contrasts or contradictions in his or her presentation of material is involved in the most useful clarification techniques. Contradictions may be noted between the patient's affect expression and the verbal discussion of a topic. Discrepancies can be noted over time when the same material is brought up. Contrasts can be seen between a statement of intentions and overt behavior, between the patient's statements of goals and the limitations of reality. In confronting the patient with contradictory statements, it is important to do this in the spirit of inquiry and not in an accusatory fashion. Contradictions can be pointed out by queries such as "Isn't it interesting that you said X, while previously you said Y?" or "What can we make of the contrast between what you just said and [what you said before]?"

Statements by the patient that imply a pervasive, unhelpful belief or thought may be restated explicitly by the therapist, who then asks the patient whether this represents the real belief. Some people, for example, have a habit of thinking in extremes—particularly when they are depressed. From a patient's discussion of his or her work, the therapist may note that the patient thinks that he or she is either a total success or an utter failure, without gradations in between, pointing this out as a depressive distortion that is likely to resolve as they work together on treating the depression. Unlike cognitive therapy, however, these irrational thoughts are not specifically catalogued, tested, and challenged. Instead, the therapist simply describes these thoughts as symptoms of the depression episode that are interfering with the patient's interpersonal functioning.

Guidelines for Using Clarification

Clarification is optimally used when the therapist has some hypothesis in mind and the patient is talking about the related subject, or as follow-through to make sure the patient has gotten the point. The point is made at a time when it is likely to be understood, not when the patient is feeling a strong, unrelated affect.

COMMUNICATION ANALYSIS

Communication analysis is used to examine and identify communication failures in order to help the patient learn to communicate more effectively. Specifically, the therapist seeks out problems in communication by asking for a highly detailed account of an important conversation or argument the patient has had with a significant other. This reconstruction of the interpersonal event should attempt both a verbatim "transcript" of the interaction and the patient's feelings and intentions at critical points.

Faulty communication may be responsible for interpersonal disputes even if those involved have mutually supportive or noncontradictory expectations of one another. When there is a realistic basis for conflict, poor communication can make a relatively minor disagreement insoluble. Communication failures may come about in a number of ways, most of which include failure of one partner to openly correct mistaken assumptions about the other's thoughts, feelings, or intentions. Some common communication difficulties include the following:

Ambiguous, indirect nonverbal communication as a substitute for open confrontation. Verbal communication has many advantages over nonverbal communication in terms of its explicitness and understandability. Many patients who either distrust verbal communication or fear openly expressing their feelings or thoughts rely on nonverbal communication or actions to get their point across to others. They may sulk when angry or make suicidal gestures when they feel lonely or deprived. The person to whom these actions are addressed cannot know what is being asked or how best to respond.

Incorrect assumption that one has communicated. Many people assume that others will know their needs or feelings without their having to make themselves clear, expecting the other person to anticipate their wants or, in effect, be a mind reader. ("Of course he knows what I think.") This often results in anger and frustration, again silent and unexpressed. Other people, having tried to communicate a message, do not bother to make sure that they have been heard or understood.

Incorrect assumption that one has understood. Many depressed patients fear massive retaliation or criticism from others and are afraid to ask if what was perceived as criticism was actually intended that way.

Unnecessarily indirect verbal communication. Many depressed patients are highly inhibited about directly expressing quite reasonable expectations or criticisms of others. As a result, they may build up resentments about being mistreated by a person who is unaware of having given offense. Instead of direct communication, the patient may use hints or ambiguous messages.

Silence—closing off communication. Many patients have discovered that silence can be an effective and infuriating way of handling a disagreement with others, but they may be unaware of the destructive potential of closing off communications entirely.

Guidelines for Using Communication Analysis

Communication analysis is aimed at identifying these and other communication failures and at guiding the patient toward learning to communicate more effectively.

Identifying faulty communication often involves listening for the assumptions that the patient makes about others' thoughts or feelings. The optimal use is when disputes are present, especially if there has been a recent argument (or unsuccessful communication). It is important to try to be as thorough as the patient's memory permits, even if the patient resists or is bored. Patients should be allowed to draw their own conclusions first before the therapist gives feedback.

It is a mistake not to follow through or pursue a particular conversation, not to let the patient draw his own conclusions, to misunderstand the patient's communications, or to fail to suggest alternatives to poor communication.

USE OF THE
THERAPEUTIC RELATIONSHIP

In this technique, the patient's feelings about the therapist and/or the therapy become the focus of discussion. Thoughts, feelings, expectations, and behavior in the therapeutic relationship are examined insofar as they represent a model of the patient's characteristic ways of feeling and/or behaving in other relationships.

In individual therapy, the relationship between the patient and the therapist is the only "live" source of data open to the therapist about the patient's style of interpersonal functioning. On the assumption that people adopt characteristic ways of approaching all personal relationships, the interaction between the therapist and the patient can be used to help the patient learn about other relationships. In IPT, the patient-therapist relationship is not the primary focus of treatment, and attempts to extrapolate from the therapy relationship the dynamics of others are used only sparingly. However, when the patient begins to think about or act toward the therapist in a way that interferes with the progress of treatment, attention must be paid to the here-and-now therapy relationship. Failure to do so will lead to premature termination or unproductive treatment.

To facilitate monitoring of this relationship, the patient should be instructed, at the onset of the treatment, to express to the therapist complaints, apprehensions, anger, and other aversive feelings that arise in the course of treatment either about the therapist or about the therapeutic process. More positive feelings (such as, for instance, an exaggerated sense of being helped by a powerful expert) need not be as systematically examined because they probably help rather than hinder the progress of treatment.

Encouraging the patient to express negative feelings about the therapist serves many vital functions. It provides a model for the patient's interactions with others, as patient and therapist negotiate around the patient's legitimate or unrealistic concerns.

It allows the therapist to correct distortions or to acknowledge genuine deficiencies or problems in treatment. In addition, analysis of unrealistic negative reactions to treatment may provide convincing data that patients can use to understand and correct their distorted view of others. For instance, excessive expectations of being attacked, ridiculed, abandoned, punished, and so on are commonly revealed when the patient begins to avoid discussing sensitive material or falls silent for periods of time.

Guidelines for Using the Therapeutic Relationship

This technique is used optimally in:

1. **role disputes**, where it gives feedback on how a person comes across to others and helps the patient understand pathological interactions

by reexperiencing them with the therapist but going one step further and solving them;

2. **grief and loss**, when reactions to the therapist may show how the patient has cut off from others or developed relationships that mirror the one with the lost person;

3. **interpersonal deficits**, as the patient develops a relationship with the therapist as a model for other relationships.

Timing Is Critical

This technique is especially useful when problems come up (e.g., when the patient is late for the appointment or has nothing to say), but it is important not to bring up the problem until some therapeutic alliance is established. The actual constraints of the relationship as well as the actual features of the patient and the therapist must be recognized.

It is a mistake to mistime this technique, to misunderstand the patient's interactions with the therapist, or to fail to take into account the patient's accurate perceptions about the therapist or the therapeutic relationship.

BEHAVIOR CHANGE
TECHNIQUES

Lasting improvement from depression usually depends on changes in the patient's interpersonal behavior outside therapy. In IPT, the therapist can use

1. directive techniques;
2. decision analysis; and
3. role playing to facilitate behavior change.

DIRECTIVE TECHNIQUES

Directive techniques include interventions such as educating, advising, modeling, or directly helping the patient solve relatively simple, practical problems. In establishing a positive working relationship in the early phases of treatment, the therapist should be alert to the possibility of directly helping the patient solve such practical problems as finding transportation, housing, or public financial assistance. Since the goal of treatment is to help the patient to function independently, heavy use of direct assistance or advice is to be avoided. Rather, patients should be taught to analyze new situations for themselves and make their own choices. As an overall strategy, the therapist should move from relatively direct helping toward relatively indirect helping as treatment progresses. When direct interventions seem warranted, the following techniques may be useful:

Advice and suggestions should be provided only when the therapist thinks the patient is unable to make a relatively successful decision on his or her own. Patients may ask for advice they do not need or help in an area the therapist cannot be expected to be knowledgeable about (income tax, for example) in order to test the therapist. In such cases, the therapist may wish to explore the patient's unrealistic expectations of the therapist. Although crucial at times, giving advice can be detrimental to treatment in that it is contradictory to the general principle that patients are responsible to themselves and for themselves, even if they choose to follow someone's advice.

Limit setting may be necessary for highly impulsive individuals whose behavior is destructive either to themselves or to the treatment. The therapist may choose to demand that the patient refrain from a given behavior if he or she is to remain in treatment.

Education is an essential function of IPT, generally and specifically. Ultimately, all the interventions of IPT are aimed at educating patients about their interactions with others. More specifically, the patient may be simply deficient in knowledge about the range of topics of importance in his or her life. The therapist may usefully educate the patient about the characteristics of depressive illness and general psychological principles, or about ways to solve practical problems. Education is preferred to advice giving in that it is aimed at providing the patient with the skills with which to make his or her own choices.

Direct help should be used exclusively for solving practical problems. For interpersonal problems, the patient should receive the message that this is an ongoing matter for which he or she, with help, is responsible.

Modeling is similar to advice giving, because it involves giving the patient examples of how the therapist has handled problems similar to the patient's. This technique is helpful in conveying to patients that they are not unique in having difficulties and that others have succeeded in solving their problems.

Guidelines for Using Directive Techniques

Optimally, with the exception of education, direct techniques should be used sparingly. They are best used in early sessions to create an atmosphere in which the therapist is perceived as a helping person. In addition, when the patient can be clearly helped by obtaining information the therapist possesses, or when the patient is grossly misinformed (for instance, about how to obtain welfare payments), direct advice may be useful. Advice should ideally be in the form of helping the patient consider options not previously entertained rather than direct suggestions. The tone would be: "One thing you might consider is ____."

Too-frequent use is a mistake; so are suggestions that are too specific and direct, or that undermine the patient's sense of autonomy, or that are based on misinformation or incorrect perceptions.

DECISION ANALYSIS

This is a technique by which the patient is helped to consider a wide range of alternative actions (and their consequences) that can be taken to solve a given problem. This is the major action-oriented technique of IPT and should be explicitly taught to the patient for use outside of treatment. It often follows communication analysis. Many depressed patients have a history of making self-defeating decisions, partly because they fail to consider all reasonable alternatives and to evaluate the consequences of their actions. The role of the therapist in decision analysis to help the patient recognize a broadening range of options and to insist that action be held off until each option is adequately explored.

Decision analysis may be used whenever the patient has an interpersonal problem to be solved. The first step is to determine a goal for the interpersonal situation at issue: "What would you want to happen? What solution to this would make you happiest?" Once the goal of the decision analysis is determined, the therapist should ask general questions: "What alternatives do you feel you have now?" or "Why don't we try to consider all the choices you have?" In the ensuing discussion, the therapist should be alert to point out useful alternatives the patient has ignored and to direct the patient to explore the probable consequences of each line of behavior. Decision analysis frequently reveals a patient's excessively restricted conceptions of alternatives or unrealistic notions about consequences. Although the therapist is highly active in decision analysis, the choice among alternatives is the patient's.

Guidelines for Using Decision Analysis

Decision analysis is used optimally if the patient has first discussed and analyzed the problem thoroughly and the therapist avoids actually suggesting what to do. There is always an option to continue discussing and thinking about the problem. There is some thoroughness in that the consequences of each action are considered.

It is a mistake if too much activity or pressuring of the patient into decisions occurs, or if the technique is used prematurely, before all information is available and has been considered. If the possibilities are too narrow, there is a failure to consider all opportunities, or to think through the consequences of behavior. For example, in a role dispute it is important to fully understand the nature of a spousal disagreement, the likely motives of both parties, the advantages and disadvantages of each course of action, and what the patient has already attempted to do, before helping the patient to decide on how to resolve a potential impasse.

ROLE PLAYING

The therapist using this technique takes the role of some person in the patient's life. Role playing can be used to accomplish two important tasks: (1) exploration of the patient's feelings and style of communication with others, and (2) rehearsal of new ways for the patient to behave with others.

For the first task, role playing can be used when the therapist feels that patients are not adequately conveying a sense of their relationships with others. When the therapist pretends to be the other person, the patient may react in fresh and revealing ways.

For the second task, role playing can be used to train the patient to interact with others in new ways, such as being more assertive or expressing anger. It is a great leap to go from thinking about acting differently to actually doing so. Often the patient has been aware for years of a desire or need to change but has been unable to do so. Role playing allows the patient to practice in a safe setting and thus may provide for a smoother transition from plans to action.

Guidelines for Using Role Playing

This technique can be useful in eliciting the patient's feelings about a subject by providing a structure for the patient's expressions. It may also be useful in helping the patient practice some difficult situations. It is an important technique for rehearsing self-expression to others, particularly with patients who lack social skills (e.g., patients with interpersonal deficits). This technique also tends to distinguish IPT from psychodynamic psychotherapy.

It is a mistake to use role playing when not necessary, to fail to follow through, or to fail to try it when the patient is not adequately getting involved in interpersonal situations.

ADJUNCTIVE TECHNIQUES

CONTRACT SETTING

This refers to the sequence of semistructured tasks in the initial session(s) that are aimed at educating the patient about IPT and obtaining the patient's cooperation as a partner in the therapeutic work. Tasks include an individualized explanation of the IPT rationale, an explanation of IPT techniques, some communication to the patient about the therapist's understanding of what brings the patient into therapy, and a discussion of the practical dimensions of treatment—length of sessions, frequency, duration of therapy, appointment time, missed sessions policy, fee, and so on (see Chapter 2).

ADMINISTRATIVE DETAILS

These interventions address the procedural or bookkeeping tasks of therapy—discussion of appointment times, vacation schedules, and so on.

EXPLAINING THE IPT
TECHNIQUES TO THE PATIENT

Patients are often curious about how the psychotherapy works, and how it may differ from friendship or counseling. This may be true both for patients new to therapy and for those already experienced in other forms of psychotherapy. Such patients may be told:

> I want to help you, although this relationship isn't a substitute for friendship. In the treatment you can talk openly about your problems, your hopes, and your fears. Your ability to be open is one indication that you are capable of intimate friendships. The relationship is an opportunity to talk to someone who won't judge you based on your feelings and wishes. Instead, my job is to help you handle the feelings and wishes that may be thwarted in your current relationships, and may be associated with your depression.

I'll be asking you questions to bring out information that should help you to understand and address the problems you're experiencing—including those that may now seem impossible to you but can probably be solved. I'll be encouraging you to express your feelings, painful as well as pleasant, about those problems. I don't intend to make you feel worse: because you're depressed, you're already feeling guilty and judgmental, and I don't want to add to that.

What we'll be exploring in this treatment is the connection between your depression and your life situation: things that have happened to you, particularly in relationship to other people, that may have contributed to your getting depressed.

Patients who want to know more about IPT can also read the IPT patient book *Mastering Depression: A Patient's Guide to Interpersonal Psychotherapy* (Weissman, 1995).

CHAPTER 9

Common Problems

Problems that arise in the course of psychotherapy may be based on the patient's social or cultural beliefs, the patient's unfamiliarity with therapy, or the inherent awkwardness of the therapeutic relationship. The problems described here are general ones, applicable to the original IPT approach, its adaptations, and probably much of psychotherapy. Problems unique to specific adaptations can be found in those chapters.

These common problems, while obviously overlapping at points, can be roughly grouped as (1) problems reflecting the patient's depression, (2) problems in the therapy itself, and (3) common patient concerns.

PROBLEMS REFLECTING
THE PATIENT'S DEPRESSION

THE PATIENT IS CHRONICALLY DEPRESSED

Some patients have an acute episode of depression superimposed upon a less symptomatically severe but chronic depression, i.e., dysthymic disorder. The acute worsening of symptoms is then termed a "double depression" (Keller et al., 1982, 1984). For these patients, defeat, pessimism, and low self-esteem have become a characteristic way of viewing the world and dealing with others. Interpersonal difficulties such as shyness, social discomfort, lack of self-assertion, and difficulty in expressing anger are hallmarks of dysthymic patients. It may be difficult to assess the chronic nature of the disorder while the patient is acutely depressed. In the acute phase, patients will appear at their worst: dependent, pessimistic, negative, irritable. They may appear quite different when they become asymptomatic. Assumptions about the personality of the patient made while the patient is acutely ill can be misleading and lead to therapeutic pessimism. Axis II diagnoses should be avoided in the presence of an Axis I disorder, and particularly a chronic Axis I disorder (Bronisch and Klerman, 1991; Loranger et al., 1991).

As we have already suggested, many depressed patients who appear to have "interpersonal deficits" may in fact suffer from chronic depression. IPT has been adapted for the treatment of dysthymic patients, incorporating an outlook more optimistic than the interpersonal deficits model (Markowitz, 1997; see Chapter 12). Preliminary data suggest the efficacy of this adaptation. Chronic discouragement can be daunting to therapists as well as to chronically depressed patients, so it is particularly important for therapists to remain hopeful and optimistic with such patients.

THE PATIENT SEES DEPRESSION AS INCURABLE

In the early stages of treatment, depressed patients often feel that their symptoms will never remit. An initial strategy is to help the patient regain a sense of mastery and hope. In some cases, reassurance suffices. Many patients, once sensing that the depression is manageable, can muster their own resources to deal with it. In addition to simply helping patients feel they are working on their problems, various supportive tactics can be useful.

The patient is educated about the syndrome of depression: the sleep and appetite disturbances, the lack of energy, the pessimism that are part of the illness. The therapist can label hopelessness as one of the more convincing symptoms that the patient is in fact depressed, but clarify that it is only a symptom:

> If you didn't feel hopeless, I would wonder whether you were really depressed. But the hopelessness is *only* a symptom of your depression, and you don't need to feel hopeless. In fact, depression is one of the most treatable of psychiatric disorders. The more you learn about depression and its treatment (with psychotherapy, medication, or both), the less hopeless I think you'll feel. Give the treatment enough time to work (at least six weeks), and don't let the hopelessness of depression discourage you from getting better.

THE PATIENT FEARS BEING ALONE

If the symptoms worsen when the patient is alone, the therapist may explore with the patient both emergency measures and long-term strategies for reducing social isolation. Alternatively, if the patient becomes depressed when associating with specific people who are hostile or otherwise unhelpful, the therapist and patient can find ways to decrease contact or to renegotiate relationships with these individuals. (See Chapter 4 on Interpersonal Role Disputes.)

THE PATIENT FEARS LOSS OF CONTROL

Patients who feel suicidal or are disturbed by hostile fantasies may fear loss of control. For these patients, the psychotherapist's extended availability may be particularly useful as treatment begins. Meeting with the patient several times a week, daily phone calls, or assurance of twenty-four hour availability by phone may reassure severely disturbed patients. These measures should be reserved for patients who really seem to need this much support. The offer of extraordinary measures may alarm less-disturbed patients, who may get the message that the psychotherapist considers them "really sick."

Many patients are reassured when the psychotherapist, in systematically taking the history of the depressive illness, seems to anticipate their symptoms. To further normalize the patient's depression, the psychotherapist should discuss the high prevalence of depressive disorders in our society, as well as the good prognosis and responsiveness of depression to treatment. It is particularly helpful to point out that people who are depressed characteristically have a negative outlook and feel that it will never end. For many patients, the current episode has been preceded by previous depressive episodes. When appropriate, patients may be told that a vulnerability to depression seems to affect their way of responding to serious life problems. And, when possible, the therapist may demonstrate that on previous occasions the patient has been able to resolve the depression.

THE PATIENT HAS DIFFICULTY ACCEPTING HIS OR HER WISHES

Many depressed patients have difficulty accepting of their wishes or hesitate to act on them, because they have learned either that their needs are unacceptable or that they are unlikely to be fulfilled anyway. Thus, for instance, a woman may meekly but resentfully accept domination by her husband if she does not believe that a different kind of treatment is legitimate or expectable. Depressed patients, and especially those who are chronically depressed, often see their wishes and needs as "selfish," and guiltily put other peoples' needs ahead of their own. To counter the tendency to suppress or deny needs or wishes, the psychotherapist may repeatedly guide patients by asking questions such as "What do you want from ____?" and encouraging them to think about their desires in a freer way. An even more basic intervention is simply to name and implicitly legitimize the needs that are expressed in the patient's behavior. Again, the therapist may remark to the patient that difficulties in recognizing the legitimacy of one's own needs and giving primacy to the wishes of others are characteristic issues of depressed patients, and often related to feelings of worthlessness.

A patient may be told:

> Try to express your wishes and needs. Let's discuss what feels reasonable, or even wishes that don't feel so reasonable. Then we can talk about what sorts of changes might be realistic.

The Patient Avoids Positive Experience

Some depressed patients are unable to respond with pleasure to any event while in an acute episode. Others may respond to pleasurable events but have difficulty in anticipating enjoyment. Patients in the latter group may fail to plan or pursue activities that they would, in fact, enjoy. They can benefit from therapeutic maneuvers in which the psychotherapist reviews their past and current sources of gratification and encourages them to increase these activities. For patients who become depressed over grief and loss, the therapist is especially active in helping the patient "fill the empty space" with new activities and relationships. The therapist might say, "Not feeling pleasure or enjoyment is a part of your depression. These painful and empty feelings should go away as your depression lifts."

The Patient Takes the Blame
for Family or Group Problems

Some depressed patients blame themselves for situations over which they have little or only partial control. Forces growing out of unrecognized family or group dynamics frequently place special pressures on particular individuals who do not necessarily experience them as coming from the group. In these cases, the patient can be taught simple principles of group or family dynamics ("scapegoating," for example), and the way these principles illustrate their role in their group constellation. The therapist can note that depression may lead patients to guiltily "scapegoat" themselves, in accord with such group dynamics. With this information, patients can be guided in changing the nature of their role in their social network. The therapist should shift the focus from the patient's perceived self-blame and sense of overresponsibility for the situation to what the patient can do to change this difficult situation.

> People who are depressed typically blame themselves for situations over which they have little or no control. Self-blame is part of depression. There may even be pressure from others on you to take the blame for things that aren't really your fault. (In the midst of a depression, you certainly don't need to be a scapegoat, if that's what's happening to you.) These are important issues for us to discuss in therapy so that you can solve these interpersonal situations.

THE PATIENT SEES
TREATMENT AS A DEFEAT

Many depressed patients see the need for treatment as an additional defeat. In such instances, the patient should be reminded that seeking treatment is the wisest thing to do in the circumstances, and that it is somewhat courageous, given the patient's negative expectations about treatment. Since IPT defines depression as a medical illness, seeking treatment is as appropriate as it would be for any other medical condition, such as diabetes, hypertension, or asthma. Seeking treatment can be framed as an attempt to take the situation in hand and to actively do something about problems that have previously been allowed to go unresolved. Thus, the psychotherapist should foster the patient's understanding that seeking help is in itself an active response to the problems.

In addition to discussing depression as a medical illness, the therapist may need to explore the patient's feelings about the stigma of depression. How do the patient and significant others view depression? How has familial depression affected the behavior of other relatives and the way that they have been viewed? As part of psychoeducation about depression, the therapist may clarify:

Although people have long been confused by and afraid of psychiatric disorders, attitudes are changing. Research shows that having just a couple of depressed symptoms can be as disabling or worse than having a variety of other medical illnesses [Wells et al., 1992]. Public awareness has been helped by the popularity of new antidepressant medicines like Prozac, and people are beginning to understand that depression is a common and treatable illness, not weakness or laziness. Since you have a depression, it's important that you understand it for what it is. It's not your fault. Seeking treatment is a positive first step out of the depression.

THE PATIENT ATTEMPTS SUICIDE

Suicide constitutes the most severe danger of depressive illness. For this reason, suicidal threats or actions must always be taken seriously.

The first task of the psychotherapist is to determine whether hospitalization is necessary for the patient who expresses suicidal ideation. This is a complex judgment that must include consideration of the seriousness of intent, the lethality of previous attempts, and the availability of others in the patient's social network. If hospitalization is not required, exploration of the meaning of suicide to the patient is in order, beginning with the assumption that suicide represents an attempt at interpersonal communication or problem solving. Attention should be paid to the circumstances in which the suicidal ideation began to develop. Thoughts about the interpersonal intent of suicide can be assessed by reviewing how patients imagine others' reactions to their death, reviewing their ideas of what death is like (there may be reunion fantasies involving deceased loved ones), or assessing what the death would accomplish. On whom would be their death have the greatest impact? Patients can often be helped to imagine a better way to achieve the results intended by the suicide.

A suicidal patient must not feel abandoned by others. The therapist will be as available as possible when a patient feels suicidal—being more reachable by phone or scheduling extra sessions. The therapist should acknowledge the potential risk of suicide but maintain optimism:

This is the symptom I'm most worried about. When people are really depressed and can't imagine life ever improving, they are at greatest risk for suicide. When the depression gets better, they almost always want to be alive. Being in the midst of a depression is the worst time to judge whether life is worthwhile.

I want to make sure we keep you alive long enough for you to feel better. I'm available to you during this crisis; I don't want you to keep these thoughts to yourself.

PROBLEMS IN THE THERAPY

THE PATIENT SUBSTITUTES THE PSYCHOTHERAPIST FOR FRIENDS OR FAMILY

Patients with poor social support from family, friends, work, or church may substitute the psychotherapist for these resources. To allow the helping relationship to be viewed as a substitute for friends or family is a disservice to the patient. Ethical psychotherapists do not confide in or share social activities with patients. The thrust of IPT always is to focus the patient on outside, "real life" relationships rather than the therapeutic relationship. If a patient begins to use the relationship as a substitute for outside resources, it is important to clarify the matter at once. The therapist might say:

> You can talk quite openly to me about your problems, your hopes, your fears. This shows me that you are capable of an intimate friendship. But we're not friends or family. What is most important for you is what your life is like outside our relationship. Who can you talk to among your friends or family the way you are talking to me? How can we help you find these people? [Or get over your fears of being open with someone?] Whom do you have to help you in your life? How can you approach them? Who have you been able to confide in?

THE PATIENT MISSES APPOINTMENTS OR IS LATE

In many other therapies, this would be considered a problem in the therapy; in IPT, with its focus on depression as an illness, it may also be considered a problem related to the depression itself.

The initial approach to this problem is simply to call attention to the behavior and to make sure trivial misunderstandings are cleared up or that realistic problems are not responsible. For instance, patients may think that coming late to an appointment is not a problem because doctors in their previous experience had a large backup in the waiting room. In this case, it should be explained that the allotted time is kept open for the patient alone and the psychotherapist has no conflicting appointments. The patient may also be reminded that the missed sessions or lateness means less time to work on problems: this uses the pressure of the time limit to motivate the patient and move the therapy forward. Other patients may be habitually late because of practical problems, such as getting baby-sitters. The therapist should make an effort to schedule times when the patient is most likely to be able to attend.

The therapist irritated by a patient's lateness should keep in mind that the depression may well be to blame. It is often helpful to attribute the patient's difficulty in getting to sessions to depressive symptoms.

> I know it's hard to get to sessions when you're feeling so bad: when you lack energy to get out of bed, you're thinking that things will not go well anyway, and it's hard to have hope or initiative. And I know it can feel anxiety-provoking to think of spending a full session here sometimes. But we need to take advantage of the limited time we have left in order to fight just those symptoms.

This avoids blaming the patient for depressive symptoms, a confusion these patients all too often make themselves.

When patients do not readily understand the meaning of their behavior (for example, "I've been coming later because I don't want to talk about ____"), the psychotherapist may examine the circumstances in which the behavior arose (coming late only after emotional sessions) and the possibly intended interpersonal consequences of the behavior (lateness shortens the sessions or angers the psychotherapist).

The therapist tries to treat the behavior as an indirect and inefficient interpersonal communication, whether or not the patient is aware that the provocative behavior has an effect on others or is aware of feeling any of the things being communicated in this indirect way. For example, patients may feel that therapy is helping and that they want to cooperate, but that for some unknown reason they just cannot remember the time of appointments. Others are quite aware of their mixed feelings and are able to discuss them when asked about missed appointments. In helping patients discover the meaning of such behavior, it may be helpful to discuss the events connected with the uncooperative actions.

For example, a patient who was punctual in the first phases of treatment, when she discussed her exasperating relationship with her hyperactive son, started missing appointments as the topic began to shift to her long-standing and previously unacknowledged resentment of her aloof, unhelpful husband. The therapist pointed this out to the patient, with an encouragement to confront the marital relationship, which possibly was not at such an impasse as the depressed patient believed.

Another technique for exploring uncooperative behavior is to begin with the idea that the patient does recognize the interpersonal consequences of the behavior or that there is at least a partial intention to have them take place. In such a situation, the first aim should be to make the patient aware of the effect the behavior has on the therapist. It frequently turns out that the patient affects family or friends the same way. For example:

CASE EXAMPLE

A patient who came for treatment with a history of short-lived, stormy relationships began early to miss appointments and then place the blame on the psychotherapist. The therapist talked with the patient about the infuriating nature of his behavior. As his behavior was examined, he revealed that he did not believe others could respond to him positively and that when involved in a dispute he felt more comfortable and engaged than when the relationship was quiet.

In applying learning that results from exploring uncooperative behavior, the therapist should attempt to point out the communicative aspects of this behavior and help the patient discover alternative, more direct methods of getting the point across. The patient's use of nonverbal means of communicating may be due to irrational fears about the outcome of more direct expression of either positive or negative feelings. For instance, a patient's feeling that angry avoidance of direct conflict is preferable to voicing complaints may be based on expectations of massive retaliation from the other person. Whenever possible, it is important to point out that depression may be responsible for, or at least compound, these maladaptive interpersonal behaviors.

THE PATIENT IS SILENT

Some silence occurs in any treatment, and in most cases does not call for discussion. In general, IPT is a treatment in which the patient and the psychotherapist share responsibility for bringing up topics to discuss and for directing the exploration of an issue. Because of the relaxed, conversational stance and activity of the therapist, silence is in fact rarely a problem. However, there may be times when it is important to allow a prolonged silence, two or three minutes or more. When emotion-laden material has been discussed, or when the psychotherapist feels that the patient may have more to reveal about an issue spontaneously than can be gained by asking questions, silence may be productive. In our experience, this is particularly true in addressing grief, where therapists who feel anxious in the presence of strong affect may interrupt the patient, interfering with their mourning process and implicitly signaling that such emotions are dangerous. Once a patient begins to mourn a complicated bereavement, therapeutic silence is often golden: a virtue, not a problem.

Occasionally patients become concerned about silences, feeling that no work is going on. In such cases, they may be told that IPT involves sharing the experiences of the time, which include silence as well as active discussion.

If silence becomes a persistent problem, its meaning may be explored by questioning the patient about possible explanations. Improvement may have been so great that the patient feels there is nothing more to talk about. In this case, discussion of termination should begin. If the patient does not believe the problems are solved, then the therapist may begin inquiring into what is preventing discussion of the issues at hand. The basic assumption here is that the patient is either avoiding recognition of conflicted thoughts or feelings about an issue or would like to bring up something but is concerned about the therapist's reaction.

The therapist may begin by asking silent patients what is on their minds or whether there is something they are refraining from discussing. This inquiry usually leads to discovery of irrational interpersonal fears connected with revealing thoughts and feelings to others. If patients can overcome their hesitation to communicate in the treatment and gain a better understanding of the assumptions they are making about others (that others will disapprove, not care, or let them down), this may lead to improved communication outside. The therapist might ask: "Are you afraid of what I might think of what you can't talk about? That I might disapprove?"

As with the exploration of lateness, the therapist may choose to point out the effect silence has in an interpersonal context. For example, the patient may use silence in a habitual, pouting way rather than voice legitimate complaints. In this case patients may be helped to see both the annoying effects of silence and the relatively unproductive nature of this communication.

Sometimes it's hard for you to talk directly about what you want in a relation-ship or about what another person does that annoys you. This is just the kind of thing it may be helpful for you to change. If you keep your needs or your annoyance inside, it's hard for other people to know what you want, and what you don't like. If you don't let people know, it's unlikely they are going to change their behavior.

THE PATIENT CHANGES OR AVOIDS SUBJECTS

Patient and therapist must have concurred on the focus of treatment for IPT to proceed into its middle phase. Thus, the therapist has the patient's agree-ment on one or more interpersonal problem areas as the central topic of dis-cussion. Most patients are willing to pursue this theme, and accept the therapist's steering the discussion back to it if the session wanders from it. Indeed, this is part of the therapist's responsibility. Even if the patient fears the topic at hand—for example, confronting a difficult spouse in a role dis-pute—the therapist gently persists: "It's better to figure out what can be done to handle the problem than to avoid it and feel more hopeless."

Nonetheless, avoiding discussion of important material may take place in a variety of ways, such as discussing only childhood events, repeatedly changing the subject, or open refusal to discuss a given problem. As in the case of silence, the psychotherapist's initial reaction should be a matter-of-fact mention of the problem. If the therapist notices that the patient changes topics only when a particular issue is brought up, this observation can be shared. (We assume here that the topic in question relates to the interper-sonal problem area. The IPT therapist may properly ignore topics of poten-tial psychological interest which are not however relevant to the interpersonal focus.) In pointing out avoidance of specific topics, it is im-portant to keep in mind the patient's relative autonomy to discuss what is of concern, as well as the identified problem that both therapist and patient have agreed will be the focus of treatment. As with silence, after pointing out the problem, the therapist should follow up with an examination of the patient's intentions in repeatedly avoiding issues and the effect this behav-ior has on others.

You can discuss anything that concerns you. We don't have to talk about every-thing. But it may be that the subject you seem to be avoiding is a key to your current problems. Perhaps you are avoiding talking about something because of shame or embarrassment. Many patients feel that way. I want to assure you that few topics you might raise could surprise me.

THE PATIENT COMPLAINS
OR IS UNCOOPERATIVE

Depressed patients often feel that nothing can help them and that their depression will go on forever. Such feelings can make them directly uncooperative. It is important to try to instill hope in these patients. They may be honestly told that the prognosis is good, since most depressed patients recover even without treatment in six months to a year. Findings about the utility of IPT in controlled studies can also be shared with the patient. Beyond reassurance, the response to persistent complaints is to use this behavior in an attempt to help patients understand their complaining in an interpersonal context. Excessive complainers may be picking on relatively trivial issues to avoid direct confrontation with central concerns. Others may have expectations of others that can never be fulfilled and may need to learn ways of caring for themselves. Regardless of the meaning of the complaints, patients can be made aware of the effects of their behavior and be provided with alternative ways of handling displeasure.

CASE EXAMPLE

Leila, a forty-two-year-old married woman with four teenagers, used more than half of each session to complain that the therapist was unhelpful, as she didn't do one of several practical tasks the patient requested: giving her the name of a private school, helping her to get a job. In the course of her complaint, it became clear that she was having a dispute with her husband, who she had seemed to idealize in her initial description. She was overwhelmed with many practical concerns and felt she could not ask for his help. The therapy then shifted to focus on the role dispute with the husband, and ways that she might get more constructive support from him.

THE PATIENT IS EXCESSIVELY DEPENDENT

Depressed patients frequently underestimate their own capabilities and feel that others must provide things that they can easily obtain for themselves.

In therapy they repeatedly ask for inappropriate advice or try to persuade the psychotherapist to intervene inappropriately in an interpersonal or other problem. Although IPT is a supportive treatment in which the psychotherapist may be realistically helpful, the sort of help offered is focused and limited. If the patient is simply misunderstanding the limitations of the therapeutic relationship, an explanation may suffice to curtail inappropriate demands. If the patient persists, this may provide an opportunity to explore the patient's unwillingness or inability to recognize personal strengths and capabilities.

The therapist might say:

> People who are depressed usually underestimate their own capabilities, and maybe that's why you're relying as you are on me. It's natural that you may feel you have to depend on others while you're depressed, and finding social supports is a good thing for you to do. We need to focus, though, on what you really *can* do to help your own situation. I want to show you that you're in fact more capable than you may feel. As you prove that to yourself and retake control of your interpersonal environment, you should start to feel better, and you may feel less dependent on other people, including me.

Following the same logic, therapists should be cautious not to diagnose dependent behaviors in depressed patients as necessarily indicative of a dependent personality disorder.

THE PATIENT IS SABOTAGING TREATMENT

Since focusing on the therapeutic relationship is not an important part of IPT, the patient's positive feelings for the psychotherapist and high expectations from treatment are not systematically explored except when they interfere with progress: when, for example, patients have such high expectations of being helped by the omnipotent psychotherapist that they make no independent effort to solve problems themselves. The therapist is careful, however, to continuously monitor the treatment for signs that the patient is developing negative or countertherapeutic feelings about the therapist or the treatment. These may take the form of relatively subtle verbal or nonverbal communication, or may be expressed in problematic behavior such as lateness, missed appointments, silence, excessive discussion of tangential material, direct uncooperativeness, or suicidal behavior, among others.

These behaviors are discussed separately later in this chapter. Here we will deal with the principles that underlie the therapist's handling of problematic attitudes and behaviors.

Confronted with such situations, the therapist has two goals: (1) to stop or mitigate the behavior, and (2) to relate the patient's disruptive behavior to problems the patient has in interpersonal relationships outside therapy. If the behavior can be brought under control, handling problems within the therapeutic relationship can provide a model for the patient's handling of problems in other relationships.

In dealing with disruptive attitudes and behaviors, the general sequence of exploration is to move from matter-of-fact mention of the behavior toward attempting to understand its meaning and interpersonal function. Thus, the psychotherapist must first make sure that simple misunderstanding or practical reasons are not the cause of the problem before proceeding to an investigation of the meaning of the behavior. In general, patients' disruptive behavior can be understood as *indirect and inefficient communication of negative feelings*, and they should be helped to find more direct and effective alternative ways of expressing themselves. One entrée into this arena is to note that many people who are depressed have trouble in directly expressing irritation or criticism to others, and to invite the patient to do so in and outside of the therapy.

> If something is troubling you about the treatment, please feel free to tell me what it is. A direct approach will help you to express yourself: as we've been discussing, confrontations with other people aren't nearly so dangerous as they feel to you, and can be much more helpful than you sometimes seem to realize. Depression often makes people feel helpless in situations where they really aren't. Since you have the symptoms of depression, it may be harder for you to express your feelings, but it should get easier as we proceed and you feel better.

THE PSYCHOTHERAPIST DEVELOPS POWERFUL FEELINGS TOWARD THE PATIENT

Psychotherapists occasionally find themselves developing strong feelings—such as anger, sexual attraction, or boredom—toward a patient. These feelings may be an extension of the interpersonal style of the therapist, or they may be a response to provocative behavior by the patient. It is important for the therapist to sort out which of the two possibilities is more likely. Response to the patient can be useful because it helps the therapist understand the response the patient elicits in others. This may help in determining the patient's strengths and weaknesses and in guiding inquiries into the patient's problematic relationships outside of treatment. In helping the patient learn about the effects of such behavior on others, the psychotherapist may tell the patient about these reactions. In fact, in instances when it is clear that the patient is acting in a provocative manner, failure to acknowledge it may cause the patient to doubt the psychotherapist's capacity to respond genuinely. For example:

CASE EXAMPLE

With a bright, argumentative patient in his early twenties, the therapist found that he was always having disagreements over a range of topics, such as appointment times or remembering what the patient had said earlier in the session. Since this man's chief complaint at the beginning of treatment was his social isolation, the therapist's reaction seemed to be an important clue to the patient's interpersonal difficulties. When the therapist expressed his annoyance, the patient seemed relieved and said he wondered why the therapist had tolerated his baiting behavior so long. Further discussion brought up the patient's long-standing belief that, since others were bound to exploit him if he showed weakness, he must approach them in an offensive, attacking manner.

Showing one's responses, especially negative ones, is a technique the therapist should use carefully and sparingly. In general, a nonjudgmental acknowledgment of the patient's difficulties is the preferred stance. Moreover, when the psychotherapist does express negative feelings to the patient, it is important that the patient's behavior, which can be changed, is what is objected to, and not the patient as a person. In gauging the timing of this kind of intervention, the therapist should be sure that the patient is provoking the response and that learning about the provocation will help the patient understand similar behavior outside of therapy. Properly used, working out conflicts between patient and psychotherapist can be a powerful tool in helping the patient learn about dispute resolution generally.

WHEN THE SIGNIFICANT OTHER
IS ASKED TO PARTICIPATE

The inclusion of the patient's significant other(s) in one or more therapy sessions is a consideration for patients with problems of interpersonal role disputes such as marital problems, and for adolescent patients. The session(s), which may be conjoint or individual, might be used to: (1) obtain additional information; (2) obtain the cooperation of the significant other; or (3) facilitate interpersonal problem solving and improved communication between the patient and the significant other. (See also Chapter 13 on depressed adolescents, and Chapter 15 on Conjoint IPT). Any involvement of other people in the treatment requires that the therapist provide assurance about confidentiality to the patient.

Family members may be guilty about the patient's illness and may blame themselves. It is useful to acknowledge that self-blame is common and to suspend judgment about the significant others' role. The medical model of depression as an illness used in IPT may serve to diminish such guilt. On the other hand, some family members may in fact be contributing to the patient's distress. If the family member is a partner in a role dispute, this should be acknowledged.

Although IPT is conceived of as an individual treatment, the therapist may choose—with the patient's agreement—to include significant others in a number of therapy sessions for either of two purposes.

Providing Information

The interpersonal difficulties of depressed patients are often exacerbated by the family's misunderstanding of the characteristics of depressive illness. For instance, one husband had interpreted his wife's apathy as willful resistance to doing housework, and a woman had been seeing her husband's loss of appetite and sexual interest as a direct criticism of her. The explanation that depression is a syndrome with predictable characteristics, a good prognosis, and unknown causes often allays relatives' apprehensions and guilt about the patient's condition. Moreover, the relatives can be told about ways to help the patient recover. They should be warned against either excessively blaming the patient or excessively excusing the patient from responsibility during a depressive illness.

For suicidal patients whose condition is serious but does not require hospitalization, relatives can be adjunctive psychotherapists with the tasks of monitoring the patient's condition and dispensing medications.

Obtaining Information

By either directly asking for information from the relative or observing interactions between the patient and the significant other, the psychotherapist may obtain information that could not be gotten from the patient alone.

> Participation of your family member will not violate your confidentiality. I will not discuss the content of your sessions with the other person, and I will discuss with you any additional contact I have with that other person. Let's discuss what you'd like to get from the conjoint sessions, and what you'd rather we didn't discuss.

THE PATIENT WISHES TO TERMINATE EARLY

The most complete avoidance of the work of therapy is premature termination. In many cases, this cannot be prevented, because the assumption of psychotherapy that talking things out should precede action runs counter to the beliefs and coping styles of many people. Early termination may also occur when patient and therapist disagree about the therapy contract or the patient feels the continuation of the contract is threatening.

Patients who express a wish to terminate should first be asked if they are satisfied that their problems have been dealt with adequately. This is seldom the case, but the question makes the point that there is still material to be worked on. The therapist should inquire about the patient's possible dissatisfactions with the therapy and try to satisfy reasonable requests or resolve misunderstandings. The tone of this inquiry should imply that the patient's plan to end treatment may be a legitimate and useful course of action. If specific insoluble problems have arisen between psychotherapist and patient, or if the patient has problems that cannot reasonably be handled with IPT methods, then referral to another psychotherapist or form of treatment is advisable.

If the psychotherapist is convinced that the patient's desire to terminate arises from confrontation of avoided issues or relates to the patient's general interpersonal problems, then the desire to terminate can be treated like any other symptom. In exploring the interpersonal meaning of threats to stop therapy, the patient should be encouraged to think and talk about feelings rather than simply acting on them. If the patient is determined to leave prematurely, it is important to communicate as strongly as possible that return to therapy is open and would not imply defeat or humiliation.

> If you want to end the treatment early, we should consider why you do. Do you feel that the problem has been adequately dealt with? Are you no longer depressed? Are there some issues you feel are too painful or frightening to confront? Is there some problem between the two of us that we haven't discussed? Are you giving up because you are still feeling depressed? Or perhaps IPT doesn't feel like the right treatment for you. If that's the case, I would be happy to help you evaluate alternative treatments and help you to find them. My main goal is to help you feel better.

From the interpersonal view, the patient's wish to terminate early is an example of unshared role expectations. The situation is a particular form of role dispute, in this case between patient and psychotherapist. At dispute is the duration of treatment, and the patient is requesting a renegotiation of the contract.

CASE EXAMPLE

A forty-two-year-old woman presented with a depressive episode convincingly related to problems in her twenty-year marriage. She agreed with the therapist's formulation of a role dispute, but became visibly anxious when certain aspects of the relationship arose during therapy sessions. She was convinced that her marriage was in "a hopeless rut," that her husband would be unwilling to change if she stated her chronic dissatisfactions with his behavior, and that in fact he would leave her. She began coming late to sessions and, by the sixth of a planned fourteen sessions, said she thought she would stop.

The therapist pointed out the patient's anxiety about "rocking the boat" of her marriage, reassured her that things need move no faster than the patient found comfortable, but also pointed out how uncomfortable she was in the current state of her marriage. How much did she have to lose by trying to improve things—attempts that, in fact, she had never made, although she had long recognized what the problems were. The patient was at least partially reassured. She subsequently took courage from some initial discussions with her husband, who was less recalcitrant than she had expected. She completed treatment in a euthymic state and with a much improved and more hopeful marriage.

The Patient Has Problems
with Self-Disclosure

In eliciting affectively charged material, timing is vital and the therapist must be reasonably certain that the patient can tolerate the feelings without becoming unproductively upset. Establishment of a trusting relationship with the psychotherapist may be necessary before the patient can deal with disclosure of suppressed topics. Moving too quickly in exploring sensitive areas can either stall progress by heightening the patient's defensiveness or lead to premature termination. It is expected that the therapeutic relationship will deepen as the therapy progresses, allowing the patient greater freedom to be open.

To help the patient be more self-revealing, the therapist is guided by the patient's displays of strong affect or, alternatively, by the lack of strong feelings when events or topics are described that would seem to warrant these feelings. If the patient begins to respond emotionally to a topic, further discussion of this material and fuller expression of feelings are encouraged. If the patient seems to be discussing material of little emotional relevance, the therapist may try to bring the focus back to important issues. (Indeed, the interpersonal focus itself—grief, role dispute, etc.—may often provide a guide to the relevance of the patient's material.) In eliciting the discussion of highly charged topics, the psychotherapist tacitly or explicitly conveys both acceptance of the affect, which in fact is not under the patient's control, and confidence that these powerful feelings need not be translated into actions, which are under the patient's control. The psychotherapist may choose to explain this in some such manner as:

Many people feel uncomfortable trying to discuss emotionally charged issues with a relative stranger. You'll need to feel you can trust me before you disclose some things. As time goes on, it should get easier to open up. And again, what you tell me I shall keep confidential.

You can't force your feelings to change, and although you find it hard to accept your [rage, fear, envy, etc.], we all have feelings like that. On the other hand, the fact that you have these feelings doesn't mean you will act on them. And if we can understand these feelings better, they may become less troubling or even make sense. Then you can figure out what to do about them.

THE PATIENT SEEKS ADDITIONAL, ALTERNATIVE TREATMENT

Patients may seek other treatment while continuing the therapy. The additional treatment may be another kind of psychotherapy and/or psychotropic medication. The therapist should maintain an open, nonjudgmental, and nonreproachful attitude about these activities, and they should be discussed in the therapy sessions. The patient should also be encouraged to discuss interest in other treatment with the therapist. Exploring alternatives and options are important themes of IPT and, for example, taking antidepressant medication or joining a group might represent productive steps the patient takes toward improved health and quality of life. During the initial phase of IPT, alternative treatment options should be discussed as part of the explanation of depression and its differential therapeutics (see Chapter 2). This discussion should set the stage for an open dialogue about other treatments during the course of IPT.

THE PATIENT RUNS OUT OF MONEY OR TREATMENT COVERAGE

This problem is generic for psychotherapy today, rather than specific to IPT. Managed care of mental illness unfortunately has limited patient benefits beyond clinical reason. And although such organizations may look with relative favor on treatments of proven efficacy like IPT, they frequently disallow even the relatively short duration (twelve to sixteen sessions) of acute treatment. In most treatments, this problem can be obviated by discussion of the fee and length of treatment at the outset.

If a patient subsequently reports that lack of money or insurance coverage is threatening the continuation of the treatment, the therapist must gauge whether this is an excuse, and the patient really just wants to end the treatment early (see above). If money is a significant issue, however—and not infrequently it is—the situation may provide an opportunity to explore interpersonal options in IPT. Are there other sources from which the patient could draw funds to complete the relatively brief treatment, from which the patient has a good chance of benefiting? Are interpersonal difficulties hindering the patient from obtaining money that is in fact available?

CASE EXAMPLE

A depressed wife in a marital role dispute felt too intimidated and worthless to ask her wealthy husband to support the treatment, not recognizing her own claim to their common property. An important aspect of treating this dispute involved discussions with the therapist leading to recognition of this disparity, role playing in the therapy to build assertiveness, and eventually a discussion with the husband about their finances, including payment for the therapy. The marital dispute, the depressive episode, and the bill were thus all resolved simultaneously.

If the problem lies with a denial of benefits by managed care or an insurance company, the therapist might use this as an opportunity to provide psychoeducation to both patient and third party payor about the treatment of depression with IPT.

IPT is a proven treatment for major depression, with numerous studies to attest to its efficacy. [See Chapter 10.] It's not an endless therapy: acute treatment requires between twelve and sixteen sessions, and in this case we had agreed on ____. For your company to allow just four sessions as "medically necessary" is unreasonable: it flies in the face of the medical literature.

This would be an opportunity for patient and therapist to work as a team to ensure that the former received maximal and appropriate benefits. The "injustice" of the denial might be treated as a social *transgression* (see Chapter 4) to galvanize the patient's anger and activity.

The therapist should act as the patient's ally in this situation, where money might distance them. If the patient has remitted and some sessions of the original contract remain, then an earlier termination might save the patient money and might serve the patient's best interest. The therapist might also reconsider the treatment fee in light of the patient's financial difficulties.

COMMON PATIENT CONCERNS

There has been a burgeoning of public mental illness awareness programs in the United States and Europe. In the U.S. these have included depression education programs such as DART (Depression/Awareness, Recognition, and Treatment), screening programs (National Depression Screening Day each October), and patient advocacy groups (e.g., the National Depressive and Manic Depressive Association [NDMDA] and National Alliance for the Mentally Ill [NAMI]). Such programs have increased patient awareness of and decreased stigma about their illness; they also have raised additional questions. We believe that an educated consumer is the best patient. Therapists can expect that patients will increasingly raise direct questions about their illness and expect direct, honest, and informed answers. Many answers are contained in the scripts in this chapter and elsewhere in the book. Some concerns that are not fully covered elsewhere are presented below.

Do I Have a "Biological" Depression?

Psychiatry once wasted energy in an ideological struggle over whether depressions are "biological" or "psychological." The debate missed the point. All depressions are ultimately biological, in that they involve (reversible) changes in the neurotransmitters and receptors in the brain; and in their physical, biological symptoms such as sleep and appetite disturbance, low energy and libido, and difficulties with concentration or memory. Beyond this biological substrate, depressions tend to occur in a psychological or psychosocial context. There may have been an upsetting change in the patient's life situation, in the patient's perception of that situation, or in the patient's ability to cope with it. Thus both biology and psychology may be said to influence essentially all depressions.

Treatment may involve medication, psychotherapy, or both. The decision to use medication usually reflects the severity of the depressive symptoms, a history of recurrence, or the patient's wishes. (It should not simply reflect the ideology of the clinical practitioner.) Patients with psychotic or delusional depression or with bipolar disorder require medication (or electroconvulsive therapy); psychotherapy might provide a helpful adjunct as their illness improves. Patients with other forms of depression often do well with psychotherapy alone.

Whether or not the patient receives medication, he or she can consider depression as a biological disorder which is often precipitated by psychosocial stressors.

CAN I GIVE DEPRESSION TO MY CHILDREN?

Patients are becoming sophisticated about the genetic basis of many of the major illnesses, including psychiatric illnesses. Increasingly, there is concern about the genetic basis of depression—or, as it may be framed by patients: "Does this mean I can give depression to my children? If I have depression, does this mean my children are also apt to have it?" Patients can be told that depression does run in families. If they are depressed, their children have a two to three times greater risk of becoming depressed when compared to children of parents who have never been depressed. However, put another way, if the normal rate of depression is 5 percent, the risk to children of depressed parents is 10 to 15 percent. The good news is that most likely their children will not get depressed (i.e., 85 to 90 percent will escape). Patients can also be told that we do not know the mechanism by which depression is transmitted in families, whether through genes and genetic vulnerability or through the stress produced by the parent's depression or through some combination thereof. Since there are good treatments, and the ability exists to detect depression very early in its course, early interventions are possible. On the other hand, if the patient is depressed and his or her children seem to be having similar problems, the patient should be instructed to pay attention, take it seriously, talk to the child about it, and get help if it persists.

CAN I DRINK MY BLUES AWAY?

There is high comorbidity between depression and alcohol abuse dependency, particularly in males. Some depressed patients may feel that alcohol relieves their symptoms, at least in the short run. In the short run, it can improve sleep and can dull painful memories and current experiences. However, patients need to be warned that alcohol is a bad treatment for depression. In the long run, it disturbs sleep and is a mood depressant. In fact, it can make the patient more depressed. Similarly, it can diminish the patient's ability to cope, create additional problems in the family and at work, interfere with treatment for depression, and increase the risk of suicide. The same case can be made with use of illicit drugs or the abuse of legal drugs. Patients must be instructed that it if they are having a drinking or drug problem, they need to be up-front about it and seek help from the therapist.

CHAPTER 10

Efficacy Data for Acute Treatment of Major Depression

IPT has developed through a progression of research trials and adaptations for further trials, each of which has tested its efficacy for a particular psychiatric disorder or a specific patient population. Here we describe the results of the acute treatment trials. The results for maintenance treatment of depression and for adaptations to particular age groups and other treatment populations are described in subsequent chapters.

BOSTON–NEW HAVEN STUDY

The first test of efficacy of IPT as an acute antidepressant treatment was a four-cell, sixteen-week randomized trial of IPT, amitriptyline (AMI), their combination, and a nonscheduled control treatment for eighty-one outpatients with major depression (DiMascio et al., 1979; Weissman et al., 1979). This study was advanced for its time in training therapists to adhere to a treatment manual. Amitriptyline was dosed at 100–200 mg. q.d., typical doses for the time but lower than might be attempted today. The nonscheduled treatment assigned patients a psychiatrist whom they were told to contact when they felt the need. No regular treatment sessions were scheduled, but patients could telephone to arrange a session if they felt sufficient distress.

Analyses of the results found that each active treatment more effectively reduced symptoms than did the nonscheduled control group treatment, and that combined AMI-IPT was more effective than either active monotherapy. (This is one of a handful of studies that has found advantages for combined psychotherapy and pharmacotherapy over monotherapies.) No significant differences appeared between IPT and AMI in symptom reduction by the end of treatment, although the beneficial effects of AMI appeared earlier. On the other hand, IPT and AMI seemed to work preferentially on different symptom clusters: medication had its initial effect on the neurovegetative symptoms of depression, whereas IPT worked mainly on mood, apathy, suicidal ideation, work, and interest (DiMascio et al., 1979). There were no differences between the treatment groups in social functioning at the end of acute treatment.

A one-year naturalistic follow-up found that many patients sustained benefits from the brief IPT intervention. Patients who received IPT developed significantly better psychosocial functioning over the course of the year, whether or not they received medication. This effect on social function was not found for AMI alone, and had not been evident for the IPT cells at the end of the sixteen-week trial (Weissman et al., 1981). Many patients from all treatments reported requiring additional treatment over the follow-up year. This suggested that acute treatment was insufficient for persistent response, a fact now recognized in many studies, which now often include a maintenance phase.

NIMH TDCRP STUDY

The most ambitious acute treatment study to date, the multi-site National Institute of Mental Health Treatment of Depression Collaborative Research Program (NIMH TDCRP) (Elkin et al., 1989), randomly assigned 250 depressed outpatients to sixteen weeks of imipramine (IMI), IPT, cognitive behavioral therapy (CBT), or placebo. This study was groundbreaking in several respects. It was the first head-to-head comparison of IPT and CBT as antidepressant treatments. It was the first time these treatments had been used away from the sites where they had been developed: the originators of IPT and CBT trained therapy teams for the TDCRP, but the study sites lacked the aura surrounding the centers (in New England and Philadelphia, respectively) where they had originated. This study thus tested whether IPT and CBT could be effectively transferred to other locations. The TDCRP was also the first time the NIMH solicited a multi-site psychotherapy trial.

Manuals were used to define each treatment, and independent adherence monitors rated tapes of sessions to ensure that therapists delivered the treatment appropriately. Imipramine and placebo were each accompanied by clinical management (CM), which represented the first research attempt to ensure that pharmacotherapists were not performing active psychotherapy. Pharmacotherapists were allowed to provide patients with a biochemical rationale for improvement, to review medication side effects, and to provide warm, supportive advice à la Marcus Welby (Fawcett et al., 1987). Therapy sessions were taped and monitored to ensure treatment adherence (Hill et al., 1992).

Most subjects completed at least fifteen weeks or twelve treatment sessions. IPT had the lowest attrition rate among the treatments. Less symptomatic patients—those with a seventeen-item Hamilton Depression Rating Scale (Ham-D; Hamilton, 1960) score of 19 or less—improved in all treatments, including placebo/CM. Because all treatments worked equally well for mildly depressed patients, no overall difference was found among the treatments. Among more severely depressed patients (Ham>D20), however, differences did appear. Imipramine/CM induced the most rapid response and was most consistently superior to placebo. IPT was comparable to IMI/CM on several outcome measures and showed a mean outcome superior to placebo. In contrast, CBT produced an intermediate level of improvement and was not superior to placebo for this group.

Klein and Ross (1993) reanalyzed the efficacy data from the TDCRP. The Johnson-Neyman technique produced an ordering for treatment efficacy with "medication superior to psychotherapy, [and] the psychotherapies somewhat superior to placebo . . . particularly among the symptomatic and impaired patients" (Klein and Ross, 1993, p. 241). The authors found "CBT relatively inferior to IPT for patients with Beck Depression Inventory (BDI) scores greater than approximately 30, generally considered the boundary between moderate and severe depression" (p. 247). The reanalysis is consistent with previously reported results (Elkin et al., 1989) but sharpens differences among treatments.

Shea et al. (1992) conducted a naturalistic follow-up study of TDCRP patients eighteen months after treatment ended. All patients had ceased treatment after sixteen weeks, including medication subjects. The researchers found no significant difference in recovery (defined as the presence of minimal or no symptoms following the end of treatment, sustained during follow-up) among remitters in the four treatment groups: only 30 percent recovered with CBT, 26 percent with IPT, 19 percent with Imipramine, and 20 percent with placebo. Among patients who had remitted by the end of the sixteen-week study, relapse over the eighteen-month follow-up was 36 percent for CBT, 33 percent for IPT, 50 percent for imipramine, and 33 percent for placebo. The authors concluded that sixteen weeks of specific treatments were insufficient to achieve full and lasting recovery for many patients.

Thus both the Boston–New Haven study and the TDCRP found that sixteen weeks of treatment could induce remission but not guarantee the maintenance of recovery from depression. This makes clinical sense: major depression tends to be a recurrent and relapsing illness for which no acute treatment, psychotherapeutic or psychopharmacological, is wholly curative. The research suggests that acute IPT can treat a depressive episode but that continuation and maintenance treatment at a monthly level may be necessary to sustain remission. An adaptation of IPT has shown efficacy, even at a low, once-monthly dosage, in preserving the gains of acute treatment (see Chapter 11).

DUTCH STUDIES

Blom and colleagues (1996) in the Netherlands found IPT effective in an open trial for patients with mood disorders. Based on this success, Hoencamp (personal communication, 1996) and colleagues are undertaking a randomized study in the Hague of two hundred patients comparing IPT alone, nefazodone alone, their combination, and IPT plus placebo for acute major depression.

NEUROIMAGING

Martin and colleagues at the University of Durham in the United Kingdom report their use of neuroimaging with antidepressant treatment (S. Martin, personal communication, 1998). They treated twenty-eight patients with DSM-IV major depression and a minimum Ham-D score of 18 who were randomized to receive either venlafaxine (n=15, mean dose 75 mg. daily) or weekly IPT (n=13). Subjects were assessed using SPECT imaging at baseline and after six weeks. Both treatment groups improved substantially but showed different patterns of SPECT change. Venlafaxine patients showed statistically significant angular gyrus and dorsolateral prefrontal cortical (DLPFC) normalization, whereas IPT patients showed DLPFC and limbic central cingulate normalization. These are the first reported neuroimaging findings involving IPT and report on a relatively large sample for such research. They require replication but are provocative results.

PREDICTORS OF RESPONSE

It has long been known that not all patients with a given disorder respond to all treatments. Comparative treatment studies with large numbers of subjects, such as the NIMH TDCRP, allow examination of which treatments work best for patients with particular clinical characteristics. This knowledge should inform differential therapeutics (Frances et al., 1984), the choice of treatment prescribed for patients (see Table 10.1).

PATIENT FACTORS

Sotsky and colleagues (1991) found that several patient factors predicted treatment outcome in the TDCRP study. Depressed patients with a low baseline level of social dysfunction responded well to IPT, whereas those with severe social deficits (probably equivalent to the "interpersonal deficits" problem area) responded less well. Patients with greater symptom severity and difficulty in concentrating responded poorly to CBT. High initial severity of major depression and of impaired functioning predicted superior response to IPT and to imipramine. Imipramine also worked most efficaciously for patients with difficulty functioning at work—perhaps reflecting its faster onset of action.

In subsequent analyses, Sotsky (1997a) reported that TDCRP subjects with symptoms of atypical depression, in particular mood reactivity and reversed neurovegetative symptoms (hypersomnia, hyperphagia, or weight gain) responded poorly to imipramine. Both IPT and CBT had significantly higher response rates for patients with atypical depression than did active or placebo pharmacotherapy. This analysis corroborates previous research findings that tricyclic antidepressants are weak treatment for atypical depression, and provides new information about psychotherapy for atypical depression.

Using the Personality Assessment Form (Shea, Glass, Pilkonis, Watkins, and Docherty, 1987; Shea et al., 1990) as a measure of avoidant and obses-

TABLE 10.1   Factors Predictive of IPT Outcome in Major Depression

Positive Prognostic Factors	Study	Notes
Patient factors		
Low social dysfunction	Sotsky et al., 1991	
Symptom severity	Sotsky et al., 1991	vs. placebo/CM
Functional impairment	Sotsky et al., 1991	vs. placebo/CM
Atypical depression	Sotsky, 1997a	vs. placebo/CM, imipramine/CM
Obsessive personality disorder?	Barber & Muenz, 1996	vs. CBT
Therapist factors		
Interpersonal focus	Frank et al., 1991	
Therapeutic alliance	Sotsky, 1997b	

Negative Prognostic Factors	Study	Notes
Patient factors		
Interpersonal deficits	Sotsky et al., 1991	
abnormal sleep EEG	Thase et al., 1997	
avoidant personality disorder?	Barber & Muenz, 1996	

sive personality types in depressed patients, Barber and Muenz (1996) reexamined the TDCRP data set. Looking only at subjects who completed treatment, they confirmed their hypotheses that IPT was more efficacious than CBT for patients with obsessive personality disorder, whereas CBT fared better for avoidant personality disorder on Ham-D. Blatt and colleagues (1995) had used a different measure, the Dysfunctional Attitude Scale (Weissman and Beck, 1979), to measure the similar concepts of perfectionism and need for approval among subjects from the TDCRP data set. Blatt et al. (1995), however, did not find significant outcome differences. Neither approach used definitive diagnostic measures for personality disorder. The role of personality traits on depressive outcome in IPT is interesting and needs further study.

Barber and Muenz (1996) also reported that IPT was more efficacious than CBT for single, separated, or divorced patients, whereas CBT did better than IPT for married or cohabiting patients (on Ham-D, not BDI). (Sotsky et al. [1991] reported similar findings within treatments.) How to interpret this is unclear. Might this mean that these patients faced role disputes, and that role disputes are a less effective problem area for treatment in IPT?

In an interesting study of "difficult," help-rejecting patients, Foley et al. (1987) found that such patients tended to drive therapists out of a neatly adherent treatment delivery, and that such patient "difficulty" had more of an effect on therapist performance than did initial symptom severity. These patient characteristics did not ultimately affect treatment outcome, however.

Another study sheds light on prognosis from a biological perspective. Thase and colleagues (1997) found that among ninety-one depressed patients, those with abnormal sleep profiles on EEG (sleep efficiency, REM latency, and REM density) had significantly poorer response to IPT than did patients with undisturbed sleep parameters. Symptom severity did not significantly predict IPT response: 43 percent of more severely depressed (Ham-D>20) responded, versus 53 percent of less severely depressed patients. In contrast, only 37 percent of patients with abnormal sleep profiles responded to IPT, versus 58 percent with normal sleep (p=.03). Three-quarters of the IPT nonresponders subsequently responded to medication trials.

THERAPIST FACTORS

Frank and colleagues (1991) found that the focal "purity" of IPT—the ability of the therapist to keep sessions focused on interpersonal themes—was significantly correlated with prevention of relapse in their maintenance study of IPT for recurrent major depression. Patients whose monthly IPT maintenance sessions had high interpersonal specificity survived a mean two years before depression recurred, whereas those whose therapy had a low interpersonal focus were afforded only five months of protection before relapse.

Sotsky (1997b) reported that the strength of the therapeutic alliance significantly influenced outcome for all four treatments in the TDCRP, pharmacotherapy included.

PART TWO
ADAPTATION OF IPT
FOR MOOD DISORDERS

Introduction

IPT's original target diagnosis was major depressive disorder without psychotic symptoms among adult outpatients. This section deals with its adaptation and efficacy for mood disorders. IPT was first developed in a continuation study treating patients recovering on medication from an acute depressive episode (see Chapter 10). Like many therapies that have demonstrated efficacy in one area, IPT has since been tested for alternative, "off-label" indications. Successful treatments are commonly extended to new diagnostic indications. Compare, for example, the use of anticonvulsant medications for the treatment of bipolar disorder; the spread of serotonin reuptake inhibitors from their initial application, major depression, to dysthymic disorder, obsessive compulsive disorder, bulimia, and other psychiatric syndromes; of beta-blockers from their original cardiovascular indications to social phobia and explosive disorders; or of cognitive behavioral therapy (CBT) from major depression to panic disorder, bulimia, and other conditions.

Usually there are theoretical reasons for expecting the treatment to work in a new area. In the pharmacotherapy of bipolar disorder, "kindling" theory justified the testing of anticonvulsant medications (Post et al., 1986). The spread of IPT probably reflects several factors. First, IPT has been proven to have efficacy for major depression. Second, CBT, similarly researched and proven, was being successfully extended to other indications. Third, patients and therapists seem to find the focus of IPT on the relationship between affective state and environment a coherent, reasonable approach to psychiatric syndromes. This linkage of emotion and environment provides an essentially ubiquitous tool for treatment of psychiatric syndromes. How important that link is, and its efficacy as a treatment strategy, may of course vary from syndrome to syndrome.

Psychosocial issues presumably vary across different diagnostic categories. Depressed patients may face different stresses, or at least react differently to them, than patients with schizophrenia, panic disorder, bulimia, or substance abuse. The four interpersonal problem areas that work for adult, nonpsychotic outpatients with major depressive disorder—grief, role disputes, role transitions, and interpersonal deficits—might or might not apply to other syndromes. It would seem to follow that IPT might need adaptation to work optimally with each treatment population.

Some of the research that follows indeed adapted the IPT manual to meet the psychosocial needs and problem areas of specific treatment populations. A listing of specialized manuals can be found in Chapter 25. Other research, however, did not alter the original IPT approach.

Investigators interested in testing IPT for a new indication would do well to consult those who have already begun down the road, so as to avoid repeating old mistakes. The general principles of adapting IPT, however, are: (1) to assess the needs of the target treatment population, usually defined by a diagnosis, diagnostic subtype, or age group; (2) to adapt the standard IPT approach to the particular psychosocial needs and issues of that population; and (3) to test the efficacy of this approach in treatment trials.

Once IPT had shown efficacy in the treatment of acute major depression, researchers wondered about its application to subpopulations of depressed patients. Just as the pharmacology of depression differs for geriatric and adolescent patients, so might the psychotherapy of depression. IPT is being tested as a primary treatment of dysthymic disorder (chronic depression), as adjunctive treatment for bipolar disorder, and for patients whose medical status complicates the use of antidepressant medication: depressed medically ill and peripartum patients.

CHAPTER 11

Maintenance IPT for Recurrent Major Depression (IPT-M)

DISORDER

Depression tends to be a recurring illness: most people who suffer a single episode will likely have a second episode in their lifetimes. The more episodes an individual has suffered, the greater the likelihood of recurrence (Keller et al., 1992). Frank and colleagues (1991) have carefully defined the terms *remission, relapse,* and *recurrence* for major depression. It is important not only to find treatments that work acutely, but to determine those that can forestall the return of a relapsing, recurrent condition such as major depression. Such prophylactic benefits have been demonstrated more clearly for antidepressant medications than for psychotherapies. Many depressed patients thus require treatment after their acute episode has resolved. Some are difficult to treat. Many have multiple marital, family, and other social problems and frequently use medical and social services (Wells et al., 1989; Klerman, 1990).

In a landmark study, Frank, Kupfer, and colleagues at the University of Pittsburgh compared pharmacotherapy to psychotherapy as prophylaxis for 128 patients at high risk of depressive relapse (Frank et al., 1989, 1990). IPT-M, a monthly maintenance form of IPT (Frank, 1991), was the psychotherapy employed. This and a parallel study in Pittsburgh for geriatric depression (Reynolds et al., 1999) are the *only* long-term maintenance studies of antidepressant psychotherapy published to date.

The development of a maintenance form of IPT opens new possibilities for extending successful acute IPT for patients who have responded but remain at risk for relapse.

RATIONALE

The rationale for continued treatment of depression after alleviation of the acute episode is based on systematic research of the natural history of depression (Angst, 1986; Keller et al., 1982a, b, 1983; Keller, 1985; Coryell and Winokur, 1994). Most patients recover from the acute episode: naturalistic data show an 80 percent recovery within one to two years (Keller et al., 1982a). Chronic depression is defined as those episodes lasting for more than two years; about 10 percent of patients become chronically depressed (Weissman and Akiskal, 1984). Remission of chronic depression still continues in subsequent years, although at a rate much reduced from that in the first two (Keller, 1985).

It was long believed that most patients would experience one acute lifetime episode without recurrence. This expectation has since been questioned (Sargent et al., 1990). Recent reports indicate high rates of depressive recurrence and relapse that have clinical significance, even when they do not warrant hospitalization.

The value of antidepressant pharmacotherapy in preventing recurrence and reducing relapse has been established. Yet efficacious alternatives to medication, including psychotherapy, are necessary. Many patients require treatment when medication may not be suitable or possible, such as during pregnancy, lactation, or major surgery. The elderly, who may tolerate medication less well, are frequently already subject to the interactions of polypharmacy; they may have a long history of recurrent depressive episodes, and thus are another population who might benefit from antidepressant psychotherapy. So are those patients who do not tolerate or respond to medication, or who refuse to take it at all. Approximately 10–15 percent of depressed patients discontinue or cannot tolerate the initial medication they receive; another 15–25 percent respond only modestly to pharmacotherapy; and 5–10 percent refuse it (Klerman, 1990).

For patients with recurrent depression, social and interpersonal problems associated with the depression may not resolve between episodes, and may trigger recurrence (Keller et al., 1992). Onset of major depressive episodes is often associated with an increase in life events, particularly after the loss or disruption of interpersonal relationships through discord, separation, divorce, or death. Thus, psychotherapy may have a role in maintenance therapy as the sole treatment, or in combination with medication, to help the patient manage the social and interpersonal consequences or triggers of recurrent depression (Frank et al., 1991).

THE CONCEPT OF MAINTENANCE THERAPY

Several terms have been used to define ongoing post-acute treatment, including "continuation," "maintenance," and "prophylactic" treatment. The distinction between continuation and maintenance treatment is somewhat academic (Frank et al., 1991). One arbitrary but increasingly accepted definition of treatment duration is that therapy in the six months following resolution of an episode constitutes continuation treatment; beyond six months, maintenance treatment.

Continuation treatment refers to treatment that persists once acute depressive symptoms have been alleviated, i.e., after acute remission. A return of symptoms following a brief period of remission (two to six months) is considered a relapse of the original depressive episode (Frank et al., 1991). Therefore, the goal of ongoing therapy is to sustain the remission brought about by short-term treatment: to *prevent relapse*. Maintenance therapy refers to longer periods of treatment, after acute patients have resolved and the patient has been asymptomatic for at least six months. Its goal is to *prevent recurrence* of new episodes, or at least to increase the time between recurrences for patients who have histories of recurrent episodes.

Prophylactic therapy refers to the efficacy of treatment in sustaining recovery after treatment has ended. Although prophylaxis has been used synonymously with maintenance treatment, the only evidence available regarding prophylaxis comes from naturalistic follow-up studies, in which investigators have attempted to determine whether an acute course of treatment somehow "inoculates" the patient against future episodes. These studies are difficult to interpret because treatments are uncontrolled and attrition rates differ. Patients who remain symptomatic tend to seek treatment—often a different treatment than they originally received. Thus naturalistic studies of patients followed up after a specific treatment has ended include a mixture, some of whom received the treatment and remained well, and others who relapsed and sought other treatments.

As maintenance treatment has not been universally defined, the evidence for the efficacy of maintenance and continuation treatment will be reviewed together. This evidence, deriving from clinical trials of depressed patients following remission of an acute episode, attempts to determine whether further treatment prevents or forestalls relapse or recurrence of depression.

The First Study

The first systematic study of IPT in depressed patients (Klerman et al., 1974; Paykel et al., 1976) would be considered a continuation study by today's standards. In the late 1960s, it was clear that tricyclic antidepressants were efficacious treatment for acute depression. It was unclear, however, how long treatment should continue and what the role of psychotherapy should be in ongoing treatment.

Attempting to answer these questions, Klerman et al. (1974) studied 150 acutely depressed outpatients who responded to four to six weeks of amitriptyline (AMI): that is, had a 50 percent symptom reduction, a criterion met by approximately 70 percent of the sample. Patients were randomized to receive eight months of IPT maintenance treatment at a high (one hour weekly) or low (fifteen minutes monthly) rate, and these two groups were further divided to receive AMI (100–150 mg./day), placebo, or no pills. The sample was restricted to women; most, though not all, had nonpsychotic major depression.

The early version of IPT used in this study consisted of individual sessions, primarily supportive in nature, that emphasized the "here and now" and focused on the current problems and interpersonal relations of the patient. Patients were assisted in identifying maladaptive patterns and attaining better adaptive responses in family and social relations. Although a draft manual was developed defining the therapy, IPT was called "high-contact" in this first study, while patients not receiving IPT were termed "low-contact." This modest nomenclature reflected the expectation that there would be no psychotherapy effect, because the few controlled psychotherapy trials to that date had not shown effects. Treatment was specified by quantity and goals, and training and supervision strove to ensure comparability among therapists. The attrition rate was generally low (less than 12 percent) across treatment groups.

Maintenance AMI therapy, regardless of whether patients received IPT, had significantly greater efficacy (p<.05) than placebo or no pill in preventing relapse. IPT combined with AMI was no more effective than AMI alone. However, as noted by Hollon and DeRubeis (1981), "high-contact" IPT alone, without placebo, was nearly as effective (16 percent relapse rate) as AMI combined with high-contact or low-contact IPT (relapse rates of 12.5 percent and 12 percent, respectively). The combination of psychotherapy with placebo (relapse rate=28 percent) reduced the overall effect for psychotherapy versus low-contact psychotherapy.

IPT alone was significantly better (p<.05) than low-contact psychotherapy in enhancing social functioning, whereas AMI plus low contact was not superior to placebo plus low contact (Klerman, 1990). Because of the differential effects of the treatments, the combination of AMI and IPT had the greatest efficacy in preventing relapse and improving social functioning. No negative interactions between the antidepressant medication and IPT were found.

IPT AS MAINTENANCE TREATMENT FOR RECURRENT DEPRESSION

The subsequent study by Frank et al. (1989, 1990) is the most comprehensive maintenance trial of IPT. It is unique in its length and sophistication. This and the Klerman et al. (1974) study already discussed represent the entire corpus of maintenance antidepressant psychotherapy studies reported to date. The subjects treated in this research had had multiple previous episodes of major depression; having achieved remission, they remained at very high risk for relapse and recurrence—as the outcome of the placebo group was to demonstrate. Hence they provided a good test of the prophylactic efficacy of the study treatments: high-dose imipramine, relatively low-dose IPT-M, and alternative conditions.

ADAPTATION

IPT-M is a maintenance form of IPT developed specifically for this study. Although based on the same general principles, it differs from acute IPT in several respects. Whereas acute IPT is usually delivered weekly, this therapy was delivered "weakly": that is, once a month. As this research entered new territory, there was no attempt at dose-finding for IPT-M. By comparison, imipramine was maintained at high doses in this treatment study.

The goal of IPT-M, similar to that of the end stage of acute IPT, was to delay or prevent relapse. Its focus was to watch for signs and symptoms of emergent episodes. Therapists sought within the broad scope of this extended treatment to develop interpersonal strategies to prevent future episodes. IPT-M was time-limited, in that it was scheduled to continue for three years, but clearly this time frame had to have a different effect than the compressed structure of a brief therapy. Because of the longer time frame, therapists and patients could choose to shift among the four IPT problem areas (grief, role dispute, role transition, or interpersonal deficits) as issues arose, rather than sticking to a specific focus (Frank, 1991).

CASE EXAMPLE

Rita, a sixty-three-year-old married artist, presented with a five-month history of recurrent depression and an initial Hamilton Depression Rating Scale score of 28. She had had four previous episodes of nondelusional major depression over a period of thirty-five years, with good intermorbid mood and functioning. History taking was involved because of the length of her illness and complexity of prior treatment, her agitation and distractibility, and her tendency to dwell on the happier moments of her youth.

Rita simultaneously announced that she didn't like to talk about her feelings and that she refused to take medications because of their side effects. The current episode, her first in eight years, coincided with her husband's retirement from medical practice. She experienced this as a diminution of the couple's prestige and spending power, but was particularly concerned at the prospect of spending more time with her "workaholic" spouse, whose career had apparently provided a useful buffer between them. "He's driving me crazy puttering around the house all day," she said. She had *not* retired from painting, and he was getting in the way, making productive work impossible. As Rita was not suicidal, had some social supports, refused medication, and presented with a clear role dispute, the therapist felt IPT was a reasonable treatment option.

Indeed, a twelve-week course of acute IPT led to symptomatic remission (Ham-D=5). This treatment focused on the role dispute, her wishes for the relationship, and how she could hope to resolve it. She confronted her husband about his anxious and intrusive pacing about the house, made her artist's studio "off limits" to him, and encouraged him to do volunteer work teaching at a nearby hospital. This allowed them both to enjoy much more fully the time they shared together.

As the twelve-week trial concluded, the therapist noted Rita's dramatic improvement and discussed the option of continuation and maintenance treatment, given her risk for further episodes. They agreed on monthly follow-up sessions for the subsequent two years. These sessions were characterized by progress reports on the marriage and retirement. Rita was pleased with her improved negotiating skills, and felt she handled her "difficult" husband well, with good results. Other issues, which had been only touched on in the acute treatment, arose from time to time: disputes in dealing with her children about the grandchildren, the role transition of a serious medical illness fifteen months into remission, and grief—uncomplicated bereavement—over the death of her best friend. She remained euthymic, with mild variation of a few points on the Hamilton scale, for the duration of the two years, at which point she pronounced the treatment helpful but sufficient, and terminated.

EFFICACY

In the Frank et al. study, a total of 128 acutely depressed patients with a history of recurrent depression (at least three previous episodes, and an average of seven [!]) responded to treatment with combined therapy: high doses of imipramine (IMI; a mean 210 mg./day) along with weekly sessions of IPT. After subjects met criteria for remission and had remained stable during four months of continuation therapy, during which IPT sessions were tapered to a dosage of once a month (IPT-M), they were randomized to one of five conditions and followed for three years. The five conditions were: (1) imipramine with IPT-M; (2) imipramine with clinical management; (3) IPT-M alone; (4) IPT-M with pill placebo; (5) clinical management plus placebo (PLA/CM). The unique feature of this study was its dosing, which included the *highest* dosage of medication and *lowest* dosage of IPT (IPT-M, monthly) ever used in a maintenance treatment trial for depression.

Patients receiving IMI had mean survival times significantly longer (p<.0001) than did patients who received PLA/CM. The mean number of weeks of survival (i.e., persisting euthymia) during the three-year study period are shown in Table 11.1. Patients who received IPT remained euthymic longer than PLA/CM patients who did not (p=.043), and a one-year trend for the superiority of combination IPT and IMI over IMI alone was observed. The authors concluded that IMI maintenance at a dosage of 200 mg. daily is an efficacious means of preventing depressive recurrence, and that monthly IPT serves to lengthen the time between episodes in patients not receiving active medication. Monthly IPT maintenance alone exhibited a median delay of recurrence of fifty-four weeks, which is sufficient to allow a

TABLE 11.1   Time until Relapse in Maintenance Depression Study

Condition	(3 year) Weeks of survival	1-year Recurrence Rates
PLA/CM	45 weeks	65%
IPT-M/placebo	74 weeks	46%
IPT-M alone	82 weeks	}
IMI alone	124 weeks	18%
IMI/IPT-M	131 weeks	8%

(from Frank et al., 1990)

woman with recurrent depression to complete a pregnancy and nurse without medication.

Reynolds and colleagues (1999) followed this study with one of similar design. They acutely treated 187 geriatric patients (sixty years and older) with recurrent major depression with the combination of IPT and nortriptyline. The 107 who remitted and then reached recovery after continuation therapy were randomly assigned to one of four three-year maintenance conditions: (1) medication clinic with nortriptyline alone, with steady-state nortriptyline plasma levels maintained in a therapeutic window of 80–120 ng./ml.; (2) medication clinic with placebo; (3) monthly maintenance IPT with placebo; or (4) monthly IPT-M plus nortriptyline. Recurrence rates were 43 percent for nortriptyline alone, 90 percent for placebo, 64 percent for IPT with placebo, and 20 percent for combined treatment. Each monotherapy was statistically superior to placebo, whereas combined therapy showed superiority to IPT alone and a trend for superiority over medication alone. Patients in their seventies were more likely to suffer recurrence, and to do so more quickly, than patients in their sixties.

COMMENT

The Frank et al. study was the first real maintenance study of the psychotherapy of recurrent major depression. It shows that even in an extremely high risk group—where more than 80 percent of placebo patients relapsed, most within the first six months of the treatment—a monthly dosage of IPT-M provided an average of a year and a half of protection against recurrence. This is sufficient time to allow a woman of childbearing age—the modal depressed patient—to conceive, deliver, and begin breast-feeding an infant off medication. The Reynolds et al. study replicates the basic findings of Frank and colleagues, with the difference that combined treatment had advantages over pharmacotherapy alone for the geriatric population.

The comparison of high-dose imipramine to low-dose IPT-M is easy to misinterpret. Had imipramine been lowered comparably to the psychotherapy dosage, recurrence in the medication group might well have been higher. Yet as there were no precedents for this research, the choice of a monthly dosing interval for IPT-M was not unreasonable, and indeed showed some benefit. This research raises the issue of dose-finding studies for psychotherapy: e.g., what might biweekly IPT-M do?

CHAPTER 12

IPT for
Dysthymic Disorder
(IPT-D)

DISORDER

Chronic depression has received less attention than its acute variant, but research suggests that it should be taken seriously. Dysthymic disorder is prevalent, affecting about 3 percent of the adult population, with women twice as likely to be affected as men (Weissman et al., 1988; Kessler et al., 1994). It has high morbidity and comorbidity. The Rand Medical Outcomes Study found dysthymic disorder had a more debilitating course than acute major depressive disorder (Wells et al., 1992). Dysthymic patients by definition (American Psychiatric Association, 1994) suffer for at least two years, more days than not, without lasting relief. By the time many present for treatment they have suffered for decades.

Dysthymic patients suffer quietly. They feel guilty, hopeless, and worthless. Because dysthymic disorder often begins early in life, patients often recall having had these symptoms all of their lives and accept them as part of their personalities. Dysthymic individuals tend to work hard out of a sense of guilt and need to justify their existence; yet they have little energy, have difficulty concentrating, and even when they achieve things they tend to think of themselves as frauds. Interpersonal difficulties are a hallmark of the disorder (Kocsis et al., 1988a; Stewart et al., 1988; Cassano et al., 1990). Dysthymic patients are reluctant to let people get close to them lest people discover how "bad" they are inside. They feel their personalities are flawed. Moreover, they are left vulnerable in the relationships they do enter by their difficulty with social skills such as self-assertion and the expression of anger. Hence they often shy away from social attention and intimate relationships, and are usually single when they present for treatment.

Dysthymic disorder is defined in DSM-IV (American Psychiatric Association, 1994) as a chronic, lingering disorder of insidious onset. Its symptoms are those of major depression, but fewer in number (at least three of seven symptoms, versus five of nine for a major depressive episode). If the patient meets criteria for a major depressive episode within the first two years of onset, the diagnosis of major depression, chronic, is made instead. Many patients, however, develop additional depressive symptoms at some juncture and thus meet criteria for "double depression" (a major depressive episode superimposed on dysthymic disorder) (Keller and Shapiro, 1982).

Dysthymic disorder historically has been underdiagnosed and mistreated (Weissman and Klerman, 1977). One explanation for this is that dysthymic disorder rarely presents alone: the great majority of dysthymic patients meet criteria for comorbid disorders, which include major depression, anxiety disorders, and Axis II disorders. Not surprisingly, these diagnoses reflect the gnawing influence of chronic depression: affectively tinged conditions such as social phobia, and avoidant, dependent, and self-defeating personality disorders (Markowitz et al., 1992a). At least some of these comorbid diagnoses may reflect the trespassing of dysthymic symptoms on other diagnostic criteria sets; accordingly, comorbid diagnoses, including *seeming* personality disorders, may resolve with treatment of the dysthymic disorder (Markowitz, 1993a, b). Dysthymic disorder has sometimes mistakenly been viewed as a secondary demoralization consequent to comorbid conditions, whereas in fact it appears usually to precede them (Markowitz, 1993a).

Open trials at Cornell University Medical College treated dysthymic patients in a sixteen-week acute individual framework. Because it seemed unfair and unrealistic to discontinue treatment for patients who had newly discovered euthymia after years of chronic suffering, subjects who responded to IPT-D were offered monthly continuation and maintenance sessions for up to two years.

This research raises questions about whether a brief intervention can efficaciously treat a chronic condition. It may be that many psychotherapists, discouraged by the chronicity of dysthymic patients' symptoms, begin therapy with low expectations for improvement and a protracted, indefinite length of treatment (Markowitz 1994, 1998). Dysthymic patients, highly sensitive to negative expectations, may well recognize their therapists' resignation and fulfill a shared, hopeless prognosis. In addition to its use as a primary treatment for dysthymic disorder, IPT-D might be useful as adjunctive treatment for dysthymic patients who respond to antidepressant medication but have residual symptoms, who feel "lost" in their newfound euthymia (Markowitz, 1993b).

RATIONALE

Prior to the publication of the DSM-III (American Psychiatric Association, 1980), chronically depressed patients were considered to have characterological disorders or "neurotic" depression (Kocsis and Frances, 1984), and psychotherapy was its preferred treatment. Since then the justice of the reclassification of this condition as dysthymic disorder in DSM-III has become apparent. Many dysthymic patients respond to antidepressant medications (Kocsis et al., 1988b, 1994; Hellerstein et al., 1993; Versiani, 1994; Bakish et al., 1993; Bersani et al., 1991) and, based on research evidence, antidepressant medication must be considered its treatment of choice. In contrast, psychotherapy has received relatively little research attention for this disorder (Markowitz 1994, 1998).

The development of an effective psychotherapy for dysthymic disorder is important for several reasons (Markowitz, 1994). About half of dysthymic patients do not respond to antidepressant medication. Others develop intolerable side effects, or refuse to take the medication in the first place. Partial responders to medication might benefit from augmentation by a psychotherapy. Other patients may have relative medical contraindications to medication. Since dysthymic individuals frequently seek treatment (Weissman et al., 1988), nonpsychiatric mental health professionals may often find dysthymic patients among their practices, and would benefit from having treatment interventions of proven efficacy.

The outcome literature on psychotherapy of chronic depression is sparse (Markowitz, 1994). No data exist on the efficacy of psychoanalytic or psychodynamic psychotherapy of chronic depression. We are concerned that these approaches might have drawbacks for dysthymic patients. Their focus on character and internal conflicts, rather than on a mood disorder, might confirm the self-blame dysthymic patients already feel. For the same reason, such patients may have difficulty with a neutral, relatively silent therapist: they need active support, even "cheerleading," to rouse themselves from the doldrums. The reflective focus on the past also may be less helpful to already ruminative patients than a present-centered, action-oriented approach. Thus, although psychodynamic psychotherapies are doubtless widely used in clinical treatment of dysthymic patients, there is no empirical justification for such treatment, and some theoretical concern.

Cognitive behavioral therapy (CBT; Beck et al., 1979) has been the best-studied modality in treating dysthymic disorder. Although the seven published studies are small and some have methodological limitations, their overall response rate of 41 percent (n=116) approaches that of antidepressant medication trials (Markowitz, 1994). Small studies have also examined social skills (Becker et al., 1987) and marital interventions (Waring et al., 1988) with and without pharmacotherapy. A multi-site study is currently comparing a variant of CBT (McCullough, 1992) to nefazodone as a treatment for chronic depression.

Given the paucity of research in this area, researchers at Cornell University Medical College adapted IPT to the treatment of dysthymic disorder. They felt that IPT might confront the interpersonal difficulties so prominently a part of the disorder and help patients to develop needed social skills while alleviating their tenacious mood disorder.

ADAPTATIONS

These are addressed at length in the treatment manual for an ongoing study (Markowitz, 1998).

1. Although many dysthymic patients deny recall of ever feeling good, it is important to search for periods of euthymia. Acutely depressed patients can helpfully be reminded that there was a time when they did not feel as bad as they now do, reframing the depression as a temporary aberration. Dysthymic patients usually do not have that luxury. Nonetheless, the therapist should seek pockets of well-being or better interpersonal functioning and present them to the patient as evidence of a capacity to feel and act better.

2. Brevity of treatment, a standard feature of IPT, has particular meaning for this treatment population. Daring to propose a sixteen-week treatment for a condition that may have lasted decades communicates therapeutic optimism and helps to shake the patient's chronically hopeless outlook. This jolt to the patient's self-view is reinforced by the next point.

3. A key difference between acute major depression and dysthymic disorder is the latter's chronicity. Standard IPT hinges on recent events in the patient's life, which the therapist links to onset of the mood disorder. Yet, by definition, dysthymic patients present years after the onset of a disorder that has an insidious onset: even if important psychosocial antecedents can be identified, they are likely to be temporally remote. In order to focus in the "here and now," the interpersonal problem area requires adjustment.

Since most dysthymic patients have been depressed so long that they see their depression as part of their personality rather than a mood disorder, this becomes the focus of therapy. The therapist diagnoses the patient as having a chronic mood disorder—dysthymic disorder—and defines the treatment period as an *iatrogenic role transition* into health. Thus IPT-D stresses the medical model with patients who are quick to characterize themselves as personality disordered. The therapist explains to the patient:

> You think that the way you feel is part of your personality, but it's really a chronic form of depression we call dysthymic disorder. (Here it is in DSM-IV.) Like other forms of depression, it's treatable. Being depressed gets in the way of how you feel and the way you handle yourself with other people. I suggest that we spend the remaining sessions focusing on what's the depression, and what you're really like when you're not depressed.

The treatment may focus on other relevant interpersonal problem areas, such as role disputes, but always in the context of the patient battling a long-standing depressive illness that tended to mold his or her view of the world and social interactions.

4. Key interpersonal difficulties for dysthymic patients usually include appropriate self-assertion, expression of anger, and the taking of so-

cial risks. The IPT-D therapist normalizes these actions ("They're hard for everyone, although harder if you've been depressed for a long time and lack confidence"), encouraging the patient first to practice them in role play during sessions, and then to try them out in real life. Anger—a bugaboo for patients who often feel too guilty themselves to justify anger at anyone else—can usefully be presented as self-defense:

> Getting angry isn't being mean, it's a form of self-defense. When someone steps on your toe, you tend to feel angry as well as hurt. If you don't tell the person, there are two problems: First, they don't know that they're hurting you and may well do it again. Second, you don't get the feeling off your chest, so it leaves you feeling doubly bad.

When patients undertake such interpersonal actions, even tentatively, for what may be the first time in their lives, they feel newly empowered. The goal is to build a "new track record" of healthy interpersonal interactions rather than continuing the depressive ones.

5. Continuation therapy helps newly remitted patients to consolidate and maintain their gains. In our experience, these sessions are more significant to the patient as evidence of the therapist's continuing availability than for the therapy that actually occurs in such sessions. It appears to take time, perhaps six months to a year after acute treatment, to integrate the new, more optimistic self-view and the confidence that the depression has really lifted.

6. Because of their chronic hopelessness and demoralization, and often a lack of any memory of euthymia, dysthymic patients can be difficult to work with. Therapists in the Cornell treatment study of dysthymic disorder agree that it takes more confidence as a therapist to treat dysthymic patients than to treat patients with major depressive episodes. Yet with therapeutic confidence and skill, successful treatment is possible. For therapists learning IPT techniques, major depression may be an easier diagnosis to start with; with experience, however, the therapist should not be afraid to take on dysthymic disorder.

CASE EXAMPLE

Barbara, a forty-year-old never-married research assistant, reported having felt depressed "as long as I can remember." She put in long hours at work in her boss's laboratory, trying to "blend in among the glassware." Because her energy was limited, she never felt she did enough. She never dared ask for a raise, always feeling sure she was about to be fired, although she had five years of excellent job evaluations. She put a "Lucite wall" between herself and other people, rarely daring to date and worrying that she was a burden on her girlfriends. "I'm a defective freak," she said: it was only a matter of time before people noticed. She reported chronic early and mid-insomnia, helplessness, hopelessness, worthlessness, and passive suicidal ideation. Her Hamilton Depression Rating Scale was 23 (normal is <6).

Barbara's therapist announced that even though she felt freakish and defective, *the problem was not really with her but with the illness that she had, dysthymic disorder.* He showed her the diagnosis in DSM-IV and reviewed relevant Ham-D items with her. Although skeptical, she agreed to the sixteen-week treatment. The therapy focused on both her occupational and her social functioning. After considerable discussion and role playing, Barbara asked her boss about a raise, expecting the worst: instead, she was delighted to receive compliments and an increase. She and her boss also discussed her taking a more advanced role in an upcoming project. For the next several weeks, she worried whether she really deserved this, but was clearly pleased and relieved.

Barbara and her therapist also reviewed her social interactions, leading her to take a more assertive role with friends, and to express overdue anger at a friend who had been taking advantage of her. Barbara anticipated that this confrontation would end the relationship, but instead it appeared to improve it. Dating was more complicated: after some false starts when she tried to meet men at bars (not on the therapist's suggestion) and in museums, she succeeded in meeting someone she liked through a personal advertisement. By the end of acute treatment, she felt shakily euthymic, pleased with her successes but unsure whether they would continue. Her Ham-D score had fallen to 5.

Barbara checked in for monthly continuation sessions over the next six months, and bimonthly sessions thereafter. Although the relationship with the new boyfriend did not work out, she did not become depressed, and in the meantime became sexually involved for the first time in her life with a coworker. After sixteen months she announced: "You know, I finally believe you. I really see that I had a mood disorder, and now I don't!"

EFFICACY

Large studies now nearing completion are starting to provide data on the efficacy of IPT for dysthymic disorder. The initial pilot data on IPT-D are promising and include three small series of subjects at Cornell University Medical College. Mason treated nine subjects: five women who had failed to respond to a research trial of desipramine, and four subjects who refused medication (Mason et al., 1993). Mean age was 37 ± 5.4 (s.d.) years; most reported protracted dysthymic disorder (mean duration 22.4 + 18.9 years, omitting the first five years of life). Subjects received 12.0 ± 4.9 sessions of IPT (range 3–16). Ham-D scores averaged 19.4 ± 5.0 at baseline and fell with treatment for all subjects: at termination, mean Ham-D was 7.4 ± 3.8. When compared in a quasi-experimental design to randomly chosen dysthymic subjects treated with desipramine, IPT response equaled that of medication.

A separate study using IPT to treat depressed HIV seropositive individuals included two dysthymic subjects. These gay white men reported lifelong depression for their forty-seven and thirty-two years. Despite the stress of HIV infection, they improved on Ham-D from a mean 20.5 at intake to 5.0 at termination of IPT (twelve and sixteen sessions, respectively) (Markowitz et al., 1992b).

Further IPT-D pilot work tested its replication with additional therapists. Two therapists treated six subjects, producing drops in Ham-D from 20.8 ± 6.4 at baseline to 8.5 ± 6.3 at acute termination (Week 16); Beck Depression Inventory (BDI; Beck, 1978) fell from 25.2 ± 9.5 to 12.7 ± 8.2. Responders generally maintained gains when seen in monthly continuation sessions with up to two and a half years of follow-up.

Thus seventeen patients at Cornell, seven of whom had failed vigorous desipramine trials, have received IPT-D. None worsened, and eleven (65 percent) remitted (Ham-D<8). Overall mean Ham-D scores fell from 21.5 ± 4.4 at baseline to 7.4 ± 4.7 at acute termination. The investigators have now received funding from the NIMH and the Nancy Pritzker Network for a randomized comparative trial of 176 subjects to sixteen-week interventions with IPT-D, supportive psychotherapy, sertraline (Zoloft) with clinical management, or sertraline with IPT-D.

Steiner and colleagues at McMaster University in Hamilton, Ontario, Canada, undertook a study of more than seven hundred dysthymic patients who were treated in the community with either twelve sessions of IPT, sertraline, or their combination for four months. Patients were then followed up over two years. Results have not yet been published, but preliminary findings have been presented at several conferences (e.g., World Psychiatric Association, Jerusalem, Israel, 1997; NCDEU, Boca Raton, Florida, 1998). Based on a 40 percent reduction of the Montgomery-Asberg Depression Rating Scale (MADRS) score at one-year follow-up, 51 percent of IPT-alone subjects improved—a substantial percentage, but significantly less than the 63 percent for sertraline and 62 percent for combined treatment. Yet in the follow-up phase, IPT, both alone and in combination with medication, was associated with significant economic savings in direct use of health care and social services. Thus, combined treatment was as efficacious but less expensive than sertraline alone.

Another study in Toronto, Canada, is comparing IPT to the short-term psychodynamic psychotherapy of Luborsky (1984) in the treatment of seventy-two patients who had either pure dysthymic disorder or "double depression." The dosage in this study is twelve weekly sessions, followed by four monthly continuation sessions. Initial results show no differences by diagnosis (i.e., between pure and doubly depressed dysthymics). Most patients show symptomatic improvement (Frey, Gillies, personal communication, 1996). Like the Cornell investigators, this group has found dysthymic disorder treatable in a manner similar to major depression, if more difficult to treat.

COMMENT

It is exciting work to pull chronically hopeless patients out of the rut of dysthymic disorder. That three independent groups are undertaking clinical trials of IPT for dysthymic disorder testifies to growing interest in both the syndrome and the therapy. In our clinical experience, the principles of IPT-D are also helpful in treating medication-responsive dysthymic patients who, though they may have improved in social and vocational functioning, still lack direction and social skills that IPT-D may help them find.

CHAPTER 13

IPT for Depressed
Adolescents (IPT-A)

BACKGROUND

IPT has been modified for depressed adolescents in general (Mufson et al., 1993) and used in unmodified format for depressed adolescents (Rossello and Bernal, 1998) and depressed pregnant adolescent girls (Gillies, Clarke Institute, Toronto, personal communication, 1999).

This adaptation of IPT incorporates adolescent developmental issues and adds a fifth problem area, *the single parent family*, which was found frequently among the adolescents Mufson and colleagues treated. Parental permission is obtained for treatment, and parents are involved in the initial phase of treatment. Telephone contacts are readily used, and the school is involved when appropriate (Moreau et al., 1991; Mufson et al., 1994; Mufson, Weissman, and Moreau, 1999). For a detailed description of these modifications, see Mufson et al. (1993).

RATIONALE

The rationale for modifying and testing IPT in depressed adolescents is based on the high prevalence and initial onset of depressive disorder in this age group, on recognition of the morbidity and precipitating stressors of depression in young people, and on the sparse evidence for efficacious pharmacotherapy. In fact, substantial numbers never receive treatment (Strober et al., 1998; Jensen et al., 1999). Clinical epidemiological, family-genetic, and high-risk studies leave no question that major depression occurs in children and adolescents. The peak age of first onset of major depression begins in adolescence across diverse cultures (Cross-National Collaborative Group, 1992; Weissman et al., 1996; Christie et al., 1989; Merikangas et al., 1994; Kessler et al., 1994a and b). For epidemiologic studies of depressive symptoms, see Earls (1980); Richman et al. (1975); Lefkowitz and Tesiny (1985); Smucker et al. (1986); Rutter et al. (1976); Kandel and Danes (1982); Kaplan et al. (1984); and Fleming et al. (1989). For depressive disorders, see Garrison et al. (1989); Rutter et al. (1976); Fleming and Offord (1990); Geller et al. (1999); Emslie et al. (1999); Ryan et al. (1999); and Jensen et al. (1999).

The symptom pattern of childhood depression resembles that of adults described in DSM-III (Ryan et al., 1987; Strober et al., 1981) and DSM-IV. It is also associated with substantially impaired psychosocial functioning (Fleming and Offord, 1990; Brent et al., 1995). For adolescents, impairment includes substance abuse, suicide attempts, school dropout, and antisocial behavior (Kandel and Davies, 1986). Depression also has significant comorbidity with other psychiatric disorders and is associated with a high degree of family dysfunction (Geller et al., 1985; Kashani et al., 1988; Kovacs et al., 1988) and high recurrence (Angst et al., 1990; Rao et al., 1995).

TREATMENTS

Clinicians treating depressed adolescents commonly use treatments found to be efficacious for adults (Hersen and Van Hasselt, 1987). Trials of tricyclic antidepressants have repeatedly failed to demonstrate efficacy relative to placebo, due in part to high rates of placebo response (Campbell and Spencer, 1988). Recent data, however, indicate that serotonin reuptake inhibitors have efficacy for depressed children and adolescents (Emslie et al., 1997, 1998). (See Geller et al., 1999; Emslie et al., 1999; and Ryan, Bhatara, and Perel, 1999.)

Several studies have examined the efficacy of psychotherapy for depressed adolescents. Wilkes et al. (1994) adapted cognitive therapy to treat nonpsychotic depressed adolescents (for review, see Dujorne, Barnard, and Rapoff, 1995). Clarke and Lewinsohn (1989) have developed a behavioral psychoeducational approach, modified for adolescents, for coping with depression.

GROUP PSYCHOTHERAPIES

Reynolds and Coats (1986) compared group cognitive behavioral therapy, relaxation training, and a waiting-list control as treatments of depressive symptoms in thirty adolescents. Treatment was conducted in ten small group meetings of fifty minutes over five weeks. The two active treatments reduced depressive symptoms compared to the waiting list; there was no difference between the two active treatments. This study used depressive symptoms, not diagnosis, as its entrance criterion, so these findings cannot be generalized to adolescents with major depressive disorder.

Lewinsohn et al. (1990) conducted a clinical trial with fifty-four depressed adolescents, comparing two different presentations of the "Coping with Depression" course for adolescents with a waiting-list control. Subjects were diagnosed using a structured diagnostic interview and met diagnostic criteria for major or minor depression. Subjects in active treatment received group therapy with or without treatment provided for their parents. The two active treatment groups improved significantly more on depressive measures than did the waiting-list group. There were no significant differences between the two active treatments, although a trend appeared for greater improvement in subjects whose parents participated relative to those whose parents did not. Although this study is large and of high quality, it does not address the efficacy of individual treatment for adolescent depression.

INDIVIDUAL PSYCHOTHERAPIES

Brent and colleagues (1997) randomized 107 depressed adolescents, ages thirteen to eighteen, to one of three manualized twelve- to sixteen-week treatments: CBT, systematic behavioral family therapy, or nondirective supportive therapy. Subjects met DSM-III-R criteria for major depression and had an entry Beck Depression Inventory score of at least 13. CBT produced more rapid and greater symptomatic relief, and had a higher recovery rate by the end of treatment, than the other two approaches.

Robbins and associates (1989a), in a pilot study of thirty-eight hospitalized adolescents with major depression, conducted an open trial of a psychotherapy that the authors described as similar to IPT. Symptoms declined in 47 percent of subjects treated. Patients who did not respond then received a combined tricyclic antidepressant and psychotherapy, to which nearly all responded. Dexamethasone nonsuppression and melancholic subtype were associated with failure to respond to psychotherapy alone. Despite the lack of a standardized manual, Robbins et al. found promising results for an IPT-like treatment, supporting the exploration of IPT as a treatment for depressed adolescents.

Kroll and colleagues (1996) conducted a six-month pilot study of continuation CBT for seventeen remitted depressed adolescents, comparing them to twelve untreated historical controls. They found a significantly lower relapse rate in the treated group: 20 percent versus 50 percent. Given the small sample and historical controls, this can at best be considered a feasibility study.

The evidence base from controlled clinical trials of individual and group psychotherapy in depressed adolescents is still sparse.

ADAPTATION

The time-limited nature of IPT fits the adolescent's reluctance to seek or stay in treatment. Its goals parallel adolescent developmental issues. The desire to focus on the "here and now," on future rather than past issues, and on the identification and resolution of disputes all seem appropriate for adolescents, who often find themselves in disputes with a parent, school, or friends. Adolescence is a time of major life choices in education, work, and establishment of intimate relationships, providing the life events on which IPT focuses.

Mufson and colleagues' modification of IPT was IPT-A for adolescents with nonpsychotic, nonsuicidal depressed adolescent outpatients who were not engaging in daily drug abuse or violent antisocial activities.

TREATMENT

The format of the initial sessions is unchanged.

Evaluation

Because of the high comorbidity of childhood depression with drug abuse, and the serious dangers of suicidal behavior (frequently impulsive in nature), both depression and drug abuse are fully evaluated. The responsible parent, usually the mother, is brought into the diagnostic process and is educated about the nature, course, and treatment options for depression. Both the parent and the adolescent are involved in discussing treatment options as part of psychoeducation about depression.

Therapeutic Contact

The telephone is used to maintain contact and ensure flexibility in timing and spacing of sessions. During the first month of treatment, the therapist may check in with the adolescent by telephone once or twice a week to support engagement in the therapeutic process. These contacts may help establish trust between therapist and patient, helping the adolescent to perceive that the therapist is concerned and involved. Telephone contacts as a substitute for sessions respond to the adolescent's need to resume normal activities with recovery.

School Involvement

The therapist develops an alliance with the school system. Therapist and school may need to develop an individual academic program to reintegrate a school-avoidant adolescent back into school and to assess the effectiveness of therapeutic interventions. The therapist can take the role of patient advocate with the educational system, educating teachers about the effects of depression on school functioning. The therapist should maintain contact with the school, obtaining information on the patient's behavior and academic performance. School may supply the most pressing problems or the strongest evidence of improvement. School personnel should be encouraged to call the therapist with questions about behavioral observations of the patient.

Parental Involvement

The therapist maintains a strong alliance with the parents, helping them to take the patient's illness seriously, to adjust to the notion of having a depressed child, and to recognize any role they may be playing in the adolescent's difficulties. If there is a dispute between the adolescent and parent(s), or the adolescent has been coerced into coming for treatment, the therapist should help the adolescent and the parent(s) see the treatment as an effort to resolve the dispute (as well as the episode of illness) in a time-limited format. This approach may also be used in sessions with the adolescent alone, depending upon the nature of the interpersonal problems.

Middle Phase

Grief.   The strategies of IPT-A in the treatment of grief are essentially the same as in IPT for adults but take into account the developmental issues of adolescents. Losing a parent during adolescence necessitates premature separation and individuation in addition to the usual tasks of mourning. Common reactions include withdrawal, depressed feelings, a display of pseudomaturity, identification with the deceased, or regression to earlier developmental stages (Krupnick, 1984). The adolescent also may feel abandoned. Depression may manifest itself in behavioral problems rather than affective symptoms. The therapist must be alert to problems of drug or alcohol abuse, sexual promiscuity, or truancy (Raphael, 1983).

Grieving adolescents are also at increased risk for suicide attempts, particularly if their loss has resulted from suicide, either of a family member or a peer (Gould and Davidson, 1988). Specific strategies to prevent their acceptance of suicide as a reasonable option for coping with problems include discussion of more adaptive ways the deceased could have chosen to address problems and development of more adaptive coping mechanisms for the adolescent.

Role Disputes.   One commonly occurring interpersonal role dispute is a struggle between a parent with traditional values and an adolescent who is trying to behave like his or her peers. These conflicting values lead to different expectations for the adolescent's behavior. This conflict can also arise in the normal adolescent's rebellion against parental authority in an effort to separate from the family.

Adolescents often act out their disputes with disruptive, antisocial, or self-punishing behavior. The therapist attempts to associate these behaviors with feelings and to encourage direct expression of the feelings.

The therapist needs to explain to the adolescent and the parents how the interpersonal role dispute contributes to depressive symptoms and how resolution of the dispute can alleviate the symptoms. It can be useful to bring in the parent(s) with whom the dispute exists and to facilitate the negotiations of the relationship in the session.

Role Transitions. Normal role transitions for adolescents include: (1) passage into puberty, (2) shift from group to dyadic relationships, (3) initiation of sexual relationships or desires, (4) separation from parents and family, and (5) work, college, or career planning. Problems arise when parents are unable to accept the changes of transitions or when adolescents themselves are unable to cope with the changes. Problems that can arise include loss of self-esteem, failure to meet one's own expectations and those of others, increasing pressures and responsibilities, inability of the adolescent to separate from the family, and vice versa.

Role transitions can be thrust upon adolescents as a result of unanticipated circumstances. Unforeseen or imposed role transitions include becoming a parent, separation from a parent, or a change in family role due to divorce, remarriage, death, illness, or parental impairment. If the role transition problems involve changes in family roles, difficulties in separation, and family pressures, the therapist may include the parents in several sessions. The therapist could include the parents to help support the adolescent in giving up his or her role or, if necessary, to help the family adjust to a normative role transition so that they do not restrict the adolescent's development or impair his or her functioning.

In addition to the adolescent, other family members may have difficulty in accepting the adolescent's role changes. Parents may need education about normal developmental adolescent tasks, the feelings these tasks may elicit in them, and ways to cope with their feelings. The therapist seeks to evaluate their concerns and fears, normalize these if possible, and put them in the appropriate context.

Interpersonal Deficits. Interpersonal deficits can impede an adolescent's achievement of developmental tasks. These tasks are primarily social: making friends, participating in extracurricular activities, joining a peer group, beginning to date, and learning to make choices regarding exclusive relations, career, and sexuality (Hersen and Van Haselt, 1987). As a result of interpersonal deficits, the adolescent may be socially isolated from peer groups and relationships, which can lead to feelings of depression and inadequacy. These depressed feelings may in turn worsen social withdrawal and compound the lag in interpersonal skills when the depression resolves.

The therapist focuses on those interpersonal deficits that appear to be a consequence of the depression rather than on personality traits that result in isolation.

Single-Parent Families. Single-parent homes arise from divorce, separation, incarceration, out-of-wedlock births, death by medical illness or violence, and social problems stemming from AIDS, crime, and drug abuse. Each of these situations presents unique emotional conflicts for the adolescent and the custodial parent. Depending on the circumstances, children of single-parent families may function well or develop significant problems, including depression.

Increased interparental conflict following a divorce or separation is associated with increases in depressed mood, anxiety, and physical symptoms in adolescents (Mechanic and Hansell, 1989). A departure often leaves uncertainty as to whether or not the parent will return, whether or not the parent is even still alive, feelings of abandonment, and difficulties in accepting the negative behaviors of the parent. The intensity of the adolescent's depressive reaction often depends upon the degree of separation, its abruptness, and whether it has happened before (Jacobson and Jacobson, 1987). The child's relationships with the absent parent and with the remaining parent are both frequently altered. Reactions to these events often include depressed mood, increased sexual behavior, and increased conflicts with the custodial parent over discipline and independence.

Therapeutic tasks of IPT-A in single-parent families include:

1. acknowledgment that the parent's departure significantly disrupted the adolescent's life;
2. addressing feelings of loss, rejection, abandonment, and/or punishment by the departed parent;
3. clarification of remaining expectations for the relationship with the absent parent;
4. negotiation of a working relationship with the remaining parent;

5. establishment of a relationship with the absent parent;
6. if appropriate, acceptance of the permanence of the current situation.

In helping the adolescent discuss feelings associated with a parent's departure, the therapist may have the custodial parent participate in a session. The focus of the session is to discuss the parent's recollection of the spouse and to correct misconceptions the adolescent may have about the parents. It may also be helpful to have a session with the parent alone to discuss parenting issues of adolescents, including appropriate discipline and restrictions on their behavior.

Final Sessions

Terminating treatment with the adolescent also means terminating with the adolescent's family. The final IPT-A session may be a family session for the patient, parent(s), and other family members who have been involved in the treatment process. This final session reviews the patient's presenting symptoms, interpersonal disputes, the identified problem area as it relates to the goals of therapy, achievement of the therapy goals, and a discussion of the changes in the family interactions and functioning as a result of therapy. The patient and family also should be made aware of the possible recurrence of symptoms after termination. Management of further treatment, if indicated, and management of future recurrent episodes of depression should be discussed.

The therapist should distinguish between a regression that will resolve in a few weeks and a recurrence of symptoms. The family should tolerate the former and support the adolescent during the transition from dependence on the therapist to independence. If the adolescent's symptoms do not resolve in a few weeks, the therapist should be contacted to determine whether further treatment is necessary. If at termination the adolescent clearly needs further treatment, appropriate referral should be arranged at that time.

Use of Medication

Mufson et al. (1993) recommend medication when depressive symptoms do not respond to a four-week course of supportive and psychotherapeutic interventions. The decision to use medication should be discussed in a joint session, as appropriate, with the psychiatrist, therapist, patient, and parents.

If the combined treatment is split, coordination of treatment between a pre-scribing child psychiatrist and the IPT therapist is crucial.

Suicidal Patients

Completed suicide in adolescence is rare, but suicide attempts and suicidal ideation are prevalent (Shaffer et al., 1988). Suicidality is a critical part of the initial evaluation and should be monitored throughout the treatment. The adolescent should be asked if he or she has thoughts about death, about wanting to die, and about killing himself or herself. The therapist should question in detail and obtain specific answers in order to assess the intent and lethality of the patient's past suicide attempts, current suicidal ideation, and future plans. Based upon this assessment, and weighing the stability of the home and family, the therapist must determine whether the adolescent is at acute suicide risk. If uncertain, the therapist should seek a second opin-ion. An adolescent at acute suicide risk is not a candidate for IPT-A and usu-ally requires psychiatric hospitalization.

The suitability of an adolescent with suicidal ideation for IPT-A depends upon his or her capacity to establish and maintain a therapeutic alliance with the therapist. The cornerstone of this alliance is the adolescent's assur-ance that he or she will not attempt suicide and will notify the therapist or go to an emergency room immediately if the urge becomes compelling. The therapist not only monitors the adolescent's suicidality but also addresses the inappropriateness of suicide as a means of communicating feelings of anger or distress, or as an attempted means of solving a conflict.

Assaultive Patients

Although adolescent patients are rarely homicidal, on occasion some ado-lescents may vent their frustration through aggressive and violent behavior. Assessment of the patient's thoughts of hurting other people should coin-cide with the assessment of suicidal behavior. As in the assessment of sui-cide, the therapist asks highly specific questions about the intent and the feasibility of going though with the action. Based on this assessment, the therapist must determine whether the adolescent is at risk of harming an-other person. If so, the therapist (by law in some, but not all, states) must hospitalize the patient and has a duty to warn the intended victim of the pa-tient's wishes.

Adolescents at serious risk for homicidal behavior are not candidates for IPT-A. An adolescent who expresses anger and hostility in vague threats to others may participate in IPT-A if he or she is able to establish an alliance with the therapist, feels capable of controlling his or her behavior, and feels capable of making an agreement with the therapist not to enact violence while in treatment. The therapist should also educate the adolescent about more appropriate methods of communicating anger or upset, and ways to diffuse the anger.

Substance Abuse

Screening and history-taking should include a complete history of drug and alcohol use/abuse. Family members should be interviewed about the adolescent's drug use. If necessary, the adolescent should be referred for substance abuse treatment before beginning IPT-A. To participate in IPT-A, the adolescent must not be abusing or using any substances and must make a commitment to staying drug-free. If substance abuse appears to be primary and the depression secondary to it, the adolescent should be referred to a drug treatment center. The therapist can help the adolescent deal with peer pressure and family dynamics that lead to drug use, and engage a family member who may be another source of support in the patient's abstinence from drugs.

School Refusal

Fatigue, poor concentration, and anhedonia may keep some depressed adolescents from attending school regularly. Having missed school for a week or two, they may feel too far behind to catch up, feel embarrassed to go back to school after their absence, and consequently remain home for an extended period of time. The therapist should ask the adolescent and parent about school attendance during the initial evaluation. The therapist's role is to stress the importance of returning to school and to enlist the assistance of the parents and school in ensuring the adolescent's return. The therapist should explain to the adolescent that although he or she may not feel like going back and may be embarrassed, the embarrassment will dissipate after the first day and he or she will feel better by being productive in school. The adolescent should be told that his or her concentration will improve as the depression resolves. Throughout treatment, the therapist should continue to check on the adolescent's school attendance and performance and be in contact with the school if necessary.

Protective Service Agencies

These agencies protect the welfare of children whose environment is harmful or neglectful. Each state has an agency to deal with reports of child abuse and neglect, and its own laws governing when and how to report a case. A child may already be in the jurisdiction of a protective service agency upon beginning therapy, or the therapist may have the duty of reporting the child to the agency if information about possible harm to the child emerges in the course of treatment. Contacting a protective service agency can disrupt the therapeutic alliance with the child or parent. The therapist must recognize this possibility and work with the patient and parent to help them understand that the service was notified in order to provide help and to alleviate a stressful situation for both the child and parent. The therapist should emphasize that the protective service agency is a means to provide the adolescent with increased social support so that the family can function better.

Sexual Abuse

The therapist should carefully inquire about any history of or current sexual abuse. Symptoms that might indicate a history of abuse include depression, suicidal ideation or behavior, sexual promiscuity, severe anxiety about sex, and conduct problems. The adolescent may not reveal the abuse initially but only later in the course of treatment, as he or she begins to trust the therapist. If abuse is ongoing, the law requires the therapist to contact the protective service agency for children so that the agency can intervene. If the abuse occurred in the past, the therapist still needs a detailed history of the interpersonal context in which the abuse occurred, so that an accurate picture of familial relationships can guide the treatment.

Learning Disabilities

Depression is commonly associated with cognitive impairments. A psychosocial history will help the therapist distinguish between long-standing learning disabilities and impairments secondary to a depressive episode.

This task is complicated when the patient has long-standing depressive symptoms or a personality style that presents with what appear to be cognitive limitations. Psychological or educational testing can be useful in identifying learning disabilities. When learning disabilities are diagnosed, the therapist will need to arrange special educational resources in conjunction with the school system. Cognitive impairments secondary to depression resolve when other depressive symptoms resolve. Psychoeducation for the adolescent and parents can explain the etiology of the child's impairments and revise their expectations accordingly.

Sexual Identity Problems

Adolescents who find that their sexual interest is homosexual can feel isolated and alone. Adolescents who feel attracted to both same and opposite-sex partners may feel confused about their sexual orientation. The role of the therapist is to help the adolescent explore sexual feelings and concerns about sexual orientation in a nonjudgmental context. It may be appropriate to identify the association between the adolescent's state of confusion and his or her depression. If the adolescent is comfortable with and has accepted his or her sexual orientation, the therapist should support the decision. It is important for the therapist to keep this discussion confidential unless the adolescent has a desire to share the information with others.

Crisis Management

The following events are considered a crisis: physical or sexual abuse, worsening suicidal ideation or a suicide attempt, suicidal behavior in a friend or family member, running away, medical illness in the adolescent, illness or death in the family, pregnancy, violence occurring at home or outside the home, drug use, legal difficulties, homicidal ideation, or abrupt termination by the adolescent or the adolescent's family. The therapist's first task is to determine the cause of the events of the crisis, the adolescent's reaction, and the family's response to the crisis. Is the crisis a response to the therapist or to issues being addressed in therapy? Did the therapist miss warning signs that such a crisis was likely, or was the patient or family concealing information that would have allowed the therapist to expect and prevent the crisis? Or was the event unpredictable and a response to events beyond the control of the therapist, patient, and family?

The second but simultaneous task in crisis management is to arrange an emergency session as soon as possible. In the case of suicidal or homicidal ideation, if an appointment cannot be scheduled soon enough, the patient should be sent to the closest emergency room. The emergency session should determine the need for and level of family involvement. When dealing with an adolescent who is under eighteen years of age, it is mandatory to notify the parent if the patient is at significant risk. The level of involvement will vary with different types of crises and the patient's relationship with family members. The therapist must carefully elicit the entire story from the adolescent regarding precipitants and accompanying emotions. After hearing the whole story, the therapist must again assess whether the risk of harm to the patient or others warrants hospitalization. In addition, the therapist must evaluate the need to involve other agencies or parties, such as medical or legal consultations or protective services.

If the therapist determines that the adolescent can remain in outpatient treatment, the IPT-A treatment contract should be reexamined and revised as necessary. Items in the contract that may change include frequency of sessions, frequency of phone calls between therapist and patient, and the identified problem area on which treatment is focused. At times, the crisis may suggest that a significant problem area, or an interaction between two problem areas, was overlooked. The therapist may choose to meet more frequently in the weeks following the crisis until it is apparent that the patient's situation has stabilized.

The most significant decisions the therapist must make are whether to hospitalize the patient and whether to terminate IPT-A in favor of another treatment. If the therapist has decided to involve the family, it is important to meet with the family separately as well as with the patient to assess their understanding of the problem and how it can best be resolved. The therapist might conduct several joint sessions with the family to assist in negotiating the crisis, then resume individual treatment with the patient.

CASE EXAMPLE

Betty was a lovely but very sad fourteen-year-old, the oldest of four children. She had aspirations to be a scientist or doctor and was doing quite well in school when her world collapsed. Her father died suddenly, leaving little insurance or savings. Her mother was forced to take a full-time job to make ends meet. Betty had to care for the younger children and cook dinner immediately after school, which meant she had no time for friends or after-school sports, and was too exhausted at night to do her homework. Added to these changes was her own grief over her father's death, and the irritability and unavailability of her grieving mother. Her school grades suffered. On several mornings she did not get up in time for school. She lost weight, had difficulty falling asleep, and felt blue.

The therapist identified both the unresolved grief over her father's death and the role transition from student to caretaker as problem areas. The mother was asked to attend a session, in which it was clear that she, too, was depressed and grieving.

EFFICACY OF IPT-A

There have been two controlled clinical trials of IPT-A in depressed adolescents. Two have been completed with primarily Hispanic patients, although this is a coincidence. One study was conducted in Puerto Rico, the other at Columbia University, which draws from the predominantly Hispanic community surrounding the hospital.

Rosello, Bernal, and Rivera at the University of Puerto Rico have completed a controlled trial comparing twelve weeks of randomly assigned IPT (n=22), CBT (n=25), and a waiting-list control condition (n=24) for depressed adolescents ages thirteen to eighteen who met DSM-III-R criteria for major depression, dysthymia, or both. The investigators did not use the Mufson modification of IPT for adolescents. They found that both IPT and CBT were more efficacious than the control condition in reducing adolescents' self-ratings of depressive symptoms (Rossello and Bernal, 1998). IPT was more effective than CBT in increasing self-esteem and social adaptation. The effect size for IPT was .73, for CBT .43.

The second controlled clinical trial, by Mufson, began with a twelve-week open feasibility study of IPT-A and one-year follow-up in fourteen depressed adolescents. After twelve weeks, the patients were significantly less depressed and functioned better than at intake. None still met criteria for DSM-III-R major depression (Mufson et al., 1994). A follow-up study found that only one patient met criteria for a mood disorder one year later (Mufson and Fairbanks, 1996). None had been hospitalized, made suicidal attempts, or become pregnant, and all were attending school. However, about a third reported having experienced serious negative life events since completing treatment, including violence, physical or sexual abuse, parental psychopathology, or death of a parent. One adolescent was hospitalized two years after completing treatment. The small sample size and lack of control treatment limited generalizability and provided the rationale for undertaking the controlled trial.

In the randomized controlled twelve-week clinical trial, Mufson, Weissman, and Moreau compared IPT-A to clinical monitoring in forty-eight clinic-referred adolescents, ages twelve to eighteen, who met DSM-III-R criteria for major depressive disorder. Patients were seen biweekly by a blind independent evaluator to assess symptomatology, social functioning, and social problem-solving skills. Thirty-two of the forty-eight patients completed the protocol (twenty-one IPT-A, eleven control).

Patients who received IPT-A reported significantly greater improvement of depressive symptoms, overall social functioning, including functioning with friends, and problem-solving skills. In the intent-to-treat sample, 75 percent of IPT-A patients met the criterion for recovery (Hamilton Depression Rating Scale score <6), compared to 46 percent of control patients. The findings support the feasibility, patient acceptance, and efficacy of twelve weeks of IPT-A with acutely depressed adolescents in reducing depressive symptomatology and improving social functioning and interpersonal problem-solving skills (Mufson, Weissman, and Moreau, 1999). Mufson will be testing IPT-A in a large-scale effectiveness study in school-based clinics and is also piloting it in a group format for depressed adolescents.

Depressed Adolescent Mothers

Gillies at the Clarke Institute in Toronto is testing IPT as a treatment for depressed pregnant adolescents (ages fifteen to nineteen). The treatment is based on observations that adolescent mothers are at high risk for depression (Rhodes and Woods, 1995; Beardslee et al., 1988) and that social supports mediate the symptoms (McKenry et al., 1990; Rhodes et al., 1995). As in the Puerto Rico study, no specific adaptations of IPT have been made.

Thirty depressed adolescents from a community support organization in Toronto for pregnant adolescents, all scoring 14 or higher on the Beck Depression Inventory, were randomly assigned to twelve weekly sessions of either individual IPT, a psychoeducational group on parenting skills, or an arts-and-crafts-activity control group. Their mean age was eighteen years, and their initial mean BDI score was 23 (SD=8). IPT participants were seen once weekly for one hour. Eleven subjects dropped out, leaving seven in IPT, seven in the psychoeducational group, and five in the control group.

Multivariate analysis of pre- and post-treatment BDI, Social Adjustment Scale Self-Report (SAS-SR), and Adult Adolescent Parenting Inventory (AAPI) scores was used to determine the relative efficacies of the three treatments. Results showed significant improvements in depressive symptomatology and social adjustment for the entire sample based on the BDI and SAS-SR scores. No statistically significant differences between the groups were found. However, BDI scores dropped nine points for the psychoeducational group and fifteen points for the IPT group. The control group and psychoeducational group went from being moderately depressed to having a mild mood disturbance, while the IPT group went from being moderately depressed to normal. The failure to find statistically significant differences between groups may be accounted for by the small sample size and high degree of variance. AAPI scores did not change with treatment, except for overall improvement in empathy toward children. The project is ongoing and further analyses will be carried out. This area clearly requires further study.

COMMENTS

The need for more efficacy data on the treatment of depressed adolescents is pressing, in the face of high rates of first onset and recurrence, high morbidity, and potential mortality through suicide. The emerging treatment data are promising but sparse. How does IPT-A compare to SSRIs in depressed adolescents? Will maintenance treatment prevent recurrence? Will treating adolescents when depressions first occur prevent long-term morbidity and reduce recurrence?

Knowledge of the treatment of depressed adolescents lags more than a decade behind that of treatment of adults. Until recently, minors were excluded from clinical trials. The recent request by the FDA for information on the efficacy of psychotropic drugs in treated populations, including children and adolescents, accelerated the numbers of clinical trials. This may lead to increased testing of psychological treatments because of their apparent importance in young people.

CHAPTER 14

IPT for Late-Life Depression

DISORDER

Major depression occurs across the life cycle, and the diagnostic criteria in older people are those of a standard major depressive episode. Elderly depressed patients, however, tend to focus more than younger patients on somatic symptoms such as physical pains and bowel habits.

As the American population ages, geriatric depression is rising (Sholomskas et al., 1983). Mood disorders are the most common psychiatric diagnoses among the elderly, with a point prevalence of 10–15 percent among the general population (Blazer and Williams, 1980; Frank et al., 1993). Geriatric depression is also associated with a disproportionate suicide rate and a major source of morbidity (Lebowitz et al., 1997).

There have been three formal trials of IPT in this population as well as a couple of clinical series. The first two, by Rothblum and colleagues (1983) and Sloane and colleagues (1985), employed a standard IPT approach based on the original manual (Klerman et al., 1984), in small, acute treatment studies. The latest, a large trial by the Pittsburgh group, used a manual developed for maintenance IPT for late-life depression (IPT-LLM [Frank and Frank, 1988 (unpublished)]). This study, comparing IPT, nortriptyline pharmacotherapy, and combined IPT/pharmacotherapy in a discontinuation treatment design, is modeled on the Pittsburgh study on recurrent major depression (Frank et al., 1989, 1990; see Chapter 11). The encouraging results of these trials are discussed below.

RATIONALE

Psychotherapeutic options are important for elderly depressed patients for several reasons. Older patients tend to have greater sensitivity to medication side effects and therefore may have difficulty tolerating antidepressant medications at therapeutic doses. Because they are likely to be taking other medications, they carry greater risks for drug interactions. The elderly are also at risk for potentially distressing life events associated with aging: retirement, physical debility, and losses such as the deaths of friends and spouses. These life changes are obvious foci for IPT. Yet, until recently, there had been little psychotherapy research on depressed geriatric patients (Thompson et al., 1987).

Psychotherapists treating geriatric patients need to fight prejudices that the elderly are untreatable, poor prognostic candidates, and that the end of life leaves them fewer options and abilities. These are prejudices that depressed elderly patients may well echo themselves. Yet why expect IPT *not* to work with the elderly, as with other ages, in treating major depression?

ADAPTATIONS

Geriatric patients almost inevitably reminisce about the past. Sholomskas and colleagues (1983) noted that some older patients needed longer than the typical fifty- to sixty-minute session to unburden themselves, while for others this duration more than sufficed. They felt that dependency needs arose more frequently with this patient population, as did the need to discuss social resources and concrete services. Therapists might respond, for example, by arranging transportation or calling the patient's physician to clarify a problem. They also noted that patients who have been in a relationship for decades might have greater difficulty in ending and fewer options in replacing it.

It is unclear whether these points in fact represent differences between geriatric and younger patients. Do they reflect therapists' preconceptions about the elderly? Many depressed patients of all ages appear helpless and dependent, and few think they have options in life. Some clinicians indeed suggest that IPT with the elderly can be conducted in much the same way as with younger patients (Miller and Silberman, 1996; Hinrichsen, 1997). Even if geriatric patients are different in some ways, it is important that the therapist not yield to pessimism and to underselling the options that remain open to them.

Hinrichsen (1997) also makes the clinically reasonable observation that cognitive impairment may preclude effective psychotherapy. The Mini-Mental Status Examination (Folstein et al., 1975) may be used as a simple screen for cognitive difficulties.

Reporting on data from the large Pittsburgh study of the elderly, Miller et. al (1998) found that, contrary perhaps to intuition, grief was not the most common interpersonal problem area in the acute treatment of the first 127 depressed elderly subjects treated with IPT-LL (Frank and Frank, 1988) in combination with nortriptyline. The focus in these cases was most commonly role transition (41 percent), followed by interpersonal disputes (35 percent) and then by grief (23 percent). It is unclear whether this distribution of interpersonal problem areas differs meaningfully from that of other depressed populations. Wolfson et al. (1997) found no association between the area of IPT focus and the likelihood or speed of recovery in the combined treatment.

CASE EXAMPLE

Alan, a seventy-two-year-old retired lawyer, developed an episode of major depression during his wife's terminal illness with breast cancer. He had had a previous episode at age sixty-four when he contemplated retirement at the time of his wife's initial diagnosis. He had responded at that time to antidepressant medication and supportive psychotherapy; she had achieved remission as well. Three months after his wife's death, Alan was brought to treatment by his son. He reported depressed mood worst in the morning; guilty and somatic ruminations; decreased sleep, appetite, energy, and concentration; and passive suicidal ideation without plans. His twenty-four-item Hamilton Depression Rating Scale (Ham-D) score was 25. He had obsessive traits but no formal Axis II diagnosis. Axis III diagnoses included hypertension, angina, and adult-onset diabetes mellitus.

Alan's agitation, ruminations about his bowels, and guilt over his wife's death prolonged history taking through four sessions of a planned sixteen-session IPT treatment. In apparent recapitulation of the themes of his previous episode, Alan characterized himself as a "workaholic" who had neglected his family for his career. This time, he felt, his lack of involvement had contributed to his wife's suffering during her final illness. He also felt unloved by family. He had in fact increasingly isolated himself from his relatively few friends and his three children as his wife's condition deteriorated.

The therapist formulated the problem as complicated bereavement. As in standard IPT format, therapist and patient explored the nature of the marital relationship, the patient's feelings about his wife as her death approached, and what had happened when she died and at her funeral. The therapist encouraged Alan to review and to bring in pictures—he responded with a videotape as well—of his wife and her illness. Discussion clarified that Alan had been more involved in caring for, and more caring about, his wife than he now believed or had related.

He had retired from the law in part to care for her—albeit a somewhat ambivalent choice—and had worked hard in his new career as her nurse. His guilt derived from his sense that he had ultimately deserted his wife at a crucial moment at her hospital deathbed. Yet a review of this moment, and the patient's subsequent interrogations of family members who had been there, revealed his behavior to have been perfectly appropriate. His guilt was labeled as a depressive symptom that seemed to arise with each depressive episode. This explanation came as a relief to him.

Pursuing the IPT strategy of facilitating mourning, the treatment explored Alan's ambivalent feelings about his wife during her onerous illness. He became increasingly tearful and sad, but less agitated, guilty, and angry, and his neurovegetative symptoms receded. Mourning also led to a discussion of his own medical problems and feelings of mortality. Alan generally took excellent care of himself, but his attention had slipped and he had skipped medication doses when he became depressed.

The therapist also encouraged this usually energetic man to find new activities and relationships as substitutes for the loss of his forty-five-year marriage. He had no interest in attending a senior citizen center, scoffing that this was for "old folks." Instead, he became more involved with his children and grandchildren, sought out old friends and colleagues, and volunteered for a legal aid society to help older Americans. By the ninth session, his Ham-D score was in the normal range at 6, and he remained euthymic thereafter, even as he continued to mourn his wife. At six-month follow-up, he remained euthymic and active.

This case of geriatric depression could pass for standard IPT. Any differences were subtle: the therapist needed to fight the bias that this older man's life, as he stated, was "over." The history taking was lengthier than in a typical IPT session, in part because there were more relationships to review in the interpersonal inventory over his long life. Alan did reminisce more about the past than younger patients might have, although this often served the therapy of the mourning process. This fiercely productive and independent man had no need of concrete services from his therapist.

EFFICACY

Rothblum and colleagues (1982) described eighteen men and women, ages sixty to eighty-five (mean=70), who met DSM-III criteria for major depression. They received six weeks of IPT in conjunction with pharmacotherapy with either imipramine, alprazolam, or placebo, administered double-blind. The medication doses are not described. The authors found that these elderly patients complied with treatment and responded rapidly to treatment, with a drop in Ham-D from 20.9 to 7.2. Eleven (61 percent) completed the trial. Because patients received combined pharmacotherapy and psychotherapy, this small study does not test the efficacy of IPT alone, but suggests it is well tolerated in combination with pharmacotherapy.

Hinrichsen (1997) described a case series of geriatric patients with mild mood disorder. Four of six unmedicated patients who completed sixteen weeks of IPT showed a mean drop in Ham-D from 11 to <2. In another small series, Miller et al. (1994) described six geriatric patients who developed major depression in the aftermath of a spouse's death: that is, late-life complicated bereavement. A mean seventeen sessions of IPT resulted in improvement of scores on the seventeen-item Ham-D from 18.5 (± 2.3) to 7.2 (± 4.6).

Sloane et al. (1985) conducted the first controlled study of IPT with depressed elderly patients, comparing IPT to nortriptyline and to pill placebo in a randomized six-week trial. They treated twenty-six men and twenty-nine women of mean age sixty-four who meet Research Diagnostic Criteria (RDC) for probable major depressive disorder of more than one month's duration. Ratings on the Ham-D and Beck Depression Inventory (BDI) indicated that all three groups significantly improved over time, with no significant differences among groups.

Mean Ham-D scores for the IPT group fell from 23.8 to 15.8 in six weeks. Only one placebo subject was judged improved at six weeks. IPT appeared as efficacious as nortriptyline in this small study and had fewer dropouts: no IPT subjects dropped out, whereas eight nortriptyline and four placebo subjects did. Baseline evidence of orthostatic hypotension predicted nortriptyline dropout (Schneider et al., 1986). The small size of the treatment cells greatly limited the likelihood of finding statistically significant differences in this study.

A key study by Reynolds and colleagues (1992, 1994, 1996a and b, 1997, 1999) in Pittsburgh assessed IPT as a maintenance treatment for late-life depression (IPT-LLM). This is essentially a geriatric version of the landmark Pittsburgh study of maintenance treatments for recurrent depression, varying principally in substituting IPT-LLM for IPT-M, and nortriptyline for imipramine (see Chapter 11). This study differs from earlier work in its larger sample size, its longer duration of treatment (most earlier reports comprise seven weeks or fewer), and the general rigor of the research design.

Geriatric patients with recurrent unipolar major depression (n=187) were acutely treated with both IPT and nortriptyline. Entry required the diagnosis of at least a second lifetime episode of major depression, determined by the Schedule for Affective Disorders and Schizophrenia (SADS-L; Spitzer et al., 1979), and a minimal seventeen-item Ham-D score of 17. Acute treatment consisted of weekly IPT-LL sessions, audiotaped and randomly monitored, and nortriptyline titrated by serum level. A brief course of adjunctive medication (four to six weeks of lithium carbonate, perphenazine, or paroxetine) was permitted for patients not responsive to therapeutic nortriptyline levels by Week 8.

A Ham-D score of ten or less on three consecutive weeks and a nortriptyline serum level of at least 50 ng./ml. were required for responder status and entry into a continuation phase. This sixteen-week continuation phase tapered clinic visits prior to randomization to monthly visits for the maintenance treatment phase. At the conclusion of this phase, patients were randomly assigned to one of four treatments—monthly IPT-LLM with placebo, nortriptyline with medication clinic, placebo with medication clinic, or monthly IPT-LLM with nortriptyline—and followed for three years.

Of the first seventy-three patients entered, sixty-one (84 percent) completed the trial. Seventy-nine percent of these completers (66 percent of all subjects entered) acutely treated with the combination of IPT-LL and nortriptyline were found to achieve full remission. Another 5 percent were deemed partial responders. Subjects whose first episode of major depression occurred after the age of sixty were just as likely to respond as those with earlier onset (Reynolds et al., 1992). In a second report, Reynolds and his group (1994) reported on thirty-two "young" elderly patients (mean age 67 ± 5 [s.d.], range 60–78) who responded to combined IPT-LL and nortriptyline, relapsed when randomized to placebo, and were subsequently re-treated with the combined approach. Re-treatment typically began within two weeks. Symptoms were milder, and the second period of treatment was briefer than the first had been for twenty-two (81 percent) of the subjects: requiring eight weeks, versus thirteen in the prior episode, to achieve remission. Thirty patients completed this second sequence of treatment, and twenty-seven (90 percent) again achieved stable remission. Their remission rate and time to remission were comparable to those of younger (nongeriatric) patients treated at the same site in an earlier combined treatment study of IPT and imipramine (Kupfer et al., 1989).

Building on this observation, Reynolds and colleagues (1996a) made post hoc comparisons of response rates and treatment outcome of 148 geriatric patients from their study (mean age sixty-eight) with 214 younger depressed patients (mean age thirty-nine) from the earlier Pittsburgh study. They found that the older sample had a comparable acute remission rate (78 percent versus 70 percent) but took slightly longer to respond and were somewhat more prone to relapse (15.5 percent versus 6.7 percent) during continuation therapy.

Reynolds et al. (1997) also reported findings similar to that of Thase et al. (1997): that depressed patients with abnormal sleep EEGs were less likely to respond to IPT. Reynolds et al. (1997) related that nine (90 percent) of ten subjects in the maintenance phase of their study reporting good subjective sleep quality remained well for at least one year receiving IPT-LLM, compared to five (31 percent) of sixteen good-sleep patients assigned to medication clinic, three (33 percent) of nine with poor sleep quality assigned to IPT-LLM, and two (17 percent) of twelve poor-sleep patients assigned to medication clinic.

They (Reynolds et al., 1996b) further documented the outcome by looking at the subset of subjects (n=29) who had received adjunctive pharmacotherapy with lithium, perphenazine, or paroxetine during the acute phase of treatment. These adjunctive medications were administered at full dosage for four to six weeks, then tapered over three to four weeks. Relative to the 119 subjects who received the standard acute intervention of nortriptyline and IPT, these patients were less likely to respond to acute treatment (64 percent versus 83 percent), much more likely to relapse during the continuation phase (52 percent vs. 6 percent), and hence less likely to attain sustained remission, or recovery (49 percent versus 77 percent). These subjects also required longer acute-phase treatment. This suggests that continuation of the adjunctive medication would have been necessary to preserve remission in this subgroup.

Opdyke et al. (1996/1997), excluding eleven relapsing cases described by Reynolds et al. (1996b) and three partial responders, looked at symptom assessments of 105 of the study patients who remained well during the continuation phase of treatment. They found that subjects generally maintained their acute gains and showed modest further improvements during the continuation interval: Ham-D scores fell from 7 (±2.3) to 5 (±3.0).

The overall maintenance results of the study are described in Chapter 11. IPT-LLM plus placebo had a lower three-year recurrence rate (64 percent) than did placebo alone (90 percent). Combined IPT-LLM and nortriptyline was more efficacious in preventing recurrence than the two active monotherapies.

COMMENT

Data on the acute efficacy of IPT for geriatric depression remain meager. The sole large study to date used combined IPT and pharmacotherapy to achieve acute remission and focuses on IPT as a maintenance treatment. Nonetheless, it appears that geriatric depressed patients resemble their younger counterparts more than they differ from them: as with depressed HIV-positive patients (Markowitz et al., 1998), it may be therapist (and patient) bias, rather than data, that has suggested a meaningful difference. Further research may be helpful to detail the acute efficacy of IPT and other psychotherapies for depressed geriatric patients. The results of the Reynolds et al. maintenance study add to the understanding of both the utility of maintenance IPT and the treatment of geriatric patients.

IPT FOR BEREAVEMENT-
RELATED DEPRESSION

IPT was originally designed to treat unresolved or complicated grief. Uncomplicated grief is not a psychiatric disorder. Yet it can be associated with significant suffering, and it might be expected that IPT would help individuals with uncomplicated bereavement, as with complicated bereavement, to deal with the issues of loss. Reynolds (personal communication, 1996) has accordingly modified IPT as an intervention for normal bereavement. Since his studies treated an older population, they are described here. The approach, however, should apply to all age groups. The modification of IPT includes more detailed information gathering in the initial phase of treatment on the quality of earlier and current relationships and roles. The therapist also explores at length the quality and practical aspects of living of the surviving spouse: bill payment, financial burden, leisure activities, and relations with children. The therapist also determines available social supports for the bereaved spouse (see Miller et al., 1994).

CHAPTER 15

Conjoint Treatment for Depressed Patients with Marital Disputes (IPT-CM)

BACKGROUND

Conjoint IPT for depressed patients with marital disputes (IPT-CM) extends individual IPT techniques for use with the identified depressed patient together with her or his spouse. It incorporates aspects of marital therapies that emphasize dysfunctional communication. This chapter condenses the unpublished manual for IPT-CM, which was developed for a clinical trial comparing conjoint to individual IPT (Foley et al., 1990). The concepts and techniques used in IPT-CM could be applied to disputes outside the marriage as well as to disputes involving unmarried heterosexual or homosexual couples. For research purposes, however, the initial formulations and clinical trial focused on disputes taking place in heterosexual married couples.

RATIONALE

Studies show a relationship between marital disputes and depression. The direction of the association can vary: research shows both that continuing marital problems delay recovery from depression and that individual psychotherapy may have limitations in treating depressed patients with ongoing marital disputes (Weissman, 1987; Bauseman et al., 1995; O'Leary et al., 1994; Gotlib, Beach, 1995). Individual psychotherapy is more likely to precipitate a divorce than couples treatment of patients with marital problems (Beckman and Leber, 1995; Berg-Cross and Cohen, 1995; Koerner, Prince, and Jacobson, 1994).

ADAPTATION

Like IPT, IPT-CM is defined by the following characteristics:

- *Emphasis on depression*. At least one party to the dispute must have clinically diagnosed depression. IPT-CM thus differs from many family or marital therapies, which deemphasize Axis I clinical disorders in the patient or spouse.
- *Time-limited goals*, with an emphasis on improving depressive symptoms and marital relations, as opposed to changing the personalities of the individuals.
- Developing a *structured and comparatively operationalized treatment plan*.
- An *active and directive therapeutic stance*.
- Fostering an *early positive relationship and alliance* with the couple.
- *Avoiding analysis of the patient/therapist relationship (transference)* as the focus of treatment.
- *Encouraging change in the couple's interpersonal relationship outside the session*.

The goals of IPT-CM are to facilitate remission of the acute depression and to resolve the marital role dispute by renegotiating role relations between the marriage partners. IPT-CM may not be applicable in cases in which one or both partners have an ongoing extramarital affair or in which both partners are unwilling to participate even in working toward the goal of a less disruptive separation. In addition, if the spouse of the identified patient has a psychotic disorder, mania, or schizophrenia, it is unlikely that treatment will be effective, especially in the absence of medication.

The basic methods and problem areas of IPT-CM are the same as in IPT, except that the spouse is involved in each session. Following the initial evaluation, managing the patient's depressive symptoms is the primary goal. Because conjoint IPT for depression is initiated by the prior identification of a clinically depressed spouse, the treatment has two complementary goals: (1) the individual goals of the depressed patient, the most important of which is to reduce depressive symptoms; and (2) the joint goals of the couple to improve their marital functioning.

THE INITIAL PHASE

Assessment of the current depressive episode requires primary history taking with the identified patient. The spouse should be present, however, during at least one session of the assessment process. The spouse may learn from this the degree and severity of the patient's depression, which the patient may previously have been reluctant to discuss.

EVALUATING THE CLINICAL STATUS OF THE SPOUSE

Because the first goal is to treat the identified patient's depression, the spouse may feel left out of this phase of the treatment. Alternatively, the spouse may feel blamed. To guard against this, the therapist should attempt to include the spouse. For example, in taking the identified patient's history, the therapist should gather a parallel history of the current depressive episode from the spouse's viewpoint, asking how the spouse has attempted to handle the episode:

> Is that how you see your spouse's symptoms? When did you think they began? What did you notice? What did you think was happening? Tell me what you did or said when you realized [your spouse] was depressed.

Evaluating the clinical status of the spouse employs the same clinical review used with the identified patient. Many spouses of depressed patients meet diagnostic criteria for a psychiatric disorder, most often major depression. The spouse of the identified patient may need an additional treatment intervention, such as psychotropic medication. Knowledge of significant psychopathology in the spouse helps the therapist set treatment goals that take this liability into consideration. The spouse's ability to change or to support the identified depressed patient may be limited if the spouse is also clinically ill.

The depressed patient typically presents for treatment alone and may not expect the recommendation of couples treatment. The patient may profess willingness to enter couples treatment but state that the spouse will refuse. If so, the therapist should at least initially pursue the possibility that the patient is reluctant to engage in couples treatment and should explore these apprehensions. The therapist may then try to motivate the patient for couples treatment by explaining its benefits or by appealing to the patient's sense of the help to which he or she is entitled from a spouse. For example, the therapist may act surprised and ask, "You mean your [husband/wife] wouldn't care enough about your welfare to help you get over this depression?"

The therapist can offer to talk to the spouse directly about the advisability of couples treatment. In many cases where the identified patient describes the spouse as unwilling, the spouse proves responsive to a direct call from the therapist.

EDUCATING THE COUPLE ABOUT DEPRESSION

Analogous to individual IPT, the therapist explains depression to the couple. The identified patient is given the "sick role" (see Chapter 2). The therapist reviews the patient's day-to-day functioning in order to help manage daily activities, taking depressive symptoms into consideration:

Tell me how you spend the day when you are feeling depressed.

ASSESSING MARITAL DISPUTES IN RELATION TO DEPRESSION

Evaluation of the marital dispute parallels IPT role dispute procedures (see Chapter 4). Complaints about the marriage are elicited. The therapist attempts to define areas in which the partners differ in their understanding and performance of marital roles. Marital role disputes often arise over responsibilities and power, finances, relations with other family members (extended and nuclear), social and work activities outside the family, sexual and intimacy roles, and communication.

Spouses frequently present long lists of grievances against each other. For each grievance, the therapist might ask the partners' role expectations and their assessment of how this aspect of the marriage is actually working at the time. Questions related to major aspects of marital functioning include the following:

Responsibilities and Power

Who is responsible for work needed to make the marriage function, e.g., housekeeping, financial management, child care, home maintenance, and socializing? How much flexibility exists to permit partners to share these responsibilities and to assist each other? How do the partners view the fairness of the division of responsibilities?

Finances

Who earns money? Who makes decisions? How are decision-making responsibilities divided? Who handles the budget and checkbook?

Family (Extended and Nuclear)

- In-laws: To what extent do relationships with in-laws interfere with interaction between the two of you? Are they too involved, or too distant and unhelpful to you?
- Children: Do you have an alliance around child rearing? Can the children play you off against each other? To what extent do you allow special relationships and alliances with children to interfere with the handling of issues that you could more appropriately manage by yourselves?

Activities Outside of the Family

How much independence do you each have? Which activities and relationships do you not share? Does the marriage permit you to pursue independent work and leisure activities to a degree that you both find reasonable and acceptable?

Sexual and Intimacy Roles

How do you show affection? Who is nurturing, and how? How satisfactory is your sex life to each of you? When and how have sexual problems arisen?

Communication

In addition to difficulties with specific roles, the couple may have communication problems that cut across roles. One of the most common marital complaints is a lack of communication between partners. Communication may be absent or characterized by too frequent quarreling. To assess the couple's communication problems, the therapist must observe how the couple interacts in therapy sessions. Although occasionally couples can articulate their miscommunications, *more frequently they demonstrate them*. As in individual IPT, the therapist must determine the stage of the dispute: renegotiation, impasse, or dissolution (see Chapter 4).

Reconstructing the History of Marriage

The marital history includes information on what was happening in each partner's life at the time they first met, how they met, why they were attracted to each other, what their expectations of marriage were, how they describe their dating and courtship, their sexual relationships, changes in roles, children, finances, disputes, and separations. At the end of the initial session(s), the therapist presents the couple with a rationale and time frame for the treatment.

This can be a therapeutic as well as a diagnostic maneuver: it may remind the couple of happier times, ways they have solved problems in the past, and the continuity of the bond they have formed together. It is often valuable to have each partner hear the other's version of the marital history in order to clarify the disputes.

Couples Who Deny or Who Acknowledge Disputes

Some partners are adamant that the problem is entirely due to their mate's depression. Others recognize that the identified patient's depression might be related to marital problems and welcome involvement in treatment in order to improve the relationship. In obtaining the history, the therapist should determine the position the spouse has taken.

If the spouse does not readily acknowledge ongoing marital problems, the therapist should not directly challenge this view in early sessions. Such a spouse is likely to feel sensitive to blame for the patient's depression and unlikely to see the therapy as having personal benefit. The therapist should shift the focus by emphasizing the couple's interaction. To motivate the euthymic spouse, the therapist should elicit information about the nondepressed spouse's dissatisfaction with the marriage—for example, by asking, "Tell me what it has been like for you. How does your spouse's depressed state make you feel? How do you respond?"

In taking the identified patient's history, the therapist may focus on the patient's view of the marital history, paying particular attention to ways that the marriage has changed and how such changes have related to the patient's depression: "How did the depression affect your marriage?"

The therapist in turn may elicit the spouse's view of the same history— "What do you feel caused the symptoms?"—attempting to direct the spouse's attention to areas where he or she would like to see improvements in the marriage. The therapist refrains from blaming either individual for marital problems, ascribing them instead to problems in role definitions the couple has chosen.

Where both partners readily identify marital disputes that preceded the onset of depressive episodes, couples treatment is explained as having two purposes: (1) to help both spouses learn to manage the identified patient's depressive symptoms; and (2) to find ways to solve marital disputes that may have contributed to the onset or perpetuation of the depression. An issue for couples who openly acknowledge marital disputes is the extent to which initial sessions focus on the identified patient's depressive symptoms. If symptoms are extremely debilitating, managing the depression may require more attention. If the depression is comparatively contained, the therapist may choose to initiate treatment with more direct work on the couple's problems.

Determining the Relationship between Depression and Marital Disputes

Symptoms of depression can disrupt even the most congenial relationships and exacerbate marital disputes. The therapist should help the spouse find constructive ways to react to the depressed patient. The therapist might ask, "How do you react to your spouse's symptoms? What do you do when she/he gets irritable or withdrawn or cries?"

The spouse might be encouraged to avoid stereotypic and destructive interactions: being overly solicitous, frustrated and critical, or withdrawing and abandoning. The spouse may have adopted one or all of these stances toward the patient and may feel guilty and bewildered by the inability to help the patient improve. As an antidote to these reactions, the therapist should encourage the spouse to seriously acknowledge the patient's depression. Being the spouse of a depressed patient may be defined as a "very difficult role," one that entails simultaneously avoiding the behavior strategies of taking over for, trying constantly to cheer, or abandoning the patient. Instead of trying to cheer up the depressed patient, the spouse should acknowledge that his or her partner is suffering: "I can see that you're sad and troubled."

The spouse may also inquire about how the patient is feeling, remark on positive changes, and encourage the patient to participate in a normal routine as much as possible.

The therapist must consider the depressed patient's limitations when setting goals and strategies for treatment. For example, it is unwise to start treatment by emphasizing shared leisure time or ways to display affection if one spouse cannot generate interest or pleasure in most activities. Preferable initial foci might be communication or authority issues.

Interpersonal Inventory

The interpersonal inventory (see Chapter 2) is obtained for each marital partner. In all cases, a detailed history of the marriage should be obtained. For young couples in their first marriage, a detailed inquiry into current and past relationships with each partner's family of origin may be desirable. For an older couple whose parents are deceased, the relationship with each partner's family of origin may be comparatively unimportant.

Individual Interpersonal Inventory of Each Partner

Within the context of marital therapy, a systematic review of major friendships, important adult and child relationships, and development of relations with the opposite sex may not be necessary. Yet it is useful to determine each partner's ties to individuals outside the marriage, to assess each partner's current social and occupational functioning, and to appraise each partner's social functioning prior to entering the marriage. This knowledge may provide clues about what each partner sought in the marriage. For example, if a husband had little dating experience prior to marriage, perceived himself as intellectually competent but unpopular, and sought marriage to solve his need to combat loneliness, this history may influence his role expectations for his spouse. Knowledge of current relationships outside of the marriage can inform the therapist of the resources and social supports of each partner.

Relationships in the Partners' Families of Origin

Learning what models for marital and family functioning a partner's family provided may generate clues to the role the partner attempts to play in the marriage. For example, if a partner's family of origin was chaotic and the partner coped by becoming overly mature and hypercompetent, the partner may attempt to play a similarly caretaking, hypercompetent role in his own marriage. This may cause difficulties if it requires others in the family to be needy and incompetent in order for the partner to take this role.

The therapist may state:

> I would like to spend the next session learning from each of you about your parents and the families you came from. To understand your own marriage, it may be useful to look at the models you had to learn from in your families.

The therapist should ask about a history of depression, other psychiatric disorders, and substance abuse in the families of origin, emphasizing particularly the family's attitudes toward the patient's and other relatives' psychiatric disorders.

Moving from Grievances to Renegotiation

Once the partners are willing to acknowledge marital disputes, they often compose lists of grievances against each other. The grievances may be long-standing and seem unmanageable to the partners. They represent unsuccessful attempts by each partner to spell out marital role expectations to the other. The therapist might say:

> The two of you disagree about _____. In this next phase of treatment, let's try to find different ways to negotiate and resolve these issues.

Sort Out the List of Grievances

To reduce the list of grievances to a workable number, the therapist may ask each partner to identify the two or three key marital problems that he or she would like to change during the course of the time-limited treatment. An alternative approach is to ask each partner to prepare at home a written list of two to four problems to discuss at the next visit. The partners are instructed not to reveal the lists to each other until the next session. Writing down goals individually may encourage greater openness about needs than might be expressed spontaneously in the partner's presence. Frequently partners are surprised by the similarity of their lists, which indicates a better mutual understanding of the marriage than either had dared anticipate.

Undoing the Role of Therapist as Judge

Partners in marital therapy often wish the therapist to sit as a judge: someone who will, after hearing the grievances of both partners, determine who is "right." The most direct strategy to avoid and undo the judicial role is simply to point out when each spouse attempts to ally with the therapist and to state explicitly that the therapist's role is not to take sides but to help the partners negotiate with each other.

Because of acute symptoms, the depressed partner may evoke greater sympathy and assistance from the therapist. The euthymic spouse on the other hand may appear as a victimizer who has "caused" the depression. To prevent this polarization, the therapist addresses comments to the couple in a way that requires both partners' participation in the problem. For example, if one partner ceaselessly complains, the therapist may ask why the other partner allows this to happen.

The therapist's formulation serves to translate the couple's statement of their goals into a workable therapeutic contract.

THE INTERMEDIATE PHASE: RENEGOTIATING THE MARITAL CONTRACT

The major goal is to renegotiate the marital roles. The treatment maintains structure and coherence by linking new material about the marriage to the central themes and targeted problem areas noted in the early sessions. As in individual IPT, nonreciprocal expectations constitute an important theme, and the options for role change are explored.

A typical middle session begins with the therapist asking:

How have you two been getting along recently? [or] What has happened between you since we last met? [or] What have you been working on this week?

The opening question typically evokes a description of one or more interactions that manifest disputes. The therapist asks each partner to reconstruct in detail the sequence of events in the interaction, including actions, feelings, and wishes. This is called the "microanalysis of recent transactions." Helping the couple to deepen their understanding of targeted problems involves moving back and forth between microanalyzing specific transactions and linking these transactions to current issues.

The couple generally responds with an edited version of events, each partner idiosyncratically supporting his or her side of the dispute. At this level, the dispute may seem unchangeable. To understand each partner's motivations and to find ways to change communication problems, the therapist needs detailed data to reconstruct the sequence of events in transactions that exemplify a particular dispute. Questions include:

What did each of you say? What did you do? Where and how did that happen? Was anyone else around? How did each of you feel? What did each of you expect? What did each of you think was happening?

The therapist persists in exploring an issue, defining a clear sequence of events and each partner's view of what took place. The therapist must avoid getting sidetracked and must undo the tendency many partners have of leaping to unwarranted conclusions about their spouse's motivation. For example, a comment intended as friendly may be regarded as nagging and provoke a counterattack. The couple may then begin arguing with no clear idea of what they are arguing about. Helping the couple to unravel and interrupt such stereotypic arguments often involves discussion of several similar arguments.

As an exploratory tool, the elaboration of specific disputes is useful because it frequently yields significant details that are clues to underlying disputed role expectations. For example:

CASE EXAMPLE

In a long-standing dispute, Mr. L. resented his wife's involvement in the management of his business. Although she had expertise in neither financial matters nor the technical aspects of the business, Mrs. L. would demand that her husband handle business issues in ways she deemed appropriate. He resented her intrusiveness and listed this as the major problem to address in treatment. In discussing this issue, the therapist asked how Mrs. L. had come to know so much about her husband's business issues. The information, it turned out, came from him. Discovering that Mr. L. had at least partial responsibility for his own problem changed the discussion from one in which he exclusively accused his wife to an exploration of the function of constant fighting in the marriage.

Although obtaining detail is vital, the larger targeted problem area should remain in focus. It is possible to lose sight of treatment goals if too many sessions are spent resolving specific disputes of minor importance. Treatment should clarify issues and behaviors that help perpetuate disputes, and develop techniques for avoiding or dealing with disputes that might arise in the future, rather than provide solutions to a specific set of problems that are likely to change over time anyway.

The therapist must ensure that solutions arise from the couple's own ideas and wishes. When the therapist attempts to engage the couple in a discussion of how they might change things, however, the couple may not be able to respond:

1. They may lack the knowledge to change because they have not been exposed to models of negotiation, compromise, sharing;
2. they may derive secondary benefits from symptomatic behavior; or
3. they may fear the consequences of getting what they ostensibly desire.

To explore why a couple is not changing, an initial approach is to ask the couple to imagine what it might be like to reach one of their targeted goals, such as spending more time together:

How would you spend time together? What new activities would take the place of the old [symptomatic] behavior? What would each of you have to do to solve the problem? Are there things that are frightening about achieving this goal?

The therapist seeks to uncover fears, including fears of intimacy, which may be perceived as suffocating or entangling; fears of angry or aggressive feelings, which might emerge if the spouses were more open with each other; or fears of sexual involvement. To get the couple to address fearful ideas, it is often necessary to approach the issue indirectly, asking about these ideas in a positive way. For a couple professing the wish to spend more time together yet unable to arrange this, "What might an ideal evening be like?" might be a preferable question to "What kinds of things feel scary about spending an evening alone with each other?"

Many couples fear change lest they be unable to find new ways to accomplish the positive goals gained by symptomatic behavior. For example, the presence of constantly bickering in-laws, while unpleasant, may yet be preferable to their absence if the couple has no other way to engage in affectively charged discussion. Fighting may be the only means to obtain a sense of closeness or intimacy. To focus on this resistance to change, the therapist may question the couple directly:

> Do you need this constant fighting, amount of distance, etc.? Have you always needed this, or have things ever been different? [or] Do you think there are other reasons you need things to stay the same? Maybe there's something that the two of you get out of this. . . . What might it be? . . . Does the old system work in some ways, so that you don't want to give it up?

The Therapist's Role in the Intermediate Sessions

Guidelines to foster productive sessions include the following:

Phrase comments in a positive way

Patients feel vulnerable to criticism and blame, particularly by the therapist in the presence of the spouse. Fear of being deemed the culprit by the therapist may lead to guarded participation or dropping out of treatment.

There are several ways the therapist can avoid sounding critical while generating change. The therapist can validate the patients' behaviors. Many patients blame themselves excessively for behaviors that result from anger, such as deliberately hurting or inducing guilt in the partner. Extramarital affairs may cause great pain, compounded by guilt and recriminations. The therapist's handling of such issues should be matter-of-fact and serious, underscoring that these behaviors are common but solvable, and indicating that the ways in which the couple has tried to solve marital problems have not been working.

The therapist can avoid blaming either partner by attributing problems not to selfish or malicious intentions or personality problems but to *lack of agreement on role expectations* in the couple's interactions. For example, ceaseless, unproductive arguments do not necessarily result from stubbornness, bad faith, or irreconcilable differences, but may stem from a failure to conduct discussions by productive rules. Such a framework assures the couple that neither partner is at fault, because both partners have been following these rules and are equally responsible for change. As always in IPT, the focus is on improving the future more than on judging the past.

By refusing to accept the partners' negative labeling of themselves, their marriage, or their actions, the therapist may elicit a complete sequential description of events or feelings. For instance, the couple may describe the past week as "a disaster" without further elaboration. By forcing the couple to give a detailed account of "disastrous" events (e.g., the first open argument in years), the therapist may render events understandable or even as signs of progress.

Remain nonjudgmental and communicate warmth and positive regard

This of course does not mean that the therapist accepts all aspects of the couple's behavior. Rather, the therapist conveys the message that the partners' problems can be resolved and do not necessarily represent permanent features of the individuals or their relationship. The therapist is optimistic and supportive, providing reassurance and giving direct advice when the patients feel most symptomatic and helpless.

Keep negative affect within bounds

The therapist should foster the expression of affect but keep it within bounds. The therapist interrupts and limits uncontrolled displays of angry feelings while keeping discussions focused on topics important to the couple, and avoiding abstract, technical, or intellectualized discussion.

Focus content on targeted problems

The therapist is responsible for keeping sessions focused on topics relevant to the targeted treatment goals. Goals are formulated and referred to in each session, as are the subgoals derived from the central treatment goals. At the beginning of intermediate sessions, the therapist should ask the couple, "What would you like to work on today?" or "What is on your agenda?" rather than "How are you doing?" or "How are things going?" The question "How did you make that happen?" replaces "How did that happen?"

Avoid alliance with one partner

Each spouse will attempt to ally the therapist with himself or herself, but the therapist must prevent this from happening. If the therapist makes interventions that seem to attack one spouse, or notes feeling an exclusive sympathy for one spouse's position and blame for the other spouse, the therapist may request to leave the session briefly, review videotapes of this and other sessions, discuss the case with a supervisor or colleague, or record and review process notes on the session. The therapist may emphasize the participation of both partners in problems, or speak of problems in terms of dysfunctional marital roles.

RENEGOTIATION OF THE MARITAL ROLE CONTRACT

How the therapist manages each session will depend on the degree to which the spouses encourage communicating with each other or through the therapist. With argumentative and angry couples, it is often pointless to allow lengthy arguments. In such cases, the therapist may insist that initially the spouses' communication take place through the therapist, with the patients speaking only when he or she questions them. With less fractious couples, spousal communication is encouraged. This is particularly important for disengaged, reticent couples who say too little to each other.

There are other instances in which the therapist may request that the spouses talk directly to each other, asking, "Can you tell [your spouse] directly now what you wish?" This should occur when the therapist wishes to heighten the impact of a partner's statements; or when one spouse is complaining about the other, stating a wish about what he or she would like the other to do; or professing affection toward or understanding of the spouse. When the couple discusses communication problems, they should be encouraged to demonstrate their difficulties in the session through role playing in order to explore them. The therapist should also be alert to instances in which one spouse is "mind reading" or speaking for the other, and might ask: "Why don't you ask [your spouse] right now what [s]he thinks or feels?"

While identifying and exploring options to achieve a more satisfactory division of marital roles, the therapist sometimes recognizes that one or both partners have role expectations derived from their family of origin that are maladaptive in the current relationship. To help the couple recognize alternatives to these expectations, the therapist points out that they have been acting as if no alternatives exist. It may be useful to review how the model of each spouse's family of origin has affected the current relationship. This model may have worked in the family of origin, but not as well as alternative models would have. Or it may have worked in the family of origin but not fit the problems or the different cast of characters in the couple's life. Finally, it may not even have worked in the family of origin.

The thrust of the intermediate phase of IPT-CM is to renegotiate roles. Questions such as "How do you wish your spouse to change?" may facilitate the process.

THE TERMINATION PHASE

Termination and the couple's feelings about it are discussed explicitly and accomplishments are reviewed. In the last few sessions, the therapist may bolster the couple's sense of their ability to handle future problems by reviewing with them areas in which they anticipate future difficulties and guiding them through an exploration of how they might handle various contingencies.

If the couple does not wish to terminate, the spouses should be instructed that they can return to therapy, but that they should wait a reasonable period of time (e.g., one month) before doing so. The exception are couples in which the identified patient is severely symptomatic and has shown little or no improvement in the course of therapy. Alternative treatment (medication and/or individual psychotherapy) should be considered for a spouse alone or for the couple, depending on their needs.

TECHNIQUES

While the techniques used in IPT-CM are similar to individual IPT, conjoint treatment allows confronting issues directly with both partners present.

COMMUNICATION ANALYSIS

This technique identifies communication failures of couples, moving them toward learning more effective communication. In a couples format, the therapist may generate samples of communication problems by: (1) asking the couple to reenact a past argument; (2) asking the couple to negotiate a current dispute; or (3) observing them in the course of transactions in any given hour. Faulty communication may generate interpersonal disputes even if the partners have mutually supportive or noncontradictory expectations of each other.

Ambiguous and Indirect Communication

a) The therapist notes that the communication has been indirect, ambiguous, or incomplete and asks the speaker to clarify it. After waiting for the other partner to respond, the therapist might ask: "Did you understand what your wife just said? . . . Well, I didn't either."

b) The therapist may restate what one partner has just said in order to help convey it to the spouse and to help check whether the therapist, too, has understood it correctly.

c) The therapist may point out contrasts between verbal and nonverbal communication. For example, "You say 'Yes,' but you don't look like you agree."

Incorrect Assumptions

Many depressed patients fear retaliation or criticism and are afraid to check whether what they perceive as critical or punitive behavior from the spouse was actually so intended. This "mind reading" often turns innocuous discussion into argument. The therapist should listen for times when one partner attributes a feeling or motivation to his or her spouse and should then ask the partner to check this assertion.

Couples should learn to distinguish between actions and intentions. A partner may act or speak in a manner perceived as hostile by the recipient. To determine the intent, each partner is instructed to monitor his or her own anger and to take responsibility for it. When one partner feels angry for something the spouse has done, he must mention this to the spouse to determine what the motivation for the provoking action was. Often the spouse is unaware that the action was offensive and had neutral or even helpful intentions.

Many patients assume that others will anticipate their needs or feelings without their having to express them. When they do attempt to communicate, there may be no follow-through to determine whether the partner has understood the intent. One way to handle this problem is to point out when it occurs. The therapist may say, "Does your wife know that this makes you unhappy? . . . How does she know?" He may then turn to the wife and ask, "Did you know that that was upsetting to your husband?"

Silence: Closing Off Communication

Many patients have discovered that silence or "pouting" can be an effective and infuriating way to handle a disagreement. They may be unaware of the destructive consequences of closing off communications. Silence is often a preferred approach to a disagreement, either because the couple has lost faith in their ability to resolve difficulties or because they feel that arguing is a sign of a bad marriage. Couples with this belief need to learn to *have arguments fairly and productively.*

This requires keeping arguments specific, focused, and clear in behavioral terms, rather than global and diffuse. If a wife is angry about her husband's habitual lateness, it is better for her to focus on this specific complaint than to make a more general accusation such as "you are inconsiderate." Focusing on a specific behavior allows the partner who is being asked to change to know what is being requested of him or her, whereas general requests like "be more considerate" are hard to respond to.

Acceptance of Painful Affect

Many patients feel overly guilty about strong hostile or sexual feelings about significant others. Patients may have only partial awareness of these feelings. In the conjoint format, it is often desirable to encourage each partner to acknowledge the other's feelings by asking questions like, "Did you know that [s]he felt so strongly about that?"

Helping the Partners Generate Suppressed Affects

Sometimes a patient will deny feeling upset by something that is obviously grossly upsetting. The therapist may remark: "I'm concerned: anyone would be upset by that. You say you aren't upset. What's stopping you from feeling that way?"

For patients who have difficulty tolerating and expressing feelings such as affection, gratitude, caring, etc., the therapist may help uncover irrational fears that lead to suppressing these emotions.

Guidelines for Using Encouragement of Affect

These techniques are used for patients who are emotionally constricted. The techniques cannot be overused, particularly when the individual seems unaware of strong feelings, such as sadness and anger. For patients troubled by intense, diffuse, and flooded affects, however, a better strategy may be to help the patient suppress these overwhelming experiences. Mere repetitions of angry, hostile, or sad outbursts are counterproductive if no attempt is made to understand these feelings. When such an outburst occurs, the therapist may interrupt the patient's affective display by asking what he or she thinks about the strong feelings. Alternatively, the therapist may explore with the patient various strategies to help him or her delay acting on impulsive feelings.

If in a conjoint session the level of mutual anger threatens to become too intense, the therapist may use several strategies to modulate the feelings.

1. The therapist may ask the couple to talk to the therapist and to use him or her as a moderator rather than speaking to each other.
2. The therapist may switch to a more neutral topic, explaining that the couple is too upset to discuss the present topic productively and should wait until they calm down. The therapist may encourage them to use this strategy on their own as well.
3. The therapist may shift the couple's attention from the content of the communication to its process, asking them to look at how angry they are both becoming and to consider the reasons for it.
4. The therapist may try to interrupt the argument by saying such things as "This hurts my ears!" Statements such as this may distract the couple and help them realize someone else is in the room.

Decision Analysis

Many depressed patients and their partners have histories of making self-defeating decisions, due either to failure to consider all reasonable alternatives or to adequately evaluate the consequences of their actions. Depression may be identified as a contributing cause to such decision making. The role of the therapist in decision analysis is to help the partners recognize their full range of options and to suggest that action be postponed until each option has been adequately explored. The therapist should begin by asking generally,

> What alternatives do you feel you have now? [or] Why don't we try to consider all the choices you have?

Assigning Exercises

Exercises are chosen that represent *partial solutions* to the major problems on which the therapy is focused. Thus, the therapist should avoid repeating past failures by reviewing ways that the couple has previously attempted and failed to handle the issue. Exercises focus on problematic aspects of marital role functioning. For example, when one or both partners are overly involved with their children to the exclusion of appropriate engagement with each other, the therapist should develop exercises that involve joint activities away from the children, such as taking a vacation together or spending a night out together.

For couples whose behavior has become rigidly differentiated, the therapist may use a series of exercises that involve taking turns. For example, if a couple has serious disagreements over disciplining the children, the therapist may instruct them to choose odd or even days of the week on which each, in turn, will take responsibility for this activity while the other does not interfere. This format often allows each partner to see the strength of the other partner's position and to adopt aspects of the other's behavior when it is his or her turn.

This format can be used for a wide range of assignments, including communication exercises (e.g., on alternate days one or the other partner is responsible for starting a brief conversation) or affection (e.g., on alternate days each of the partners is instructed to make a request for a show of affection from the other). These exercises are powerful because they are not intended to solve the whole problem. When trying to implement an exercise, the therapist's task is to help the couple feel successful at their work. Exercises require having established at least the beginning of a working alliance with the couple. At minimum, both partners must profess interest in working on the marriage.

Start with small, manageable exercises to ensure that they will be performed. Simply instructing a couple to curtail problematic behavior is futile. If the couple could do this, they might have solved their problems on their own. Each partner should be helped to limit his or her expectations for change to behaviors under the partner's volitional control. Hence, changes in relatively permanent attributes (height, handsomeness) or emotional states ("I want him to love me more") are not reasonable goals. Change in love and caring can be discussed by stating that the therapy will attempt to help the couple solve problems that have gotten in the way of feeling more loving toward each other. It will help the partners behave with each other in ways that will make them want to show more affection, etc.

An aspect of choosing an exercise is to emphasize the implementation of new, positive behaviors and to deemphasize old, negative behaviors. It is more difficult to learn to curtail a bad habit than to learn a new one that replaces it. It therefore will seem less onerous and punitive to the partner whose behavior is to change.

Exercises should be described explicitly and the therapist should obtain feedback from each partner to be sure that each understands them. This includes choosing specific days and times on which a behavior is to be performed and assigning time limits. For example, in a typical early communication exercise, the therapist might help the couple find half an hour when they will be free from distraction. The format of the task might be that one partner begins talking while the other listens and agrees not to interrupt. The partner is instructed to talk about himself or herself, and about his or her wishes, indeed anything other than complaints about the spouse. In the next fifteen minutes, the roles are reversed. To ensure that the couple understands the nature of the task, the therapist can help them practice in the session.

Partners should have roughly equal roles in each assignment. For example, if an exercise involves one partner making a concession to the other (e.g., doing the dishes), the other should make a reciprocal concession (e.g., having the meals ready on time). In the "taking turns" format described above, each partner has an equal number of days "in charge" of a given behavior, while the other partner is a watchful observer. When focusing on what both partners agree is dysfunctional behavior of one spouse, the other spouse's role may be to help him or her perform the assignment. For example:

CASE EXAMPLE

Mrs. R. complained that her husband did not show enough interest in their children. He agreed: he felt that he wanted to do more in this area, but did not know how to. In devising an exercise for them, the therapist gave Mrs. R. the role of "teaching" Mr. R. how to approach the children, while Mr. R. took the role of trying to play with them in a limited but specific format.

Several steps can increase the couple's motivation to attempt the exercises. To counter excessive pessimism, the therapist can emphasize that performing the assignments will differ from methods that the couple has previously used in attempting to solve problems: they have not had as large a repertoire of techniques as they will now develop working with the therapist. Exercises should also include some reward or benefit for each partner, even if this is not readily apparent. How an assignment is described may influence the likelihood of its being undertaken and accomplished. For example, to a resistant couple, the exercise can be purposely described as important but small. For other, more crisis-oriented couples, it may be valuable to label it as "major" in order to instill the belief that the couple is accomplishing something just by completing the assignment.

The therapist should explore with the couple the possibility that the assignment will not be accomplished. An aspect of anticipating the possible failure to carry out assignments is making each partner aware that he or she is responsible for part of the work, even if the other partner does not perform his or her part properly. In addition, the therapist attempts to ensure that one member of the couple will not punish the other for failure to perform the exercise. After an exercise is assigned, the therapist discusses it in the next session.

If the couple has carried out the exercises, the therapist should foster a sense of accomplishment. He or she may congratulate them or even express surprise that they were able to do it. This can take the form of praise. When the couple has not tried to carry out the assignment, the therapist should avoid criticism. It is equally important to take it seriously and hold both spouses responsible for failing to perform the exercise. Frequently it is difficult to engage a couple in a discussion of why they did not do an assignment. They may simply repeat their initial statement that they "forgot," etc. The therapist must not accept this explanation. One way to develop the discussion is to use the "false choice" technique, where the therapist poses a complex question with multiple possible answers but phrases it as a simple, forced choice with a small number of alternatives. For example, the therapist might say,

> There are usually only three reasons for not doing a task: (1) either you don't know how to do it; (2) you're getting something important from the old way of doing things that you don't want to give up; or (3) you find something frightening in trying to do something new. Which one of these things do you think is happening? Let's go through each possibility.

Seldom is any one of these possibilities exclusively correct, yet posing the question in this manner can facilitate discussion.

Following discussion of failed or partially accomplished exercises, the therapist attempts to choose and implement revised assignments, following the guidelines described above but avoiding the difficulties discovered in the discussion of the previous exercise. This sometimes involves simply reassigning the same exercise. Examples of exercises include:

Leadership Exercises

a) Making decisions about money, vacations, in-laws, etc.
b) Assigning different areas of expertise to each spouse.

Communication Exercises

a) Learning how to have arguments that will resolve (learning "rules of fighting").
b) Learning how to talk together for a defined time period about unsavory aspects of the day.
c) Exploring how to communicate more directly.
d) Learning how to acknowledge the feelings of the spouse.

Intimacy Exercises

a) Spending time together alone: going out for dinner, to the movies, away for a weekend; watching TV together; having a candlelight dinner at home.

b) Showing affection to each other (doing something nice that the spouse would not expect, surprising the other person, cuddling in the living room and holding hands, having a date).

c) Sexual exercises (changing the setting and hour of sex in order to enhance it; changing the ritual of sex: who initiates it, longer or shorter foreplay, greater awareness of how to satisfy the spouse).

CLARIFICATION

Examples of therapist interventions include:

a) Asking a partner to repeat or rephrase what has been said. This is useful if the patient has made a misstatement, said something in a surprising or unusual way, or contradicted previous statements.

b) Rephrasing what a partner has said and asking whether this is what was intended. The rephrasing should place the patient's statement in an interpersonal context. For instance, when discussing an incident in which his wife had come home late, one patient described his feelings by saying, "There was anger," to which the therapist responded, "You were angry at her?"

c) Calling attention to the logical extension of the statement or pointing out implicit assumptions. A useful clarification technique involves calling the couple's attention to *contrasts* or *contradictions* in the presentation of material. Contradictions may be noted between the partner's affective expression and the verbal discussion of a topic. Contrasts may be seen between an initial statement of intentions and overt behavior, between statements of goals and the limitations of reality. In confronting the couple with contradictory statements, the therapist should approach them in the spirit of inquiry, not accusation:

Isn't it interesting that you said [A], when previously you had said [B]? [or] What can we make of the contrast between [A] and [B]?

PROBLEMS ARISING IN THE
COURSE OF CONJOINT THERAPY

EXCESSIVE PESSIMISM OF ONE OR BOTH SPOUSES

Although coming to treatment may itself be considered evidence that the couple is interested in working on their marriage, either partner may wish treatment to fail. Early in treatment it is vital to assess the couple's commitment to their marriage and to working in treatment. For example, one or both partners may have already determined that the marriage cannot last and may enter treatment to extricate themselves from the relationship. Although the therapist is willing to work with the couple regardless of their goals, it is essential that the partners be truthful about their intentions. The therapist may pose three alternatives to the couple:

1. They can stay the same: What would happen if neither person changes and the marriage continues?
2. They can work on the problems in treatment: What would this accomplish? and
3. They can separate.

Few couples will choose options 1 or 3 at the outset of treatment. This understanding is vital in dealing with later resistance to the work. Whenever a partner seems to "go on strike," the couple can be reminded that they have chosen option 2: to work on the marriage. It is sometimes useful for the therapist to be very literal. For example, the therapist may say,

> Oh, let me clarify this: we're changing the contract. We are no longer working on trying to change things but instead have decided to take the option of moving toward a breakup. Is that what you're saying?

A more specific source of pessimism and obstruction early in therapy may be rage that one partner feels toward the other related to feelings of being irretrievably "wronged." This frequently arises when one or both partners have had an extramarital affair. The therapist's stance toward past extramarital affairs is that they are nothing more or less than a sign of marital problems. If the affair is over, the work at hand is to solve the problems so that affairs will no longer seem attractive or necessary. If a spouse expresses interest in working on the marriage but cannot stop berating the partner for past wrongdoing, the therapist may say:

> You're really mad at each other. Maybe we need to get this anger out before we can move on.

Then the therapist may instruct the spouses to each take three minutes to tell the other what they are angry about. During this time, the other is instructed to simply listen. This technique usually stops the argument from escalating, as it is the give-and-take that keeps the fights going.

Another tactic is to tell the couple that while anger is very important, it cannot be allowed to take up so much time in the therapy. Instead, the therapist may instruct the couple to choose a half-hour period each night during which the "wronged" spouse will berate the victimizing one while the victimizer listens and does not respond. They are told not to mention the issue any other time. This maneuver usually brings blaming to a halt because very few people can keep up an unaccompanied tirade for that long.

Another manifestation of excessive pessimism is when one partner declares that he or she is unwilling to work or change because he or she knows that the partner has no intent or ability to change. There are several options for handling this stance. First, the therapist may state tasks in terms such that each partner is responsible for changing only him- or herself, as follows:

> In my experience, people don't have much success at changing other people directly. Rather, they can work on changing themselves in ways that might make the other person want to change. You've been trying to get your spouse to change for years and you feel as though you've been beating your head against the wall. Maybe it's time to try another tactic, to try changing yourself instead.

Another option is to take the complainer at his or her word. If, for example, one spouse says that the other will not cooperate with a task, check it as follows:

> There are only two possibilities. Either she's right and you're not going to do it, or she's wrong and you are.

By describing the two possibilities bluntly, the therapist gives the accused partner the option to acknowledge a problem with compliance if he or she has no intention of following a prescription. If this partner has doubts and is forced into saying that he or she will go along with it, it will be harder to back out. The therapist then can say to the complainer, "Give him [or her] a chance to do it or not."

A variant on this intervention places the responsibility for change on both partners. When the accused spouse states a willingness to change, the therapist responds: "You're going to have to work to convince your wife, because she doesn't believe you."

To involve the complainer, the therapist may say: "You know, maybe your husband doesn't know how to change. Perhaps you can help him out with this by teaching him how to [listen to you, show his interest in the children, etc]."

ONE OR BOTH SPOUSES ARE EXCESSIVELY CRITICAL

It is important for both partners to feel that treatment will help them. When one partner uses the therapy to repeatedly complain about the spouse, this is not only unproductive but can escalate disputes and sabotage treatment. There are several techniques for managing this problem. The therapist can ask the patient to address comments to the partner and/or encourage the partner to respond:

What's your reaction to what your wife is saying? What's your view of this?

Criticisms about the spouse should not go unanswered. The therapist may use the opportunity to educate the couple on how to fight fairly. For example, the therapist may set rules against "hitting below the belt" or encourage the complainer to rephrase the complaints so that they focus on specific things that the partner can change.

The therapist may ask the accused partner if he or she knows how the complaining spouse feels. The therapist may also ask whether the accused spouse knows how to make the complaining spouse happy. If the answer is "No," the therapist may say to the accused spouse: "Get her to teach you what you need to do to make her happy," and to the complainer, "You'll have to work hard to teach him how to change."

The therapist may try to relabel the complaining in a positive light while also encouraging the complainer to cease. For example,

You really are working hard, taking on the job of talking and figuring out the problems for both you and your partner. That protects your spouse from having to work on things. I wonder whether [s]he really needs so much protection and help from you, and whether you have to work so hard?

The therapist may then say to the criticized spouse, "Do you need to have your wife talk for you all the time?" The spouse will say no. Then the therapist can continue: "Well, you're going to have to work to convince her that she doesn't need to."

A final possibility is to banter by exaggerating the complainer's criticism:

> You say that you're married to a [wo]man who is a hundred percent bad. How do you manage? Is there really not even a speck of good?

ONE OR BOTH SPOUSES
INTERRUPT OR MONOPOLIZE

The most direct and practical way of handling excessive interrupting or monopolizing is to set a rule against it or to simply intervene by saying something like, "Let your partner finish; you'll have your turn," or "I can't hear when both of you are talking at once."

THE PARTNERS ENGAGE IN INCESSANT
ARGUMENTS IN AND OUT OF THERAPY

Repetitious, angry arguments are counterproductive and may increase the couple's pessimism about the benefits of treatment. One response is to insist that the couple talk though the therapist. A second is to set limits and rules on arguments: the therapist may set a time limit for a particular argument either at home or in the session. At the end of the time limit, in order that neither partner gets the last word, both can end by saying, "I'm sorry that you feel this way."

A third option is to coach the partners in the arguments. One simple directive is to eliminate the word "you" from each partner's discussion and to restate problems in terms of "I" statements. "I am hurt that . . . ", "I would like. . . ."

THE THERAPY IS STALLED

Treatment can stall. Patients may repetitiously rehash the same material, proclaim themselves cured when obvious problems remain, be unable to talk or to generate affect about an important issue, or deteriorate symptomatically. Handling of each of these situations varies, but the common assumption is that *something important is being avoided*. One or both partners may be withholding a secret from the therapist or from each other. Alternatively, the therapy may be conflicting with individual motives or marital rules that have not clearly been recognized. A third possibility is that the couple is genuinely better and no longer needs treatment.

When treatment stalls, the therapist determines which of these situations is occurring. The therapist can explore whether or not the couple wishes to continue treatment:

> I've noticed that there hasn't seemed to be much to talk about the past few sessions. I wonder if we've reached our treatment goals and don't need to continue to work on them. Let's review the goals we set in Session 4. [Or, more simply,] Is the reason why you're not talking that you're feeling better?

This latter possibility is seldom the case, but verbalizing it points out that work remains to be done and helps to refocus the patients on the treatment goals.

To explore possible secrets, the therapist might say:

> We seem to be going back and forth on the issue of the in-laws without making much progress. When things slow down in therapy, it's often because something more important isn't being discussed. Sometimes it's a third party, like an extramarital affair, or sometimes it's something that's been hard to talk about before. Do you think that something like that is happening here?

If other possibilities are ruled out, the therapist must assume that the treatment has run into key forces that have maintained the symptomatic behavior in the marriage. The therapist can explore this possibility by evaluating the context in which the treatment got stalled, including when the problem began.

DEALING WITH TRANSGRESSIONS

(See Chapter 4.) Some marriages contain a "secret" based upon wrongdoings. These secrets often involve marital infidelity, misuse of funds, or other violations of trust. Situations frequently arise in clinical practice where one party acknowledges some wrongdoing to an individual therapist but refuses to share this transgression with the spouse in couples therapy. The presence of the secret makes renegotiation of the marital dispute difficult. When this situation arises, individual therapy must continue until the individual feels ready to share the secret and make it the subject of the couple's psychotherapeutic work.

In the interpersonal context, the individual who has committed a transgression must confess to the other, ask for forgiveness, offer to do penance, and receive forgiveness. Only then can renegotiation of the relationship take place. A corresponding process occurs for the victimized individual. He or she must recognize having been injured, assert his or her rightful request for knowledge of the wrongdoing, hear the confession, offer forgiveness, suggest means by which penance can occur, and resolve the issue by renegotiating the relationship.

CASE EXAMPLE

Martina, a thirty-five-year-old married housewife, lived with her thirty-eight-year-old husband, Fred, and their two boys, aged seven and ten. In the first session, Martina presented as an attractive, well-dressed woman who appeared sad and was frequently tearful. She tended to describe her life in dramatic terms. Fred was attentive but undemonstrative, speaking softly in a controlled, distant manner.

INITIAL PHASE

Session 1

Depressive History and Social Context.   The hour began with the therapist explaining that he would meet with Martina and Fred for sixteen weeks. The history of depression was elicited from Martina while Fred listened. Martina described feeling depressed for four years, beginning when the family moved from her hometown near Martina's parents, with whom she had had frequent contact. They moved to a rural, comparatively isolated area with only one good friend from Fred's college days and no nearby relatives. Shortly after the move, Martina's mother developed breast cancer, which was successfully treated but caused Martina considerable anguish because she could not help out.

After the move, Fred started a law practice and Martina functioned as his secretary. This arrangement was stressful because she felt torn between her job and her desire to care for her two young children. Two years later, Fred changed his practice and Martina began to stay home full-time, feeling increasingly isolated from her husband. He was working twelve hours daily and frequently on Saturdays as well. She had total responsibility for child care and housekeeping. Although Martina had made some friends through church and her children's schools, she did not feel part of a community. Since she had felt greater self-confidence while working, she decided to pursue a career, but her college degree did not equip her with marketable skills. She had felt torn between the arduous educational course that would qualify her for law and the less demanding road for teaching. She had chosen the latter and in the past year had been taking education courses at a local community college.

Martina's major depressive episode developed over the six to eight months prior to presentation. She described a pervasive dysphoric mood characterized by apathy and guilt, which was worst on weekdays and improved on weekends when her husband was home. She felt irritable, snapping at the children, and had frequent crying spells that felt uncontrollable. She had some difficulty concentrating but could do her classwork and housework. She reported pervasive feelings of guilt over her performance as daughter to her ailing mother, mother to her children, and wife to her husband. She had lost interest in sex and in most pleasurable activities. She felt continuously apprehensive and had numerous headaches. She had withdrawn from many social contacts. She had occasional suicidal ideation but denied any real intent, given her religious upbringing and family obligations. She denied early morning awakening, agitation, or retardation but reported loss of appetite and a weight loss of fifteen pounds.

Spouse's View of Depression

Fred had become aware of his wife's depression only in the past six to eight months; he had not recognized the degree of her unhappiness prior to this. While aware of some marital problems, he was reluctant to engage in treatment of what he saw as primarily his wife's problems.

Spouse's Response to Depression

The couple described numerous interactions that left both partners discouraged and exhausted. Fred typically came home to find Martina in tears. When he attempted to draw her out, discussion centered on her mixed feelings about her career plans. He would attempt a thorough review of the options available to her, paternalistically guiding her to the correct choice. Martina would then accuse him of being unsupportive and selfish, of caring only about his own career and not for her or her family. Martina's tearful diatribe would lead Fred to react with initial tightness, and later anger. On other occasions, rather than taking this "sympathetic" but controlling approach, he instead berated her about her failure to "get her act together." At other times he would try to distract Martina when she was in a bad mood, or would avoid any discussion with her.

Martina described feeling ashamed of her outbursts but wished her husband would devote more attention to the family and wanted his support as she chose her career. For his part, Fred reported concern about spending so much time and energy away from the family, but also felt compelled to by the demands of his career. He was drained by the emotional outbursts and did not know how to respond.

Psychoeducation

The therapist educated the couple about depression and common problems families face in dealing with it. The couple was told that although what had precipitated Martina's depression was unclear, she had been under many stresses and, once depressed, found them overwhelming. She met criteria for major depression. Although she tried to shake it, she had limited control over the depression. The couple had been doing the best they could to cope, with Fred sometimes acting supportive but being rebuffed. He then reacted with anger and complaints, exacerbating Martina's depression and withdrawal, which further compounded her feeling of isolation. His responses were described as "the natural responses of a concerned husband." These did not succeed because depressed people have limited control over their symptoms. It is futile to tell them to "cheer up" or to change; these interventions only disappoint or anger both partners.

The spouse should not feel that he or she can make the depression go away. On the other hand, an available and sympathetic spouse can be helpful, and it is not constructive for the spouse to withdraw. Being available but not overwhelming is the fine line the spouse must walk.

Martina and Fred were told that depression has a good prognosis, and they were instructed about the available treatment options and the details of IPT. The therapist noted that the first sessions would be devoted to learning more about the couple and about Martina's depression.

Session 2

The session was devoted to taking a *history of the marriage* from both partners, who alternated in supplying details. The couple had begun dating in college and had been married for sixteen years. Martina described her husband as a "big man on campus" whom she idolized. By contrast, she was a poor girl, and lonely away from home. He was strong, supportive, and rescued her. He was attracted by her good looks, her admiration for him, her warmth and emotionality. Martina described having difficulty in asserting herself in the relationship from the start, giving the example that the couple never made formal dates; instead, he independently decided whether to come to her dorm on weekend nights. She was always ready for him and did not complain if he did not appear or came very late. She felt so lucky to have him that she did not feel she could make any demands.

The couple moved many times during the marriage and had spent much time apart because of Fred's educational and occupational demands. There was only one brief time during which he did not either work two jobs or attend school while working. The couple more or less agreed on the necessity of his educational and financial mobility, but also agreed that it exhausted them. Martina had been responsible for housekeeping and child care while Fred provided income. At one period, Martina had held a relatively important job. She described feeling best about herself during that time but could not manage both working and mothering. She described long-standing internal conflicts about how to balance the desire for a career with raising her children and supporting Fred in his career.

Reviewing their marital functioning, the couple denied significant disputes in handling finances, relationships with in-laws, disciplining the children, or sexual activity. Major areas of disagreement arose in decision making, division of labor, and communications. Martina felt she nearly always acquiesced to her husband's demands and had little share in major decisions, including the latest home move. She resented it, but also blamed herself for being an unassertive "dishrag." In contrast, Fred felt that Martina had had a major share in many mutual decisions and methodically listed half a dozen.

Regarding division of labor, Martina complained primarily about her husband's absence from the home and lack of involvement in family life. She resented having all the household duties but was unwilling to either get a maid or ask her husband to help because she felt it her duty to support his career. More important than housework was Fred's lack of temporal and emotional involvement with Martina and the family. The couple agreed that these were critical problems. Regarding communication, Martina felt that she could get through to her husband. He, on the other hand, described himself as being as attentive as he could be, but admitted that he was frequently exhausted and did not know how to respond to his wife's confusing, emotional, and contradictory demands. While discussing this issue, Martina became frustrated and declared her hopelessness that anything could change.

The therapist reviewed the problematic areas of current marital functioning and announced that, while the couple did not see any way out of their dilemmas, the work of therapy would be to explore options, including those they had not previously considered.

Session 3

This session focused on a *history of each partner's family of origin and interpersonal inventory*. Both spouses came from working-class families that emphasized hard work. Martina described her parents' marriage as a model she wished to avoid. Her immigrant father worked two jobs and was seldom home. Her mother was moody and bitter about the family's socioeconomic level and her husband's absence. Although the parents did not quarrel openly, they displayed little affection and heavily emphasized religious morality. The patient became a dutiful, unassertive daughter who attempted to rise above circumstances through school achievement. Her role within the family was to cheer others up through emotional liveliness. The patient recognized the similarity of her own bitterness, hard work, and isolation to her mother's and felt all the more hopeless about being able to change.

Fred was the oldest son in a large farming family. Both his parents were extremely hardworking and strict, with few leisure-time activities or displays of affection. He was the only family member to get a higher education and become a professional. Fred also recognized that his family provided him with a stern and joyless model of married life.

The therapist summarized the session by pointing out that both spouses were trying to build a marriage with new roles. They did not wish to follow the models provided by their families, but had had difficulty in finding alternatives. The task of the current therapy was to explore alternative models that might yield greater happiness. The therapist asked each spouse to prepare a list of three to four treatment goals to work on, and to think about what both partners could do to reach the goals.

Session 4

This session reviewed treatment goals. Martina listed two: (1) the need for more "quality time" together; and (2) the need for better communication and for her to feel included in decision making. In elaborating these goals, Martina vacillated, especially on the "quality time" issue. On the one hand, she said that her husband had to spend more time with her and the family or that there were would be "no marriage." On the other hand, she said in a self-deprecating way that she had no right to demand time from someone with so important and busy a work schedule. The therapist pointed out her mixed message: that it was difficult for her to make a clear, legitimate request of her husband. Moreover, this "mixed message" problem might be behind the communication issue. Martina then burst into tears and said that she was so miserable and worthless that she had no right to demand anything and that her husband would be better off without her. She felt that she was the "weak" one. The therapist responded that Martina was not the weak one but the "emotional" partner, who was carrying the pain in a marriage that involved serious deprivations for both partners. Both partners had been driving themselves and not providing for mutual and individual rewards. Their roles had become overdifferentiated, with Martina expressing all the painful emotion and Fred expressing less and less in response.

In reviewing his treatment goals, Fred readily agreed that he was overly devoted to his work and spent too little time with the family. He also acknowledged frustration in talking with Martina. He stated, however, that the "burden" was on him to change and that it would be "painful." The therapist attempted to help him identify how he might benefit from this change. Did he enjoy being with his family and wife? He answered yes. What made it difficult to find time for them? He admitted being "driven" about his work and said that this had begun with the birth of the first child. He felt that being a good father meant being a superior provider. He admitted that he would have difficulty changing. Martina began to cry, asserting that he would never change. The therapist then pointedly asked Fred, "Is she right, or is she wrong? Can you find time for the family or not?" He said that he could. The therapist then turned to Martina and asked, "Will you give him a chance to change?" She said yes.

The therapist noted that the couple had identified similar areas of dispute and had the same treatment goals. The primary one was to create more quality time together and the second to find ways to communicate more freely. All agreed that the next session would be spent working on the first goal.

Intermediate Phase (Sessions 5–12)

Session 5

Two weeks intervened between sessions, and two other visits had been canceled and rescheduled in earlier weeks. The therapist pointed out the attendance problem. Both spouses professed interest in coming, saying that therapy had been eye-opening. The scheduling problems arose from Fred's erratic work schedule. The therapist pointed out the parallel between the therapy and the marriage generally, and Fred's need to find time for both. Much of the session was spent developing a plan to achieve the goal of trying to spend more quality time together.

Both partners recognized the limitations of Fred's work schedule. The therapist suggested that they consider scheduling one specific time during the week to spend together without the children. This time would be reserved for their shared activity; should emergencies prevent its use for that purpose, it would be rescheduled for the same week. The couple was intrigued. After discussion, they chose Friday nights. They then discussed how they might spend their time together. At the therapist's suggestion, they decided to take turns choosing how to spend their Friday nights and made a plan for the following Friday. The therapist asked them to anticipate what might go wrong with this plan; they felt that it would work. They claimed they enjoyed time they spent together. Martina pointed out that her depression improved on weekends when Fred was home and grew progressively worse during the week as she spent less time with him.

The couple was then asked why they had not thought of this plan before. Fred responded that he was unable to give himself a break like this because he felt duty-bound to devote all his energy to work. When asked how Martina could help him to relax and enjoy the time, he felt she did not need to do anything special. For her part, Martina acknowledged that her husband's work involvement was sincere and less glamorous than she had supposed. She based this comment on having attended a public hearing he was involved in and noted how boring it had been.

Session 6

This session followed up on the plan to spend an evening together. This had gone very well: the couple had gone out to dinner alone for the first time in years. Both had enjoyed the time and felt little strain during it. Martina felt buoyed. The therapist congratulated them but continued to voice skepticism that they could change so rapidly. The subsequent discussion focused on Martina's difficulty in asserting herself. She tended to make no demands because she did not feel deserving of attention. When she did make demands, they usually took the form of angry, histrionic, tearful outbursts. Her husband interpreted these as evidence of her being "overtired" and tended to ignore their content. She angrily accused Fred of "not caring" about the family or her, then recanted and apologized. For his part, Fred had no interest in hearing demands that involved his changing his own priorities. He took advantage of the confused messages he received from his wife by ignoring them.

Sessions 7–8

Session 7 was canceled because the couple took a spur-of-the moment vacation at Fred's initiative. They came to Session 8 tanned, fit, and in good spirits. Fred had left his legal work entirely in his partners' hands. He had never done this previously (although the partners had left him in charge on many occasions) and was surprised at his freedom from worry during the vacation. The therapist congratulated them on creatively finding another way to spend quality time together and again encouraged them to consider what had kept them from doing this previously. The therapist asked them to try to articulate what they were doing differently now in order to prevent a reversion to old patterns when the therapy ended. They were reminded that they had completed half of the therapy. The communication issue arose again, with an acknowledgment of the different styles of the two partners.

Session 9

Between Sessions 8 and 9, Martina had called the therapist because she had what Fred had told her was her individual problem, not the couple's issue. This problem was the couple's continued social involvement with a man who had been Fred's best friend, and with whom Martina had had an extramarital affair two years previously. Martina was uncomfortable about continuing to see this man, while Fred denied any discomfort. The therapist told Martina that this seemed to be the couple's issue and that they should discuss it at the next session.

This session began with an explication of the suppressed part of the marital history. The affair had taken place two years earlier because, in Martina's words, "Rick showed me the affection and interest that my husband did not." After several months, she had confessed the ongoing affair, whereupon Fred threatened divorce. She considered returning home to her family, but they refused her when they learned the circumstances. Martina felt desperate and guilty. She now felt that she had never entirely recovered from this stormy one-month period after the affair.

Afterward, things settled down, and the couple attempted to return to life as usual, which included monthly socializing with Rick. He had been Fred's best friend in college and had been one reason why they had moved to this neighborhood. Martina felt that Rick competed with her husband and wanted to break up their marriage. She was also attracted to this wealthy, handsome playboy. Continued contact with Rick was painful because Rick teased and ridiculed her, while Fred made no attempt to intervene.

Although there were several unanswered questions about the couple's involvement with Rick (e.g., Martina's continued attraction, and the possibly homosexual nature of Fred's attraction to him), the therapist decided to focus the inquiry on one of the two central themes of the therapy: how Martina could learn to articulate her needs and how Fred could respond to her. The problems were reframed as communication issues: Martina's unwillingness to articulate her wish to limit contact with Rick, or at least to have Fred stop Rick's teasing. She had mentioned these issues before, but Fred tended to minimize the difficulties, and Martina had backed down. As the session was ending, the couple was encouraged to discuss their options for handling their relationship with Rick by themselves between sessions.

Session 10

This session pursued the communication theme. The couple had decided to "play it by ear" in dealing with Rick. Both partners reported an interest in keeping up the relationship. The therapist questioned in detail what this meant and assisted Martina in articulating her wish that Fred protect her from Rick and attend to her more when the couple frequented social gatherings. She felt abandoned by him at large parties, which they frequently attended. He expressed surprise that she felt this way. The couple discussed remedies to the problem. That Martina had never previously articulated this issue was tied to the theme of Fred's having trouble hearing her. Both partners were encouraged to consider the simplicity of solutions once problems were clearly articulated.

Session 11

This session clarified that the marital dispute had moved from impasse to active renegotiation. The couple described having had a loud, heated argument the previous Friday. Fred had come home late on their scheduled "together" night after Martina had taken pains to ready herself for the evening. She complained bitterly and an argument ensued, with the couple at first deciding to cancel plans for the evening. They discussed the matter for fifteen to twenty minutes, then went out and spent an enjoyable evening. Both partners reported the occasion as upsetting at first but indicative of their having more open communication. They had had a brief, productive fight rather than several days of suppressed, smoldering resentment. The therapist congratulated them and reinforced the importance of negotiating actively but fairly.

Session 12

In this session, Martina was visibly upset and made vague complaints about Fred, such as his lack of chivalry. On examination, however, Martina reported that his behavior had improved greatly. She herself had been in unaccountably bad spirits for the past several days, tearful and irritable; this frequently happened to her premenstrually. The therapist took a thorough history of her moodiness while Fred listened. She had been moody premenstrually all of her adult life. The therapist recommended that she take this seriously and consider a gynecological consultation.

The therapist then described Martina's moodiness as an individual issue that affected the couple's communication problem. Martina had difficulty in distinguishing whether her discontent with Fred was related to realistic problems or exaggerated by her premenstrual mood, and thus hesitated to articulate legitimate problems or demands. Her husband was asked if he could assist Martina in making this distinction. He said he was aware of the issue.

Comment on Intermediate Phase. :The middle sessions focused on the two themes of the therapy: (1) increased shared time, and (2) communication with more opportunity for Martina to make herself heard. These themes were promoted by the initial exercise of finding a night to spend together as a couple, and sticking to this throughout the therapy. The exercise became a successful new marital institution and provided material for discussion in sessions. The persistent focus on a limited number of themes also protected the therapy from getting stuck in a morass of recriminations and pathological secrets when Martina's extramarital affair was revealed. The communication issue was the least charged in that session and allowed the organization of material so that it did not interfere with the progress of treatment.

A feature that may distinguish IPT-CM from other marital treatments was the focus on Martina's individual problems as the identified patient. The therapist was careful with the couple to distinguish between individual problems of each partner and conjoint problems of their marriage. When Martina reported premenstrual dysphoria, the therapist focused on her as the identified patient after previous sessions of exclusive focus on the couple's issues. A return to a focus on the couple's problems took place in the next session.

TERMINATION PHASE (SESSIONS 13–15)

Session 13

The couple described attending a wedding at which Rick was present. Both spouses enjoyed themselves and Martina commented on Fred's attentiveness. The therapist congratulated them on making progress and reminded them that the end of therapy was approaching. They were asked to review the experience. Fred described taking a different view of the importance of family and leisure time and expressed surprise and delight that his life could be as full as it was becoming. The communication issue was reiterated, using the examples of Martina's desire for (1) more of Fred's time, (2) greater attention to her problems with Rick, and (3) greater attentiveness at social gatherings. In all three instances, Fred had responded willingly and at little cost to himself. What had been missing previously were clear requests from Martina to which Fred knew how to respond.

Session 14

The couple described a "normal" week, including several small arguments that they were able to resolve. The most important concerned Martina's wish that Fred speak to their elder son. He had at first tried to brush off the request, but she persisted in telling him that she considered it important. He complied and ultimately welcomed the opportunity to get closer to the boy. Both partners felt satisfied. In addition, Fred had become newly involved in family activities. He became more involved in attending church with Martina. They found this mutually satisfying. The couple also kept up their Friday nights together and described the success of this practice.

The therapist encouraged them to consider their future together. Martina professed less conflict over her career than before. She described having felt the need for a career only because she was convinced Fred was going to leave her and that she needed job skills to support herself. She reported greater confidence in the marriage and felt no need to pursue training beyond teaching certification until the children grew older.

Session 15

Final Session

The couple described their joint struggles with adversity in the past week. A rainstorm had flooded the basement and Fred had had a particularly difficult work week. Instead of these circumstances causing conflict, as in the past, the couple had shared their tribulations at the end of each day and profited from mutual support. Fred had discovered that he enjoyed talking about work problems with Martina even though she was not a lawyer, and Martina felt greater intimacy with him and greater inclusion in his life when he did this. Their conversations had deepened and covered issues other than household catastrophes and problems with money or the children. They described greatly increased satisfaction in the marriage and faith that they would continue to do well.

Martina reported improvement of her depression, which was now limited to brief periods of "moodiness." She no longer met diagnostic criteria for major depression. She averred no interest in further individual therapy at the time. Fred stated that the therapy had changed his life by allowing him to seek satisfaction from family and leisure-time activities. He felt that he had started to become three-dimensional and regretted the many years during which he was obsessed with work at the expense of other things. The communication issue was again briefly reviewed and the couple was encouraged to identify danger signals for the marriage and for Martina that might indicate a need for further treatment.

EFFICACY

In addition to one pilot study of IPT-CM, two published clinical trials have compared individual with conjoint marital therapy for depressed patients with marital problems. Jacobson et al. (1991) studied sixty married depressed women who were randomly assigned to either conjoint behavioral marital therapy (BMT) alone, individual cognitive therapy alone, or combined individual cognitive and conjoint BMT. Results suggested that BMT had less efficacy than individual cognitive therapy for depression in couples without marital distress, whereas for maritally distressed couples the two treatments had equal efficacy. Only BMT had a significant positive impact on the marital relationship in distressed couples, and only cognitive therapy combined with conjoint BMT enhanced marital satisfaction of nondistressed couples. The small sample size and absence of a control group limit conclusions. In follow-up six months and one year after treatment ended, no significant difference among treatments was found. High levels of the husband's facilitating behavior after treatment was related to the wife's recovery (Jacobson et al., 1993).

O'Leary and Beach (1990) studied thirty-six maritally discordant couples with depressed wives randomly assigned to marital therapy, cognitive therapy, or a waiting-list control for twelve weeks. Women given marital or cognitive therapy showed statistically significant and clinically meaningful improvement in their depression. Marital therapy yielded greater increases in marital satisfaction than did cognitive therapy or no treatment, differences that persisted at one year follow-up. The findings thus suggest that marital therapy may be more effective than individual treatment for clinically significant marital discord with comorbid depression.

EFFICACY OF IPT-CM

A pilot study of IPT-CM examined its feasibility and patient acceptance and provided preliminary evidence of efficacy. It compared individual IPT to conjoint IPT in treating symptoms, social functioning, and marital adjustment (Foley et al., 1989).

Eighteen couples participated. The marital partner who originally sought treatment for major depression was assigned the identified patient status. The patient sample consisted of five male and thirteen female married, nonbipolar, nonpsychotic, depressed outpatients, ages twenty-one to sixty. The patients met Research Diagnostic Criteria (RDC; Spitzer et al., 1978) for a current episode of major depressive disorder based on a diagnostic interview (SADS-L; Endicott and Spitzer, 1978). Only patients who identified marital disputes as the major problem associated with the onset or exacerbation of their depression were admitted to the study. Prospective patients were excluded if a clinician judged them or their spouses to be at serious suicide risk.

Patients were randomly assigned to sixteen weekly IPT or IPT-CM sessions. In IPT-CM, the spouse was required to participate in all psychotherapy sessions, whereas in individual IPT the spouse did not meet with the psychotherapist. Treatments followed the IPT and IPT-CM manuals. Patients and spouses in both treatment conditions were asked to refrain from taking psychotropic medication during the study without prior discussion with their therapists, who were discouraged from prescribing. Only two prescriptions were written by psychiatrists during the study: one patient in individual therapy and one in conjoint marital therapy received sedatives to treat insomnia.

Three therapists (a psychiatrist, a psychologist, and a social worker) administered individual IPT. Three others (social workers) administered conjoint marital IPT. All had extensive prior experience in treating depressed patients and were trained using the manuals. Quality of therapist performance was monitored by expert raters who reviewed videotapes of entire therapy sessions. All therapists were judged adherent to their treatment during the study.

Symptom status, social functioning, and marital adjustment of patients and spouses in both treatment conditions were evaluated at intake and at termination of the sixteen-week course of therapy by a clinical evaluator blind to treatment condition. Social marital functioning was assessed on the Social Adjustment Scale (SAS; Weissman and Bothwell, 1976). Marital adjustment was measured on a forty-four-item version of the Locke-Wallace Marital Adjustment Test (Locke and Wallace, 1976), a self-report scale. The Spanier Dyadic Adjustment Scale (Spanier, 1976) contains four empirically verified subscales: *dyadic satisfaction,* which measures a subject's feelings of happiness and contentment in the marriage; *dyadic cohesion,* which reflects the strength of the union between the marital partners; *dyadic consensus,* which assesses the extent of agreement or disagreement between marital partners on a wide variety of issues; and *affectional expression,* which characterizes a subject's view of affection and sexual relations in the marriage. On both scales, higher scores indicate better marital adjustment.

The eighteen patients had a mean age of forty, were predominantly Catholic, white, and had been married an average of fifteen years. Eighty-nine percent reported previous episodes of major depression. Seventy-eight percent of spouses had a lifetime history of some psychiatric disorder, with 50 percent reporting previous episodes of major depression, and an additional 17 percent reporting histories of RDC minor depression. At intake, two spouses met criteria for major depression sufficiently severe to qualify for patient status in the study. The high prevalence of major depression among spouses of depressed patients is consistent with other reports (Merikangas, 1982; Weissman et al., 1982).

Patients were easily recruited for the study and accepted randomization to the two treatment groups. Two patients in IPT and one in IPT-CM terminated treatment prior to completion. One IPT patient left treatment after Session 12 because of a serious physical illness. Another terminated IPT-CM after Session 13 because of symptomatic deterioration. Spouses of all subjects agreed to participate in the study and cooperated with periodic assessments. In IPT-CM, only two therapy sessions were missed and three sessions were rescheduled. In IPT, no therapy sessions were skipped and two sessions were rescheduled. Patient evaluations of the quality of treatment did not differ by treatment cell. Patients in both groups expressed satisfaction with treatment, felt they had improved, and attributed improvement to the therapy.

Outcome Assessment of IPT-CM

Patients in both treatments had significantly reduced depressive symptoms and social impairment by the end of therapy, with no significant difference between treatment groups in degree of improvement in depressive symptoms or social functioning by endpoint. Locke-Wallace Marital Adjustment Test scores at Session 16 were significantly higher (indicating better marital adjustment) for patients receiving IPT-CM than for patients receiving IPT. Scores on the Spanier Dyadic Adjustment Scale also indicated more improved marital functioning for IPT-CM than for IPT patients. At Session 16, IPT-CM patients reported significantly higher levels of improvement in affectional expression (demonstrations of affection and sexual relations in the marriage) than did IPT patients.

Although spouses exhibited some symptoms of depression and social maladjustment, their overall symptoms were not severe enough to allow for marked improvement over the course of the study. While the Locke-Wallace Marital Adjustment Test scores of spouses in both treatment groups improved, there was no significant difference in degree of spousal improvement between treatment groups.

In summary, attendance of both patients and spouses in treatment sessions was excellent. Only two patients (one from each treatment group) dropped out. Patients in both treatments improved equally in symptoms and in social adjustment, but patients receiving IPT-CM had greater improvements in marital adjustment and affectional expression than did patients receiving IPT. The results should be interpreted with caution due to the pilot nature of the study, the small sample size, the lack of a no-treatment control group, and the absence of a pharmacotherapy or combined pharmacotherapy-psychotherapy comparison group.

COMMENT

Future research on IPT-CM should address the following issues that emerged during the pilot study. Because some spouses of the identified patients were also depressed, it appears important to examine systematically the psychiatric status of spouses and to develop a strategy for managing their symptoms. The IPT-CM study therapists found it difficult to focus on marital issues if their patients were severely depressed. The therapists felt that managing marital disputes would be more effective if the patients' depressive symptoms were initially controlled (either by medication or by psychotherapy), and marital issues addressed subsequently.

The results of this pilot study are promising enough to warrant further testing on a larger sample in a design including a no-treatment control and a pharmacotherapy group. Such a clinical trial might provide useful information on the best treatment for patients experiencing depression in the context of marital disputes.

CHAPTER 16

Bipolar Disorder

DISORDER

The DSM-IV definition of bipolar disorder requires at least one manic episode. Some patients have had a previous depressive episode and most will have subsequent episodes, either manic or depressive. Hypomanic or mixed episodes can also occur, as can significant mood lability between episodes. Assessment includes both current state and prior course.

MANIC EPISODES

- A distinct period of abnormally and persistently elevated, expansive, or irritable mood lasting at least one week.
- During the period of mood disturbance, at least three of the following symptoms have persisted to a significant degree:

1. Inflated self-esteem or grandiosity.
2. Decreased need for sleep.
3. More talkative than usual, or pressure to keep talking.
4. Flight of ideas or subjective experiences that thoughts are racing.
5. Distractibility.
6. Increase in goal-directed activities, either social, at work, at school, etc.; psychomotor agitation.
7. Excessive involvement in pleasurable activities that have a high potential for painful consequences (for example engaging in un-

restrained buying sprees, sexual indiscretions, or foolish business investments).

[Adapted from DSM-IV, 1994]

Bipolar disorder, sometimes called manic depression, is an episodic illness with a variable but impairing course. It should always be considered in the differential diagnosis of patients presenting with major depression. The lifetime prevalence across diverse countries is approximately 1 percent (Weissman et al., 1996), with similar rates in men and women. The average age of onset is in the early twenties. Although it can begin in childhood, prepubertal onset is uncommon. First onset over the age of sixty is usually associated with general medical conditions such as cerebrovascular disease. As many as five to ten years may elapse between onset of the illness and its first treatment.

Pharmacology is the basic treatment for bipolar disorder and has demonstrated efficacy for both acute and recurrent episodes. Since its introduction circa 1969, lithium has represented a treatment breakthrough (Schou, 1997). Mood-stabilizing anticonvulsant medications such as valproate and carbamazepine have been in increasing use since the late 1970s. The consensus reflected in the American Psychiatric Association treatment guidelines (American Psychiatric Association, 1994) is that patients with bipolar disorder require maintenance and probably lifelong pharmacologic treatment.

Compliance with pharmacotherapy is a major issue, both because of medication side effects and because patients miss the highs of the manic phase of the disorder. Although pharmacotherapy reduces the frequency and severity of episodes, there is good evidence that even with prophylactic treatment most patients relapse over the course of two years. Some of this relapse has been related to lack of medication adherence. Since suicide is a too-frequent outcome of untreated bipolar disorder, close management of patients is essential (Gitlin and Altshuler, 1997; Gershon and Soares, 1997).

RATIONALE

Effective psychotropic medication has markedly improved the treatment and prognosis of the bipolar patient, but the social and personal sequelae of the illness remain. In the premedication era, psychoanalysts made heroic efforts to treat bipolar patients. These psychotherapeutic pioneers were frustrated by their results and did not consider bipolar patients good psychoanalytic candidates. Abraham called them "impatient, envious, exploitative"; Fromm-Reichmann described them as "lacking in complexity and subtlety, dependent, clinging" (Goodwin and Jamison, 1990, p. 727).

The introduction of efficacious medications made psychopharmacology the primary treatment and psychotherapy adjunctive. Yet the pharmacologic revolution was also a renaissance for the psychotherapy of bipolar patients. Symptom reduction and maintenance treatment with medication permitted handling the social and interpersonal problems associated with the illness in psychotherapy. There are still few published controlled clinical trials of the efficacy of psychotherapy added to medication in pure samples of patients with bipolar illness. However, some well-designed clinical trials on the efficacy of psychotherapy have included bipolar patients.

Cognitive, behavioral, interpersonal, and family psychotherapies have been modified to address the problems the illness poses. Clinics specializing in treatment of bipolar illness have developed psychosocial strategies to improve the prognosis of bipolar patients, which include maximizing medication compliance, charting moods, educating patient and family, and employing self-help programs. Practice guidelines (APA, 1994) include psychotherapy in their management. Frank has modified IPT as an adjunctive maintenance treatment for medication-stabilized bipolar patients, adding to it the monitoring of social rhythms.

The rationale for psychotherapy as adjunctive treatment for bipolar disorder is based on the following factors: (1) the high relapse rate of bipolar patients, even with medication; (2) patient noncompliance with medication; (3) the social and personal events that may trigger manic or depressive episodes; and (4) the devastating social and interpersonal consequences of the illness. Among the issues often treated in psychotherapy are developmental delays and deviations from life patterns as a result of the illness; compliance with treatment (denial, anger, ambivalence); fear of recurrence; the effects of the illness on work, marriage, childbearing, family, friends; pregnancy; fear of genetic transmission; countertransference; and stigma (Goodwin and Jamison, 1990).

Giving up the "high"—the euphoria, creativity, and cognitive sharpness of hypomania, however transient—is a serious issue for bipolar patients and must be dealt with to improve compliance with medication or with psychotherapy. This may be a realistic loss, a decrease in sexuality, energy, productivity, and possibly creativity, or an increased need for sleep; or an unrealistic and symbolic loss, as when patients blame personal failure on treatment. The sacrifice of that high must be weighed against the often catastrophic damage and suffering associated with manic and depressive episodes and the risk of developing refractory or rapid-cycling illness.

The 1994 APA practice guidelines for bipolar disorder noted that "psychiatric management and pharmacologic therapy are essential components of treatment. . . . Specific psychotherapeutic treatments may be critical components of the treatment plan" (p. 15). The APA guidelines' recommendations for psychotherapeutic management suggest that the therapist:

- establish a therapeutic alliance,
- monitor symptoms using life charts of events and moods,
- educate about bipolar illness,
- enhance treatment compliance,
- promote regular daily activities and sleep, and
- promote understanding of psychosocial effects of the illness.

The boundaries between general clinical management and specific psychotherapies are unclear. The new psychotherapies for bipolar disorder contain components of clinical management, including education, compliance, and addressing current interpersonal issues. None involves a regressive transference, interpretation, dream analysis, or exploration of personality. The neurobiology of the disorder—e.g., kindling theory—suggests that it is best viewed as a hardwired, biological disorder rather than a personality trait. Hence uncovering, regressive therapies may not be appropriate approaches to bipolar disorder.

SPECIFIC PSYCHOTHERAPIES
FOR BIPOLAR DISORDER

Specific psychotherapies for bipolar disorder and evidence for their efficacy have been slow to emerge, but the situation is changing. Psychotherapies specific to bipolar disorder and based on research findings are now being tested. Most completed studies have small treatment samples and might be considered Phase 1 or 2 studies that provide the basis for more ambitious current undertakings.

PSYCHOEDUCATION

The purpose of psychoeducation is to educate patients about the illness and its treatment, including types of treatment (especially pharmacology) and side effects, in order to enhance understanding and compliance. Peet and Harvey (1991) randomly assigned sixty bipolar outpatients to either a twelve-minute video lecture on lithium, with a written transcript, or standard treatment. They showed that knowledge about lithium improved in the education group and resulted in increased lithium levels and fewer missed doses.

FAMILY THERAPY

There are several anecdotal reports on family therapy for bipolar patients. Its purpose is to improve communication among family members, reducing interpersonal crisis and noncompliance. Miller et al. (1991; cited in APA guidelines, 1994, p. 16) compared standard treatment (medication and clinical management) to family therapy combined with medication in a study of fourteen bipolar patients. Treatment continued for eighteen weeks after hospital discharge. At two-year follow-up, the family therapy group had lower rates of family separation, greater functional improvement in patients, and higher rates of recovery. Glick et al. (1985) reported positive results in twelve families with a bipolar patient in group therapy compared to eight subjects in standard care, finding better patient functioning and fewer hospitalizations in the family-therapy group at eighteen months. The same group reported positive effects for female bipolar patients after a six-session psychoeducational family intervention (Haas et al., 1988).

BEHAVIORAL FAMILY MANAGEMENT (BFM)

Miklowitz and Goldstein (1990) have shown that negative family attitudes (high expressed emotion, criticism, overinvolvement) predict relapse in bipolar patients independent of medication compliance. BFM follows from these observations. Therapy includes a diagnostic procedure, education about bipolar illness, and training for the patient in communication skills and problem solving. Pilot results in nine recently discharged patients indicate that patients receiving lithium alone without BFM had a 61 percent relapse, compared to 11 percent of patients receiving BFM and lithium.

COGNITIVE BEHAVIORAL THERAPY (CBT)

CBT, which helps patients understand and change depressed negative cognitions, has demonstrated efficacy in numerous acute clinical trials for major depression. Cochran (1984) treated twenty-eight outpatients on lithium to determine whether CBT altered cognitions and behavior that interfere with medication compliance. Half the patients received medication and standard clinical care; the rest received six sessions of CBT aimed at enhancing medication compliance. Patients given CBT had enhanced compliance at both three- and six-month follow-up, were less likely to terminate lithium against medical advice, and had fewer hospitalizations during the course of the study.

Basco and Rush (1995) also adapted CBT for bipolar patients. Their adaptation, incorporating elements of CBT and psychoeducation, aims to enhance medication compliance and to help patients understand the dysfunctional patterns of information processing that may lead to relapse.

SELF-HELP

Although they are not specific psychotherapies as such, excellent self-help programs have been developed under the auspices of the National Depressive and Manic Depressive Association (NDMDA). These self-help groups were nationally organized in 1986. There are now more than one hundred in existence, with more forming each year. NDMDA provides personal support and educational services to people with depression or manic depression and their families; educates the public about the nature and management of these treatable medical disorders; and promotes research. Other organizations, such as the National Alliance of the Mentally Ill (NAMI), also offer educational programs for patients and their families and self-help groups for patients and families. These groups work in collaboration with clinicians. Bipolar patients should be encouraged to seek support from their local groups. These services enhance the primary care of the patient by a physician and psychotherapist by providing supplementary support in addition to other benefits.

IPT

Frank and colleagues (1994, 1997) have modified IPT for bipolar disorder in what is perhaps the most radical reworking of IPT. This adaptation re-

Respondent # _____ **Week of:** _____

			PEOPLE 1 = Other just present 3 = Others very stimulating 0 = Alone 2 = Others actively involved						
ACTIVITY	**TIME**	**PM** **AM or**	**DAY OF WEEK**						
			MON	**TUE**	**WED**	**TH**	**FRI**	**SAT**	**SUN**
OUT OF BED	Earlier								
	8:00								
	8:15								
	8:30								
	8:45								
Mid-point of your	9:00						0		
normal range ➤	9:15								
	9:30		0		0	0			
	9:45			0					
	10:00								
	10:15								
	10:30								
	Later							0	0
	Check if did not do								
FIRST CONTACT	Earlier								
(In person or by phone)	9:15								
or with another person	9:30								
	9:45								
	10:00								
	10:15								
Mid-point of your ➤	10:30								
normal range	10:45				2				
	11:00		2	2		2	2		
	11:15								
	11:30								
	11:45							3	3
	Later								
	Check if did not do								

tains the main components of IPT: the focus on psychosocial factors known to relate to the onset of depressive episodes, and the four interpersonal problem areas. A new component has been added, however, to manage symptoms by regulating social rhythms. Disruption of social rhythms by social demands, tasks, and personal relationships may result in instability of biological rhythms, triggering onset of a bipolar mood episode in vulnerable individuals. Behavioral techniques such as self-monitoring, goal setting, guided task assignments, and cognitive restructuring are utilized in order to regulate the patient's lifestyle and stabilize social rhythms. A randomized controlled trial in medication-stabilized patients is under way to determine the efficacy of this approach (Ehlers et al., 1984; Frank et al., 1995).

This therapy is a hybridization of IPT with behavioral Social Rhythm Therapy (SRT) to form "Interpersonal and Social Rhythm Therapy" (IPSRT) for bipolar disorder.

The SRT component introduces the Social Rhythm Metric (SRM), a self-report instrument that measures the regularity of seventeen daily activities, such as getting out of bed, having breakfast, beginning the day's work; whether they occurred alone or in company; and how stimulating they were. The instrument helps patients recognize patterns and changes in timing for each activity during the week and their relationship to mood change. A high score on the metric indicates a high level of regularity in the timing of activities; a low score indicates high variability. Patients are encouraged to monitor and avoid instability in daily routines. The investigators hypothesize that regularizing routines will lead to greater regularity in circadian rhythm, which may reduce relapse or recurrence rate in bipolar patients.

Frank et al. (1994) describe four phases in conducting IPSRT. The initial phase is weekly, either while the patient is still recovering from an acute episode or during an euthymic state. Patients learn principles of IPT and then therapy moves to biweekly and then monthly visits. The initial phase, as in IPT, involves history taking, completing the interpersonal inventory, identifying the problem areas, and educating the patient about bipolar disorder. The Social Rhythm Metric is introduced in these early sessions.

The history of the illness covers symptomatic and interpersonal aspects of the index and earlier episodes, with emphasis on the most recent episodes. Following the social zeitgeber hypothesis (Ehlers, Frank, and Kupfer, 1988) that a close relationship exists between disruption in social rhythms in the patient's life and the onset of episodes, the therapist in taking the history seeks evidence of disruption in the patient's daily life routines preceding the development of symptoms. Family members and close friends may be involved in the history-taking phase, especially if the patient has limited recall of the period prior to developing mania. For example, a reduction in total sleep time over the course of several days may either represent an early sign of the illness or—if caused by external demands, such as studying for an examination or taking a child to the emergency room—instead be the trigger of mania.

The therapist develops a time line that includes episodes of illness, important life events, lifestyle alterations, and any other information patients may find relevant to understanding their vulnerable periods (Frank et al., 1994). The interpersonal inventory proceeds as usual. Psychoeducation about bipolar illness is conducted in the usual IPT manner, with added emphasis on the way lifestyle disruptions may affect the onset of illness episodes. Hence the goal is to determine events and patterns in the patient's life that lead to increased or decreased sleep or social stimulation. The patient is educated about the risk associated with rhythm disregulation. This may help to reduce denial of illness and to facilitate changes that the patient may need to make. The discussion includes identifying situations such as meetings, or movies, or parties where the patient may become overstimulated.

The tasks of the second phase of treatment are to resolve the interpersonal problem areas and to develop the management plan: to search for typical triggers of rhythm disruptions, finding and maintaining a healthy balance of activity and stimulation, and adapting to changes in routine. The search for rhythm disruptions uses SRM data and current information provided during the session. In each session, patient and therapist review the SRM, seeking rhythms that seem unstable. The therapist tries to determine whether the instability is due to symptoms of the disorder or represents a self-imposed lifestyle that might be disregulating. The goal is to work with the patient to stabilize social rhythms: for example, to go to sleep at a regular time rather than to stay up all night working on a project, to eat meals at a regular time, etc. Preserving sleep is paramount, as lack of sleep can induce mania. Patients are helped to manage the affective symptoms, and to find and maintain a healthy rhythmic balance to avoid triggers of disruption in their life and usual activity.

Social rhythm aspects of the treatment occur in conjunction with treatment of the interpersonal problem areas identified during the early phases of the treatment.

- *Grief:* In addition to unresolved grief as described in IPT, symbolic losses are discussed, including grief over the loss of the "healthy self." Frank et al. (1994) describe this as the self that might have been in better control of moods and behavior. Grief may also result from the contemplation of lifestyle changes required by the illness. The reader will note that this redefines the usual IPT sense of "grief" as complicated bereavement, which requires an actual death of another person close to the patient. Symbolic losses in IPT for unipolar disorder are typically treated as role transitions.
- *Interpersonal Disputes:* Interpersonal disputes are common for bipolar patients and may be exacerbated by the manic phase of the ill-

ness. Bipolar patients often need help to modify argumentative and critical impulses.

- *Role Transitions:* Role transitions are by definition a disruption of normal rhythms. As such they may leave the patient vulnerable to recurrences of illness and may require considerable interpersonal management.

- *Interpersonal Deficits:* Frank and colleagues (1994) remark that bipolar patients often have numerous but unsatisfying relationships, particularly when the patient has alienated close friends and family during prior episodes. Helping the patient to see others in perspective and to temper demanding expectations is part of the work of IPT. A new form of interpersonal deficits for bipolar patients identified by Frank et al. (1994) arises in the aftermath of manic episodes. Patients may be unwilling to resume old friendships or to seek a job. Again, this would usually be characterized as a role transition in standard IPT.

In the third phase of treatment, the therapist works to establish the patient's confidence in using the method to address the relationship among symptoms, rhythm disruption, and interpersonal issues. When termination seems appropriate, it is addressed over four to six months in monthly sessions with a review of vulnerabilities and of early signs and symptoms of recurrence. This review in the fourth, termination, phase serves to develop an ongoing plan for the future.

CASE EXAMPLE[1]

Stuart, a thirty-seven-year-old divorced man, entered IPSRT following his fourth manic episode. In Session 2, he and his therapist reviewed the events that led up to his manic episodes. Although he had never previously made the connection, Stuart recognized that the common thread connecting his episodes was sleep deprivation, often combined with missing a single dose of lithium. Working as a technical writer, Stuart was often required to work late into the night in order to complete his projects. On the night prior to three of his onsets of mania, his boss insisted that he work all night to meet a deadline. On each of these occasions he also neglected to take his evening dose of lithium.

His fourth episode followed a night during which he had been kept awake by persistent nausea and vomiting related to an intestinal flu. Although he had taken his lithium that evening, in all likelihood little had remained in his system after the vomiting began. Although the similarities among events preceding each episode were obvious when Stuart reviewed them, he had previously failed to connect his sleep deprivation and the onset of his manic episodes because of the different settings and the different individuals he had worked for on each occasion. The IPSRT approach underscored the need to maintain good sleeping habits as protection against future episodes.

EFFICACY

Frank et al. (1997) describe their study of maintenance treatment of bipolar patients using interpersonal psychotherapy and social rhythm therapy in medication-maintained patients. Their preliminary report comparing IPSRT as adjunctive treatment to conventional medication-clinic treatment found comparable changes in symptomatology in the two groups over the fifty-two-week treatment period: that is, in the sample treated to date, there was no advantage in treatment outcome for IPSRT. Ultimately, more than fifty patients will be studied in each condition. The first eighteen patients assigned to IPSRT did show significantly greater stability of daily routines as treatment proceeded. Patients assigned to the medication-clinic condition (n=20) showed essentially no change in social rhythms as measured by SRM. The authors conclude that IPSRT influenced lifestyle regularity in patients with bipolar disorder, possibly providing protection against future episodes. Data about the interpersonal problem areas remain to be analyzed.

WHEN PSYCHOTHERAPY
MAY BE ESPECIALLY IMPORTANT

Psychotherapy has been recommended as adjunctive treatment to medication for bipolar patients. This recommendation is based more on clinical judgment than on existing outcome research. However, in intervals when medication is either contraindicated or discontinued, psychotherapy may be useful. For example, for noncompliant patients there is evidence that changing attitudes by using education or CBT can help compliance in pregnancy (Cochrane, 1984; Zaretsky and Segal, 1994–1995).

Bipolar disorder affects women in their childbearing years. Women with bipolar disorder may exhibit significant affective symptoms during pregnancy and carry a high risk for postpartum episodes: there is an eightfold increase in mood episodes in the postpartum months. During the first trimester, exposure to any of the three mood stabilizers—lithium, valproic acid, or carbamazepine—is associated with increased risk of birth defects (Goodwin and Jamison, 1990, pp. 679–681), although the teratogenic risk of lithium is controversial and may have been overstated. But for such patients effective psychotherapy may have particular importance.

COMMENT

This work is important for several reasons. First, it takes the difficult step from unipolar to bipolar affective illness, a disorder for which the optimal use of psychotherapy remains far from clear. Second, Frank and colleagues (1994) have made a dramatic shift in combining IPT with a behavioral approach. Whether this combination has therapeutic benefit will be determined by the complete results of their large-scale study, but preliminary results do suggest some benefit (E. Frank, personal communication, 1999). IPSRT also raises interesting theoretical questions about psychotherapy. Can IPT and a behavioral approach with different theoretical underpinnings be efficaciously combined? And is there a contradiction between the usual IPT approach, which emphasizes the benefits of change and encourages patients to make appropriate changes, and the tenor of this adaptation, which tries to standardize and regularize the patient's life, in many respects suggesting that change may exacerbate symptoms?

Frank (personal communication, 1999) emphasizes that IPSRT does encourage patients to make important interpersonal life changes while simultaneously urging regularity of routines and management of social stimulation. For example, a therapist might encourage a patient in an unsatisfying job to seek a new one, but not a job that required rotating shifts and unstable hours.

NOTES

1. This material is provided by Ellen Frank, Ph.D., from the Western Psychiatric Institute and Clinic, Pittsburgh, Pennsylvania.

CHAPTER 17

Primary-Care and Medically Ill Patients

Many patients with psychiatric symptoms and diagnoses present to primary-care and medical settings. Their treatment commands considerable interest and controversy in the current fiscally cautious health-care climate. The prevalence, health impact, and cost of depression for medical patients has been well documented (Barrett et al., 1988; Higgins, 1994). The point prevalence of depression in primary care is estimated at 6–8 percent (Regier et al., 1993). Untreated, depression produces significant medical health costs, social and vocational disability, and adverse effects on the family (Weissman et al., 1997; Wells et al., 1989; World Health Organization, 1996). Official guidelines on the treatment of depression in primary-care settings include psychotherapy (AHCPR guidelines: Depression Guideline Panel, 1993). Recognition and treatment of depression in primary care, evidence for effectiveness of standard approaches, and training of medical personnel to diagnose and treat depression remain scant (Schulberg et al., 1996; Frasure-Smith et al., 1997).

Yet there has also been increasing interest in the treatment of psychiatric disorders complicating medical conditions. This is based on recognition that depression comorbid with cardiovascular disease (Frasure-Smith et al., 1993; Musselman, Evans, and Nemeroff, 1998) and other disorders (Cohen-Cole and Kaufman, 1993) may complicate the course and outcome of the medical condition (e. g., Musselman, Evans, and Nemeroff, 1998; Pratt et al., 1996;

Van Hermert et al., 1993). An important focus of research on psychiatric-treatment delivery to primary-care patients has been its cost-effectiveness: whether the intervention pays for itself ("cost offset") or saves money by reducing other medical costs.

IPT is among the treatments recommended for treating depression in the AHCPR primary-care guidelines. IPT has been tested with little adaptation as a treatment for primary-care patients with major depression, dysthymia, and depressive symptoms (Schulberg et al., 1996; Browne and Steiner, 1996; Lave et al., 1998). IPT has also been adapted and simplified as Interpersonal Counseling (IPC) for use by professionals outside the field of mental health, and tested in primary-care patients (Klerman et al., 1987) and in elderly depressed patients following surgery for hip fracture (Mossey, Knott, and Clark, 1990; Mossey et al., 1996). A further adaptation is being planned by Judd in Melbourne, Australia, which incorporates the use of the *Patient Guide* (see Chapter 24 for a description of the *Patient Guide*).

ADAPTATION FOR PRIMARY CARE

Schulberg et al. (1993, 1996) in Pittsburgh used IPT to treat patients with major depression at academically affiliated ambulatory health centers. Psychiatrists and clinical psychologists provided the treatment. The authors selected IPT for study because their depressed medical outpatients described troublesome interpersonal relationships. No specific adaptations were made to IPT (Weissman and Klerman, 1993).

Browne and Steiner (1997) used IPT to treat dysthymic patients coming to medical health services in southern Ontario and surrounding areas. Therapists were social workers and nurses who had received training in IPT. No adaptations are described. The manual for dysthymic disorder (Markowitz, 1998) was not available at the time of their study, hence its suggested adaptations of IPT for dysthymic disorder (see Chapter 12) were not used. Since marital disputes were frequent in this population, spouses were often involved in sessions, and portions of the conjoint marital IPT manual were used (see Chapter 15).

EFFICACY

The Schulberg et al. study (1996) compared IPT (n=93), nortriptyline (n=91), and physicians' usual care (n=92) over eight months. Patients in IPT were seen weekly for sixteen weeks followed by four monthly continuation sessions for patients showing some response. The time period was selected to conform with AHCPR guidelines for patients with major depression. Depressive symptoms decreased more rapidly and fully among patients randomized to either of the active treatments than among those randomized to physician's usual care. Approximately 70 percent of patients receiving medication or IPT, compared to 20 percent in usual care, were judged recovered at eight months. Patients with comorbid anxiety in all groups took longer to recover but generally showed similar responses to patients diagnosed with major depression alone. Patients with comorbid panic disorder had poorer overall response to all conditions (Brown et al., 1996), although the number of patients with panic disorder was too small to draw definitive conclusions. Antidepressant medication might have been a better choice for patients with comorbid panic disorder and major depressive disorder. IPT has not been used for patients with panic disorder (see Chapter 22). Perhaps CBT, whose efficacy has been demonstrated for panic, would have been more effective, although efficacy studies with this medical population are limited as well.

The cost-effectiveness of the study treatments, nortriptyline and IPT, was evaluated in terms of depression-free days, quality-adjusted days, and cost of care in this study (Lave et al., 1998). On both economic cost and quality-of-life measures, nortriptyline was slightly more cost-effective than IPT, and both did better than usual care. No meaningful cost offsets were found. The cost-effectiveness measures were based on many assumptions and were limited to health-care costs within the medical center. The study by Browne and Steiner illustrates the potential significance of this limitation.

The Steiner et al. study (1996) was even more ambitious (see Chapter 12). More than seven hundred dysthymic patients presenting to medical clinics received either sertraline (n=229), IPT (n=231), or the combination (n=247). Patients received up to twelve sessions of IPT during the first four months of the study. Preliminary results at six months showed that sertraline alone had better compliance than IPT alone, and was equally effective as sertraline with IPT and more effective than IPT alone, as measured by symptom reduction. However, patients who received IPT either alone or in combination with sertraline had economically important containment of or reduction in expenditures from use of health and social services, and there were lower expenditures for those on social assistance. One- and two-year follow-ups are planned to assess the enduring nature of these effects and the impact, if any, on family functioning.

COMMENT

These two studies demonstrate the complexity of determining the cost-effectiveness of treatment. Both clearly demonstrate the value of medication for rapid symptom reduction. This outcome needs to be tempered with the fact that women of childbearing and rearing age constituted the large majority of their patient samples. This demographic fact has two implications. Effective alternatives to medication are needed for many depressed women during pregnancy and nursing. And, since the entire family is usually covered by the primary-care system, studies of health-care costs should take the whole family into account. For example, there is evidence that children of depressed parents have increased rates of early-onset depression, as well as other behavioral problems and substance abuse, in later adolescence (Weissman et al., 1997). Moreover, these offspring have an increased risk of medical problems (Kramer et al., 1998). It is possible, although it has never directly been shown, that successful treatment of the parental depression would reduce the problems in their offspring. Finally, the Browne and Steiner (1997) six-month follow-up showed that cost containment occurred outside the medical system, in a domain absent from the Schulberg study's assessment of cost.

Both studies made valiant efforts to consider long-term effects and costs of treatment, which are important issues for any treatment under consideration for primary care. The use of medically trained or even doctoral-level therapists, as in the Schulberg study, may prove simply too costly for real-world health economics.

There is interest, especially outside the United States, in testing psychological interventions for depressed patients coming to primary care. A large study in Edinburgh, Scotland, is comparing IPT, CBT, and treatment as usual in patients with anxiety and depressive disorders (C. Freeman, Royal Edinburgh Hospital, personal communication, August 1998). An interesting feature of this study is that the effects of early versus late interventions of IPT and of CBT will be evaluated. While all patients will receive sixteen sessions over twenty weeks, sessions in the early-intervention group will start three weeks after referral, and in the late group six months after referral. All patients will receive standard care throughout. The study will include forty patients in each treatment condition and 160 in the usual-care condition.

INTERPERSONAL
COUNSELING (IPC)

Klerman et al. (1987) adapted IPT for routine use in medical settings, employing existing personnel who may not necessarily have mental health training, and treating patients with milder depressive symptoms. To differentiate it from IPT and suggest a lower level of interventions and severity of patients' symptoms, this treatment is called interpersonal counseling (IPC).

ADAPTATION

IPC is a brief treatment of six fifteen- to twenty-minute sessions, with the initial session being longer. Focused on the patient's current psychosocial functioning, IPC is administered by a health-care professional, usually a nurse practitioner without special training in mental health treatment. It is designed for nonpsychiatric patients who are in distress, have symptoms related to current stresses in their lives, but do not have serious concurrent psychiatric disorders or medical conditions. The therapist attends to recent changes in the person's life: events; sources of stress in the family, home, workplace, and friendship patterns; and ongoing difficulties in interpersonal relations. In IPC, it is assumed that such events provide the interpersonal context in which physical and emotional symptoms related to distress, anxiety, and depression occur. Although designed for use in primary-care facilities, IPC may suit other medical settings.

IPC is briefer than IPT in number and duration of sessions. To facilitate use by professionals outside the field of mental health, actual scripts for each session are outlined, and homework has been added to accelerate the process. The IPT manual was used as a general guide in developing the IPC manual (Weissman and Klerman, 1988). Thus, the three phases, the interpersonal inventory, and the problem areas remain unchanged. Forms from the *Patient Guide* workbook (Weissman, 1995) can be used to structure the homework (see Chapter 24). While offered six sessions in the initial contract, patients are not encouraged to use all six sessions if they can work out the presenting problem or feel sufficiently improved with fewer. The IPC manual addresses issues likely to occur in medical settings; for example, differentiating between IPC and ongoing medical responsibility for the patient, and dealing with the emergence of a medical illness.

Treatment requires a recent physical examination to rule out medical illness as the explanation of symptoms and a psychiatric diagnostic interview to rule out serious depression, other psychiatric disorders, and suicidal risk. Scripts describe engaging patients who, despite a negative physical workup, insist that their symptoms are due to a still-undetected physical illness. After a medical illness is ruled out, the nurse or counselor begins:

> Your symptoms [state symptoms: e. g., headaches, sleep problems, fatigue, etc.] don't seem to have a physical basis. The tests are negative. How are you feeling now? Just because there is no physical basis doesn't mean that your symptoms—[your headache, fatigue, etc.]—are not real and that you are feeling well. Stress in your life can also cause these symptoms. Let's review what has been going on in your life.

Patient reactions to this type of exploration may be as follows:

1. The patient may insist that he or she has an undetected physical illness.
2. The patient may remain focused on distressing symptoms—for example, sleep disturbance or fatigue—and deny any possible connection to life stress.
3. The patient may acknowledge a current life stress.

If the patient denies an association, the nurse or counselor avoids coercion or lecturing. If the patient's denial persists, it may be necessary to review the results of physical and laboratory examinations. As in usual clinical practice, a second opinion may reassure the patient. The nurse or counselor is advised to proceed gently, not to get into an argument, and to follow the patient's lead, never denying the reality of the symptoms and the real discomfort they produce. A second visit is offered.

In some cases, it may be appropriate to enter into a negotiation with the patient about perceptions by saying,

> We both agree that you have problems with [state symptoms], but we have different ideas about what is producing them. Can we, working together, see how things go for you and see what we find out over the next few weeks?

CASE EXAMPLE–ROLE DISPUTE
(2 SESSIONS)

Todd, a fifty-two-year-old business executive, came to his doctor with vague somatic complaints including headache, dyspepsia, and muscle and back aches. Physical examination and laboratory tests were negative. A counseling session revealed that symptoms had begun three months before, when a newly hired manager had begun to merge three departments, including Todd's, into one. Todd disagreed with this managerial strategy, felt it reflected poorly on his own performance, but was unable to speak up at staff meetings or individually with the manager. He was at an impasse, largely due to his own reluctance to speak out.

After the first session, when the counselor identified the onset of the symptoms as possibly being related to the hidden dispute with the manager, Todd arranged a meeting with the manager and expressed his concern. In the second session, he expressed relief at knowing that he didn't have a serious physical illness. He reported details of the meeting with the manager, which he felt clarified many issues, and announced that the problem seemed resolved, at least for now.

EFFICACY

Two clinical trials of IPC have been completed, at Harvard and in Philadelphia.

HARVARD STUDY

IPC was first tested treating medical patients with stress symptoms presenting to the Harvard Community Health Plan (Klerman et al., 1987; Weissman and Klerman, 1993). More than five thousand consecutive new enrollees at the Harvard Community Health Plan were sent a General Health Questionnaire (GHQ), a measure widely used in primary-care studies to assess symptoms of distress and mild depression (Goldberg, 1980). Sixty-four patients with elevated GHQ scores were randomized to IPC and compared to sixty-four untreated patients with similarly elevated GHQ scores. Subjects were primarily female (approximately 60 percent), young adults (average age twenty-eight years old), and in good physical health. The GHQ was readministered at the completion of treatment. Patients in IPC were offered a maximum of six sessions. The average number of completed IPC sessions was 3.4. Using previously established scores of 4 or below on the GHQ as an indicator that the patient had no significant emotional symptoms, 83 percent of the IPC group reached this criterion, compared to 63 percent of the comparison group. The difference in these proportions was highly statistically significant. Initial severity of symptoms did not account for these observed effects. The statistical model accounted for 20 percent of the variance in final score, and two-thirds of the final score could be attributed to the IPC intervention.

IPC proved feasible in this primary-care environment. Non-mental-health nurse practitioners easily learned IPC in an eight-hour training program conducted over several months. Nurses were able to counsel several patients whose level of psychiatric stress would normally have resulted in direct referral to specialty mental health care. Over an average of three months, often involving only one or two sessions, IPC patients had significantly greater symptom relief than controls, particularly improvement of depressed mood. However, the following year, IPC led to *greater* rather than reduced use of mental health services by patients newly attuned to the psychological source of their symptoms. The differences in utilization of healthcare services were not statistically significant, and it is possible that the delay in referral to mental health care in the first three months may have yielded initial cost-effectiveness. The findings suggest that IPC did not have a cost offset.

"Subdysthymic" Hospitalized Elderly Patients

Mossey (1990) observed that physical recovery in elderly women surgically treated for hip fractures was impeded by the presence of depressive symptoms that do not meet the threshold criteria for major depression. Accordingly, Mossey and colleagues (1996) conducted a trial of IPC in Philadelphia with elderly hospitalized medically ill patients who had some depressive symptoms. They modified the original IPC manual by increasing the number of sessions from six to ten and their duration from twenty to sixty minutes. They also eased the flexibility of scheduling, shifting from once weekly to a schedule that reflected the medical status of hospitalized patients.

Seventy-six hospitalized patients over the age of sixty, who did not meet criteria for major depression but had depressive symptoms on two consecutive assessments, were randomized either to treatment with IPC, administered by clinical nurse specialists, or to usual care (UC). A control group of euthymic hospitalized patients was also followed. Primary outcomes were reviewed in terms of depressive symptoms, measured on a scale designed for a geriatric population; physical health ratings; and social functioning.

At three months, IPC patients showed greater improvement than UC patients on all outcome variables, although between-group differences did not reach statistical significance. At six months, results revealed a statistically significant difference in the rate of improvement of depressive symptoms for IPC (60.6 percent) relative to UC (35.1 percent). Multivariate analyses controlling for a variety of possible social and medical confounds confirmed a positive treatment effect for depressive symptoms. Similar multivariate analyses showed a statistically significant positive treatment effect on self-rated health but not on physical or social functioning.

IPC appears feasible, acceptable to patients, and effective in reducing mild depressive symptoms and improving self-rated health status. Mossey and colleagues recommended IPC as an intervention for "subdysthymic" hospitalized elderly patients. They felt, however, that ten sessions were insufficient, and that maintenance treatment would be helpful to patients.

COMMENT

IPC, a "slimmed down" version of IPT, has demonstrated efficacy in the treatment of two groups of medical patients. Therapists need not be mental health professionals. While patients with defined psychiatric disorders may well need more intensive treatment, IPC appears to be a helpful brief intervention for patients who may not want formal mental health interventions. The cost-effectiveness of IPC needs to be determined. Like other psychological interventions in primary care, it will probably not demonstrate cost-effectiveness unless investigators include a broader assessment of the cost of nonmedical services and of the effect on the patient's family, particularly on offspring.

Chapter 23, describing IPT for somatization and for patients with physical disabilities, may have related interest to readers.

CHAPTER 18

IPT for Depressed
HIV-Positive Patients
(IPT-HIV)

In 1987, the Centers for Disease Control estimated that more than a million Americans were infected with human immunodeficiency virus (HIV), the virus that causes acquired immunodeficiency syndrome (AIDS) (Centers for Disease Control, 1990). The virus has clearly spread since. When the HIV epidemic emerged in the 1980s, young adults died acutely, at first mysteriously. There were no effective treatments. Thus there was concern that depression would be rampant among those infected: "Who wouldn't be depressed, being HIV-positive?" A group at Cornell University Medical College, including the late Gerald L. Klerman, M.D., the late Samuel W. Perry, M.D., John Markowitz, M.D., and Kathleen Clougherty, M.S.W., tested the efficacy of IPT as an antidepressant treatment for this at-risk population.

The epidemiology of depression among HIV-infected people can only be guessed at. The reason for this is that the epidemiology of HIV infection is itself unknown: there have been no large-scale studies, and most people who are HIV-positive do not yet themselves know it. The prevalence of depression among HIV-positive individuals cannot be known without knowing first who is HIV-positive.

Studies of small samples of HIV-positive patients suggest that most people infected with the virus do not become depressed. Moreover, most of those who do become depressed have histories of depression that predate HIV infection (Markowitz et al., 1994a). Hence, HIV infection seems to be a stressor comparable to other serious medical illness—albeit a severe stressor, with significant social and interpersonal consequences—that may push vulnerable individuals into a depressive episode. In many respects, the treatment of depressed patients with HIV infection thus resembles that of other consultation-liaison interventions for depressed patients with cancer or other medical illness.

Yet HIV infection differs from other medical illness in important respects. No other illness currently carries the stigma of HIV, a stigma probably related to its sexual and injection-drug transmission, and to prejudices against the gay and drug-using subcultures in which it first appeared in this country. It is further feared because of its grim prognosis. Patients with HIV tend to be young, otherwise healthy individuals who discover that their life has suddenly been cut short, that their career and social situation have been irrevocably altered. People with HIV infection have faced discrimination at work and in housing, life insurance, and socialization. Even protease inhibitors, which have furthered the transformation of HIV from an acute death sentence to a chronic and treatable illness, have not erased the fear and stigma surrounding HIV.

DISORDER

Patients treated in the Cornell program who had a minimum twenty-four-item Hamilton Depression Rating Scale (Hamilton, 1960; Ham-D) score of at least 15 were judged clinically depressed. The diagnostician must be careful to rule out HIV-related medical problems that mimic mood disorder (Markowitz et al., 1990). Secondary infection by toxoplasmosis or cryptococcus may present with symptoms resembling a mood disorder, as can medications for the treatment of HIV and its sequelae. HIV itself can cause loss of appetite, weight loss, fatigue, insomnia (due to pain, night sweats, etc.), somatic preoccupation or hypochondriasis, and thoughts about death, items that appear on the Ham-D. Thus, medical and neurological assessment is warranted to rule out medical causes of depression. In practice, however, depressive disorders are usually easy to distinguish from medical syndromes. Indeed, HIV-positive patients often mistakenly attribute to the infection symptoms that in fact reflect depression and that clear with antidepressant treatment.

RATIONALE

Given the scope of the HIV epidemic, there has been shockingly little outcome research on the psychotherapy of HIV-positive patients. Antidepressant medication has demonstrated efficacy for HIV-positive patients with mood disorders (Markowitz et al., 1994a). The work at Cornell, however, is the only individual psychotherapy research addressing depression in HIV-positive individuals. (There are scant reports on group therapy [Kelly et al., 1993; Targ et al., 1994].) The working hypothesis was that since IPT had been efficacious in treating depressed HIV-seronegative patients, it would work for depressed HIV-seropositive patients as well.

A corollary was that IPT dealt with real-life events, of which most HIV-positive patients reported a plethora. HIV creates interpersonal problem areas. HIV-positive patients by definition have a role transition: knowledge of HIV infection alters their life trajectory and perspective on their lives. Most of the study patients came from communities devastated by the HIV epidemic, and had lost so numbing a number of friends, colleagues, and business associates to AIDS that they were at high risk for complicated bereavement. If they had told friends or family of their own infection, they were often rejected; if they had not, there was often tension in the relationship over this secret. Thus, role disputes were also commonplace. Finally, some of these patients also had interpersonal deficits: e.g., some gay men who lacked any intimate relationships had contracted HIV infection through anonymous sex.

At the outset of the study, HIV was an acutely lethal disease rather than the chronic and treatable illness it has become. The investigators were unsure that IPT would treat depression in HIV-infected patients. To their relief, IPT proved to be an efficacious and gratifying treatment.

ADAPTATIONS

Based on work with pilot cases, the Cornell research group developed a treatment manual adapting IPT as a sixteen-week individual treatment for treating HIV-positive patients. Features of this adaptation included:

1. Recognition of the multitude of life events and stressors that accompany HIV infection. Many subjects offered three or even all four interpersonal problem areas as potential foci. Given a surfeit of choices,

therapists focused the therapy on the problem area that appeared most salient to the patient. Because HIV infection inherently provided a role transition, therapists were able to ignore the alternative of interpersonal deficits, the least developed of IPT problem areas.

2. In presenting the IPT formulation to the patient, the therapist linked mood to interpersonal environment as usual. But, having defined depression as a medical illness, the IPT therapist offered this formulation:

> You have *two* medical conditions: depression and HIV infection. Both are treatable, although depression is the easier one to treat. In this sixteen-week treatment, we can work to help you solve your [interpersonal problem area] and at the same time relieve your depression. It's important that you become expert about both these conditions and do what you can to protect yourself from them.

The "sick role" (Parsons, 1951) was thus adapted to encompass both the psychiatric disorder and HIV.

3. As the above formulation suggests, psychoeducation extended beyond depression and its treatments to include HIV and its treatments as well. Although the primary focus of IPT-HIV was depression, not medical treatment of HIV, it was important that therapists know about HIV and its treatment. HIV-positive patients vary in their knowledge of HIV and its treatment, but even individuals with sophisticated knowledge frequently harbor distortions about their condition. For background reading, a text such as Kalichman's (1995) is recommended.

4. Within the framework of the interpersonal problem areas of grief or role transition, therapists helped patients to address anticipatory mourning of their own deaths, whether imminent or not. *Mourning of one's own AIDS-related death was almost inevitably an issue, even if not the focus of therapy: as such, role transitions were unavoidably present for seropositive patients.* At the same time, IPT was used to mobilize some patients who had prematurely given themselves up for dead:

> You're acting as if you're mourning your own death, as if your life is over. Yet you have no symptoms of physical illness, and may not have

any for years. What you're suffering from is depression, which is making your life seem hopeless and ended. But in fact you have options, and depression is treatable. Let's talk about what you can do to make the most of your life.

5. Role disputes not infrequently raised the issue of social transgressions (Markowitz et al., 1993; see Chapter 4): instances where people break written or unwritten social codes. A transgression, usually a breach of trust, gives its victims the right to some sort of justice, or at least an apology. Some patients reported lethal instances of transgressions, wherein a sexual partner had known of his infectious status but failed to inform or to change behavior patterns that endangered his mate. Therapists addressed this as a moral outrage, using the situation to mobilize depressed patients to express appropriate anger at the transgressors. This often helped to resolve the role dispute and to relieve the depression.

6. Although HIV infection represents a serious and seemingly objectively bad role transition, IPT-HIV still focused on the positive possibilities that any role transition provides. One silver lining to the lethal cloud is the increased value HIV infection places on however much time the patient has left in life. IPT-HIV therapists encouraged patients to "live out your fantasies," which many of them did. Many were willing to take the sorts of chances in their lives that therapists generally encourage patients to take, but which the patients are often reluctant to risk.

7. IPT therapists had to address their own concerns about conducting a treatment that would terminate after sixteen weeks with fatally infected patients who might shortly die. In fact, however, most HIV-positive subjects who entered treatment felt a time pressure that fit with the brief therapy model. They wanted quick results, not long-term therapy. This time pressure seemed to catalyze treatment, as patients, feeling they had little to lose, made extraordinary changes in their lives in a matter of weeks.

The explicit goal was to "make the most of however much time you have left": to make precious time count. Although longevity varies widely, the average individual survives for more than a decade after HIV infection. Therapists encouraged subjects to live out their fantasies; the latter were often willing to try, and often delighted by their success.[1] Sicker subjects often spoke of leaving a mark on people or institutions they were involved with, and developed realistic strategies to pursue this aim.

8. Although most subjects entered treatment protocols with few current HIV-related symptoms, some became ill and required medical hospitalization during the sixteen-week intervention. When this occurred, therapists made every effort to call and visit them in the hospital. When possible, they conducted IPT sessions despite the hospitalization. This therapeutic support, at a moment when the patient's worst fears appeared to be materializing, tended to cement the therapeutic alliance.

CASE EXAMPLE

Benjamin, a thirty-three-year-old commercial artist, reported having been depressed for more than a year and a half. He had had a meteoric career, achieving early professional and financial success. He had a monogamous relationship with a seronegative younger man with whom he practiced safe sex. After testing HIV-positive, Benjamin made halfhearted attempts to continue his career, but he and his lover soon retreated from city life to a house in the country. There he spent the next year, accumulating debt and awaiting death, although he was physically asymptomatic. He smoked marijuana daily. He reported a depressed and anxious mood worst in the morning, early and mid-insomnia, decreased appetite with weight loss, low libido, poor concentration, hypochondriacal concerns that every skin freckle might be Kaposi's sarcoma, and passive suicidal ideation. His Ham-D score was 26.

Benjamin generally felt comfortable with his lover, but some tensions in the relationship had been exacerbated by knowledge of his HIV infection. He also reported having lost more than a hundred acquaintances to AIDS, including most of his business contacts: feeling "numbed," he had ceased attending funerals. He felt hopelessly cut off from what had been a satisfying life.

Benjamin's therapist formulated his case as a role transition, a difficulty in navigating the changes that knowledge of HIV infection had brought. Therapy focused on his marijuana use, which he ceased, and mobilizing from avoidance to action. Benjamin assembled his remaining friends to provide needed emotional and financial support. After some preparatory role play, he spoke to his lover about their difficulties and particularly about the role of HIV in their serodiscordant relationship. He also developed a new artistic portfolio and began to reestablish business connections. His Ham-D score fell to 4. He also took an interest in his medical status and, still asymptomatic, looked into appropriate treatment trials for his future.

EFFICACY

In an initial open trial in the mid-1980s, Markowitz, Klerman, and Perry treated twenty-three subjects who met clinical criteria for DSM-III-R (9) major depression or dysthymia. Most were white (70 percent) men (78 percent) whose risk behavior was gay or bisexual unprotected sexual contact (74 percent). In sixteen sessions, twenty (87 percent) subjects remitted. Five patients whose cases were videotaped for supervision with Dr. Klerman significantly improved on the Ham-D: from 25.8 (± 7.5 s.d.) at baseline, to 13.0 (± 6.5) at mid-treatment, to 6.8 (± 5.3) at termination (p>.01). Not only did symptoms abate, but many subjects made dramatic changes in social situations, careers, and lifestyles. And, rather than becoming demoralized by their subjects' dismal situations, therapists were gratified by what turned out to be deeply moving work with brave, daring patients.

The pilot study led to an NIMH-funded, four-cell study based on the model of the NIMH Treatment of Depression Collaborative Research Program (TDCRP, Elkin et al., 1989). Led by the late Samuel Perry, M.D., this study randomized HIV-positive depressed subjects to treatment with (1) IPT, (2) CBT (Beck et al., 1979), (3) supportive psychotherapy (SP), or (4) SP with the antidepressant medication imipramine (IMI/SP). All treatments were codified in manuals, and therapy sessions were audio- or videotaped to assure adherence (Markowitz et al., 1994b). Supportive psychotherapy was a non-interpersonal, non-cognitive, quasi-Rogerian psychotherapy (Rogers, 1951) delivered by empathic, skilled therapists. It was envisioned as an active control, not a nontreatment.

A preliminary report comparing subjects in the IPT (n=16) and SP (n=16) cells found IPT clinically and statistically superior on both Ham-D and BDI scales (Markowitz et al., 1995). The researchers hypothesized that both therapies would reduce depressive symptoms, but that IPT-HIV, as a specifically antidepressant psychotherapy, would have greater efficacy than the more generic SP. It should be noted that comparisons between two effective treatments have rarely yielded significant differences, particularly with the relatively small cell sizes involved here.

The thirty-two subjects, sixteen in each cell, were demographically similar. As in the pilot study, they were mainly male (88 percent) and gay or bisexual (84 percent); but, reflecting changes in the HIV epidemic, only 56 percent were white, with 25 percent Hispanic and 19 percent Black. Inclusion criteria required known HIV infection for at least six months (to rule out adjustment disorders resulting from learning of seropositivity), a score of at least 15 on the twenty-four-item Hamilton Depression Rating Scale (Hamilton, 1960), and clinical impression of DSM-III-R major depression or dysthymic disorder. Physical health had to permit attending sessions; most but not all subjects were in CDC stages II–III (Centers for Disease Control, 1987), i.e., relatively asymptomatic at entry. Exclusion criteria were: significant non-HIV-related medical disease, schizophrenia, bipolar disorder, other contraindication to imipramine, current substance abuse, significant cognitive impairment (assessed by Mini-Mental Status Examination [Folstein et al., 1975] score >24) or disability, inability to speak English, and concurrent psychiatric treatment aside from HIV-related self-help or support groups.

Analyses using last-observation-carried-forward and completer analyses showed that scores decreased significantly on Ham-D and BDI for both treatments. Statistically significant differential improvement for IPT appeared by mid-treatment (Week 8) on Ham-D and BDI and persisted at termination. For IPT-HIV, Ham-D fell from 19.8 (± 4.8) at entry to 9.9 (± 6.2) at midpoint and 6.4 (± 5.7) at termination; for SP, comparable scores were 20.7 (± 5.8) at baseline, 14.3 (± 4.5) at midpoint, and 11.9 (± 6.2) at termination. On the BDI, entry, midpoint, and termination scores were 27.6, 11.8, and 10.6 for IPT-HIV, versus 26.1, 21.3, and 19.5 for SP.

Serum CD4 count fell nonsignificantly for both groups. On the 100-point Karnofsky scale (Karnofsky, 1949), administered by independent raters to assess subjects' physical functioning, scores of physical functioning increased significantly for IPT subjects (n=13), from 80.7 ± 4.0 at baseline to 91.8 ± 4.7 at termination (p>.001), while remaining essentially unchanged for SP subjects (n=14, baseline 79.1 ± 4.8; termination 81.2 ± 6.4).

Data on the full sample of 101 randomized subjects indicate that IPT and IMI/SP tended to cluster with similarly low outcome scores, whereas CBT and SP alone showed less improvement. In the intent-to-treat analysis, IPT and IMI/SP were each superior to CBT, with SP a distant but not statistically different third. On BDI, IMI/SP was superior to CBT and SP, and IPT superior to SP. Similar findings were found for the completer cells (Markowitz et al., 1998). Neither Axis I nor Axis II comorbidity, route of infection, nor other demographic factors affected treatment outcome. Inasmuch as most study participants (85 percent) were men, the efficacy of IPT-HIV for women remains unknown. HIV-positive women, a growing subset of individuals with HIV, may face different psychosocial stressors than men (Swartz et al., 1997; see note 1).

COMMENT

This study is the only published research on individual psychotherapy of depressed HIV-positive patients. Its findings resemble those among more severely depressed patients in the NIMH TDCRP study (Elkin et al., 1989), on whose design this research was based. This is the rare study that finds differences among active psychotherapies, even when the less efficacious therapies were associated with diminished symptoms over time. The somewhat surprising disparity between IPT and CBT in this study may reflect the fact that IPT acknowledges the patient's distress at painful life events but then optimistically and pragmatically helps the patient to move on and make the best of the future. This approach may address perfectly the dilemma in which depressed HIV-positive patients find themselves. In contrast, CBT therapists faced the awkward task of, in essence, encouraging patients not to exaggerate cognitive and emotional responses to an extremely difficult situation.

IPT appears useful as a treatment for HIV-positive depressed patients, a severely stressed population with a stigmatizing illness. IPT produced statistically and clinically significant gains over and above those of other helpful therapies—an unusual finding in itself. The results also indicate utility of brief interventions for a medically at-risk population, and the ability of the optimistic, action-oriented IPT approach to find a silver lining in even such a grave situation.

NOTES

1. The idea of living out fantasies seems benign so long as it does not jeopardize the lives of others. For gay men, this mainly requires attention to "safe sex" procedures. For HIV-positive women, however, another dilemma arises.

One important fantasy, and perhaps an attempt at immortality, is to have a child. Women from constrained educational, economic, and social circumstances, infected through injection-drug use or sexual relationships with injection-drug users, may have few other opportunities for self-expression. Yet to have a child who may inherit HIV via vertical transmission, or who even if HIV-negative may grow up an orphan, presents a complex moral dilemma. Research indicates that mothers who follow an AZT protocol can reduce the risk of vertical transmission by two-thirds (E. M. Connor, et al. 1994. Reduction of maternal-infant transmission of human immunodeficiency virus type 1 with zidovudine treatment. *N. Engl. J. Med.* 331:1173–1180).

See also Chapter 19 for case description.

CHAPTER 19

Depressed Ante- and Postpartum Patients

DISORDER

DSM-IV recognizes childbirth as a possible precipitant of major depressive episodes, using the specifier "... with postpartum onset" if the episode begins within four weeks of delivery (American Psychiatric Association, 1994). There is no separate classification for depression occurring during pregnancy. IPT has been adapted for depressed women during pregnancy and the postpartum period, but not to other postpartum disturbances such as bipolar disorder or brief psychotic disorder.

Although conventional wisdom deems pregnancy a time of calm expectation and happiness, about 10 percent of pregnant women develop a major or minor depressive episode (Spinelli, 1997a). Predisposing factors include a personal or family history of depression; marital problems; single parenthood; a large number of children; young age; and low education. Depressed pregnant women are at increased risk for poor health habits, including drug, alcohol, and nicotine use, and failure to obtain adequate prenatal care. Pregnant depressed women have an increased risk after childbirth of child abuse and neglect and postpartum depression. Numerous studies have shown that the offspring of depressed mothers face high risk for onset of prepubertal anxiety disorders, major depression in adolescence, substance abuse in late adolescence and young adulthood, as well as greater medical and school problems (Weissman et al., 1997; Wickramaratne and Weissman, 1999; Kramer et al., 1998). These problems persist over generations.

RATIONALE

Psychotherapy is a potentially important treatment for depression during pregnancy and postpartum periods because women of childbearing years are the group at highest risk for depression across diverse cultures (Weissman et al., 1996—Cross National Study; O'Hara et al., 1984). The postpartum period further increases the risk of depression (Murray and Cooper, 1997; Gotlib and Whiffen, 1989; Whiffen, 1988). Pharmacotherapy during pregnancy has potential teratogenetic risk (American Academy of Pediatrics, 1994), as most antidepressant medications cross the placenta; the few studies examining their fetal effects have been inconclusive (Chambers et al., 1996; Pastuszak et al., 1993; Koren, 1994; Nulman et al., 1997). Moreover, medication may carry the risk of behavioral morbidity for the fetus. The fetus develops behavioral responses quite early in gestation. It responds to external sounds from at least twenty weeks, and can produce its own hormonal and other stress responses from mid-gestation (Glover, 1997). We know little about the long-term effects on the offspring of maternal stress or depression during pregnancy.

Depression during pregnancy and the postpartum period may be related to dramatic somatic and endocrinological changes or the presence of a newborn, either of which can be major life stressors. Like pregnant women, mothers who wish to breast-feed their babies have reason to avoid antidepressant medication, again indicating the potential utility of psychosocial treatments such as IPT. In IPT terms, the peripartum period is a major role transition in which role disputes often occur.

ADAPTATION FOR
ANTEPARTUM DEPRESSION

Spinelli (1997b) has developed a manual for IPT in antepartum depression at Columbia University. It makes few changes to the basic IPT approach, but its content relates specifically to pregnancy. For example, role transition focuses on the pregnant woman's evaluation of herself as a parent, the physiologic changes of pregnancy, and altered relationships with spouse, significant other, or other children. A fifth problem area, "complicated pregnancy," has been added. Women with unplanned pregnancies may mourn their loss of freedom to work or finish school, or may have a dispute with a spouse or significant other. Timing and duration of sessions require flexibility around bed rest, delivery, obstetrical complications, and child care. Young children may be brought to sessions, and postpartum mothers may breast-feed during sessions. Telephone sessions and hospital visits may be necessary. During the initial phase of therapy, in addition to the review of depressive symptoms, a review of symptoms and discomfort associated with pregnancy is undertaken. The therapist inquires about hostile feelings toward the fetus, including thoughts of infanticide: "Do you worry that you might hurt your baby?"

In pursuing the interpersonal inventory, the therapist inquires about the circumstances of the conception and pregnancy, feelings about the pregnancy and about the baby's father. Problem areas are the same as in standard IPT. Grief reactions can include grief over perinatal loss, either in the past or currently. Maternal grief over the lost fetus is facilitated by a review of her wishes, expectations, and fantasies about the baby. For example, the mother may blame herself for the death of the fetus.

CASE EXAMPLE

Karen was a healthy thirty-six-year-old married woman whose first and much-desired pregnancy had resulted in a miscarriage at four months. She presented quite depressed in the fourth month of her new pregnancy. She reminisced about the circumstances of the miscarriage, blamed herself for continuing with her job, for getting insufficient sleep, and for waiting until her late thirties to conceive. She felt she would never be a good mother. Hidden in her grief reaction at the loss of her first pregnancy was a dispute with her husband, who had wanted to delay having children until they had greater financial stability.

Pregnancy can be framed as a role transition characterized by both physical transformation and the life changes pregnancy produces. Role disputes often involve the baby's father, disorders of the mother-infant relationship, and recall of old disputes with the family of origin. Role disputes also encompasses difficulty in bonding with the fetus, particularly in the case of an unwanted pregnancy. Interpersonal deficits may address situations leading to an unwanted pregnancy or anticipated problems in interacting with a child. A fifth problem area, complicated pregnancy, includes problems arising from concurrent life events, obstetrical difficulties, physical illness (e.g., diabetes, HIV, cardiac disease), gestational circumstances such as rape, abandonment, or unwanted pregnancy; or alternatively, infertility and use of new reproductive technologies.

CASE EXAMPLE

Lanie, a forty-two-year-old primipara, finally became pregnant after six years of infertility treatment, including artificial insemination and in vitro fertilization. The highly valued fetus was the source of great anxiety: would it survive? While she presented depressed, anxious, and concerned about the viability of the fetus, Lanie's underlying worry was about the technology. Since the sperm was not her husband's, what effect would this have on her marriage? Would her husband bond with the baby?

EFFICACY

Spinelli (1997a) completed a sixteen-week open trial with thirteen pregnant women meeting DSM-III-R criteria for major depression. Mean depression scores on both clinician and self-rating instruments decreased significantly in treatment. Timing and duration of sessions required flexibility around issues of bed rest, delivery, and child care. Young children were often brought to sessions, and after delivery the infants were brought as well.

Based on this open study, Spinelli has undertaken a controlled clinical trial comparing IPT to a didactic parent education group, treating fifty depressed pregnant women weekly over sixteen weeks of acute treatment, then monthly for six months. This study will provide an empirical basis for treatment guidelines for depressed pregnant women who might otherwise need medication (Spinelli, 1997).

Swartz and colleagues (1997) reported the case of a depressed pregnant HIV-positive woman who received four months of IPT. Her major problem areas were role transition (pregnancy, unemployment, HIV infection) and a dispute with the baby's father. IPT concentrated on the role dispute, which was at an impasse. IPT helped the patient to focus on her current situation and to obtain more help from the child's father, easing her burden and helping her plan for the baby's future in the event of her own death. Anger toward the boyfriend who had infected her was framed as a transgression (see Chapter 4): he had violated the rules of their relationship by not disclosing his HIV status. She explicitly discussed this with him and refused to have unprotected sex. She thus gained mastery over a difficult situation and was able to enjoy her child. Depressive symptoms improved: Ham-D score fell from 18 at intake to 2 at termination. The patient remained euthymic at three-month follow-up, but showed recurrent symptoms a year later, despite continuing interpersonal gains.

ADAPTATION FOR
POSTPARTUM DEPRESSION

Emotional problems following childbirth are common. Blues in the first few weeks after childbirth are so common—it has been estimated that about half of new mothers experience them—that they have been termed "the new-baby blues." About 10–15 percent of new mothers experience a more serious and enduring depression. They may worry excessively about their newborn and feel inadequate as caretakers. Some fear they will harm their baby. About one in a thousand new mothers has a psychotic episode with confusion, delusions, and rapid mood shifts, usually occurring in the first few postpartum weeks and often requiring hospitalization. Delusions usually center on the baby. The causes and distinctiveness of postpartum depression and psychosis are unclear. Depression in the postpartum period is associated with both family and personal history of unipolar and/or bipolar depression.

O'Hara and Stuart at the University of Iowa have adapted IPT for postpartum depression. They report that depressed postpartum women often attribute mood changes and symptoms such as anhedonia and low motivation to "normal" changes after childbirth, or to "difficult" children. As a consequence, many postpartum women with significant symptoms of depression underreport their difficulties. As in pregnancy, depressive symptoms such as insomnia and lack of energy resemble changes that women normally experience postpartum. The clinician must also assess the patient's expectations about motherhood and her feelings regarding her child and their relationship. History obtained should also include the planning and course of the pregnancy and the labor and delivery process.

O'Hara and Stuart have found it useful to conceptualize most cases of postpartum depression as role transitions. This problem area provides a rationale for postpartum patients to understand their problems and makes intuitive sense to most patients. In addition, it implies that the depression will be time-limited.

Role transitions in the postpartum period typically involve the need to develop new parenting skills and manage new responsibilities while attempting to maintain old relationships. A patient may find herself having to juggle several different roles, each with increasing demands. Decreased self-esteem often results, as well as confusion over which relationships and responsibilities deserve priority. Although the patient rarely loses her familiar social supports entirely, they often must be greatly modified.

An example of a role transition in the postpartum period is a working woman who now faces the role of mother in addition to her previous roles of spouse and employee. The patient may become overwhelmed if she is unable to reconfigure her priorities, time, and emotional commitments. A difficult spouse or employer could easily exacerbate the problems such a patient faces. O'Hara and Stuart's strategy is to help the patient to understand the types of relationships she has with her spouse and her employer, and understand her expectations about those relationships. The patient develops a balanced view of her needs and the degree to which they are to be met. The therapist then assists the patient to clearly communicate her needs to significant others and to renegotiate the relationships.

The patient must recognize that others in her interpersonal sphere have also undergone significant role transitions. The husband or significant other may also make substantial adjustments in assuming the role of father. The same is true to a lesser degree for extended-family members. As the patient begins to appreciate that others face a transition as well, she is able to shift from a blaming stance to one of active negotiation with her significant other.

Interpersonal disputes are frequently associated with depression in postpartum women. Typical conflicts involve disputes between the patient and her husband regarding child care responsibilities, and conflicts with extended-family members over the patient's management of her newborn. Therapists should thoroughly explore the expectations the patient had prior to delivery as well as examining the communication patterns in the conflict.

O'Hara and Stuart suggest including the patient's husband or significant other in one or two therapy sessions when role transitions or interpersonal disputes are the treatment focus. The purpose is to obtain ancillary information about the patient's behavior, examining in detail the point of view of the other party in the dispute, and allowing the therapist to examine "in vivo" interactions between the partners. Conjoint sessions provide an opportunity for psychoeducation of the partner as well. This often involves information not only about depression but about normal sexual changes and sexuality during the postpartum period.

CASE EXAMPLE

Margaret, a twenty-nine-year-old primiparous woman, sought treatment for depression after a normal pregnancy and delivery. She complained of a depressed mood, difficulty sleeping, poor appetite, low energy, guilt feelings, and low self-esteem. During her pregnancy, she had held a teaching position and a research assistantship, had begun work on her doctoral dissertation, and had anticipated continuing all of these after delivery. Following the birth of her child, she could no longer keep up the work on her dissertation and felt great pressure from her adviser. Her method of coping was to pour her energies into her relationship with her child.

Treatment focused initially on educating Margaret about normal postpartum experiences and helping her to appreciate that her expectations might have been unrealistic. The therapist defined her problem as a role transition and suggested that she could gradually adapt to the situation and resume her previous high level of functioning, albeit with some modifications. She was encouraged to adjust some of her interpersonal relationships: she negotiated with her husband over child care and housework responsibilities she had previously managed alone, freeing time for herself and for her dissertation work. She was also able to confront her adviser about the pressure she felt, arranging a more realistic schedule for completion of her academic work.

EFFICACY

O'Hara and Stuart compared IPT to a waiting-list control in 120 women with postpartum depression. The acute treatment trial lasted twelve weeks, with an eighteen-month follow-up. They assessed both the mothers' symptom states and their interactions with their infants (Stuart and O'Hara, 1995). Preliminary results indicate the superiority of IPT: 44 percent of the IPT group, but only 14 percent of the waiting-list group, showed remission on the Beck Depression Inventory (BDI) (Stuart, O'Hara, and Blehar, 1998; Stuart, personal communication, 1998). Sixty percent of IPT patients, versus 16 percent of controls, showed a greater than 50 percent reduction on the BDI. Women receiving IPT also showed significant improvement in measures of social adjustment relative to the control group.

See Chapter 13 for a description of an IPT study of depressed pregnant adolescents.

ADAPTATION FOR POSTPARTUM DEPRESSION
IN A GROUP FORMAT

Klier at the University of Vienna in Austria has adapted IPT in a twelve-session group format for women with postpartum depression. The content of IPT is unchanged, but it focuses on problems linked to the postpartum period. The initial evaluation period, the first two sessions, and the last session are held individually. In the initial phase, the mother is educated about the course of depression occurring during this period. There are nine additional ninety-minute weekly group sessions. There are three-, six-, and twelve-month follow-ups.

Thus far, seventeen women ages eighteen to forty-five with a diagnosis of major depression during the past year have been enrolled. Role disputes were the most common interpersonal problem area, followed by role transitions. Themes that emerged during the sessions included birth trauma, body changes and sexuality, breast-feeding, disputes with parents, stigma of depression, and negative feelings toward the infant. Klier notes the reluctance of postpartum depressed mothers to enter treatment, a problem that may be unique to Austria. The work is ongoing (Klier, Muzik, and Rosenblum, 1998), but 65 percent of subjects (n=17) completed the group treatment. Endpoint analysis revealed a significant decrease in mean Ham-D scores, with full remission reached by 58 percent of the women, and partial remission by 35 percent (C. Klier, personal communication, 1999).

Stuart and O'Hara in Iowa used group IPT as a preventive treatment for pregnant women who had either depressive symptoms or a family or personal history of depressive episodes. Forty-five pregnant women were assigned to either five sessions of group IPT, starting in late pregnancy and continuing until one month postpartum, or to a no-treatment control group. At one month postpartum, none of the IPT patients and 25 percent of the controls were depressed; at six months postpartum, 15 percent of the IPT patients and 24 percent of the control patients were depressed. Yet when measured by the patients' self-report, depressive symptoms did not differ at either assessment (Stuart, O'Hara, and Blehar, 1998).

COMMENT

These studies of depressed women during and after pregnancy reach women at a time when they are vulnerable but also amenable to change. These interventions have the potential to prevent depressive episodes. If successful, treatment of depressed mothers could influence the care and well-being of newborns as well as other offspring. Weissman at Columbia is conducting a pilot study of IPT treatment for depressed mothers who are bringing their children for treatment. The study will directly test the hypothesis that treating the mother has beneficial effects on the next generation. Many of the IPT studies of depression have treated women of child-bearing years. The high risk and serious consequences of depression on their own functioning and that of their offspring deserve notice. Routine assessment for depression and treatment when needed should be a routine part of care for these women.

NOTES

The authors acknowledge the assistance of Drs. Margaret Spinelli, Michael O'Hara, and Scott Stuart, who provided their expertise and case examples on antepartum (Dr. Spinelli) and postpartum (Drs. O'Hara and Stuart) depression.

PART THREE
ADAPTATION OF IPT FOR
NON-MOOD DISORDERS

CHAPTER 20

Substance Use Disorders

DISORDER

Substance-related disorders are divided into two groups: *dependence* and *abuse* of substances such as alcohol, opiates, cocaine, and nicotine. DSM-IV (American Psychiatric Association, 1994) defines substance *abuse* as maladaptive use that leads to clinically significant impairment or distress. Substance *dependence* escalates the problem to include tolerance and withdrawal, and involves impairment of major role obligations, physical danger, legal problems, and the like.

BACKGROUND

IPT has been tested in two controlled trials for patients suffering from substance abuse or dependence. One used IPT to reduce psychopathology in methadone-maintained opiate addicts, the other to try to achieve cocaine abstinence. Both trials had negative outcomes for IPT relative to a standard comparison treatment. These are the only negative studies of IPT to date. Other applications are possible, however. Markowitz and colleagues are currently comparing IPT to supportive psychotherapy in conjunction with Alcoholics Anonymous (AA) attendance as a treatment for patients diagnosed with comorbid dysthymic disorder and alcohol abuse.

Because opiates and cocaine are illegal, it is difficult to estimate the precise epidemiology of their abuse, but estimates exceed 2 million Americans.

311

Only one-third or fewer are dependent or addicted, and still fewer are receiving treatment for their substance problems. Most individuals who seek treatment have failed in numerous attempts to stop on their own. Treatments include inpatient programs, which sequester the patient from access to drugs; and pharmacotherapy, including maintenance on an agonist similar to the abused drug (e.g., methadone or levo-alpha-acetyl-methadol [LAAM] for opiate-addicted patients), taking an antagonist that blocks drug effect (e.g., naltrexone), medications that produce aversive symptoms with drug-taking (e.g., disulfiram), and medications that reduce withdrawal symptoms (e.g., clonidine). Psychotherapy of some type is usually part of the treatment program as at least an adjunct to pharmacotherapy (Bigelow and Preston, 1995).

RATIONALE

The rationale for using IPT for these patients is based on the assumption that substance abuse either represents an attempt to compensate for inadequate interpersonal skills or may erode existing skills. Substance abuse often leads to—and is partly defined by—interpersonal difficulties in social and vocational functioning. Helping patients to solve interpersonal problems and to develop new skills might be expected to alleviate distress and perhaps reduce the need for substance use. In the IPT/methadone study, the investigators hoped that patients whose craving for opiates was reduced by methadone would be more likely to engage in psychotherapy.

ADAPTATIONS

Rounsaville and Carroll (1993) distinguish between using IPT as an adjunctive treatment, as they did in their first study with opioid-addicted patients maintained on methadone, and using it as a sole intervention or combined treatment aimed at achieving abstinence, as in their treatment of intravenous cocaine abusers. They describe their adaptations of IPT for substance abuse as relatively minor. The context of the sessions was geared to the particular problems of substance abusers. The focus was switched from treating depressive symptoms to the reduction or elimination of substance abuse. The emphasis on developing better social and interpersonal coping strategies was retained.

Three goals were developed for stopping substance abuse: (1) acceptance of the need to stop; (2) management of impulsivity; and (3) recognition of the context of drug use and supply. The first goal addresses the patient's denial of the severity of the problem and his or her ambivalence about stopping drug use. It requires the therapist to catalogue in detail and to point out to the patient the costs and destructiveness of drug use. The second goal requires new skills and social supports in order to delay immediate gratification. This may involve support from twelve-step programs as well as from the therapist. The third goal is to confront the patient's involvement in a substance milieu: the need to avoid certain individuals, social situations, and other triggers of substance use.

Seeing substance abuse as an attempt to cope with social problems, the IPT therapist points out both the importance of substance abuse in handling interpersonal situations and its limitations. For example, drugs might be used to escape the dysphoric affect of a difficult role transition or difficulty with social skills. Understanding how the patient uses drugs to handle feelings about significant others is expected to provide a rationale for developing alternative coping strategies. The interpersonal inventory includes exploration of the history of drug use, the context of use and family reaction to it, and the influence of drugs on the patient's perception of sexual behavior and intimacy, as well as the behaviors necessary to obtain and finance drug use, and illegal behaviors and risks. The usual IPT problem areas were used.

Since most patients in drug programs relapse during the course of treatment, this possibility is discussed early in IPT. IPT does not terminate with drug relapse. Rather, while viewed as undesirable, the relapse is framed as an opportunity to understand problem areas that can be worked on in treatment.

CASE EXAMPLE

Jenny, a fifty-six-year-old married woman, presented with the symptoms of dysthymic disorder and chronic alcohol abuse. She reported having been married for twenty-four years to her second husband in a relationship that was intellectually stimulating but emotionally and physically distant. Jenny's husband, Harry, a recovered alcoholic, spent most of his day apart from her. This had been less problematic when she worked as a fashion industry executive, but had bothered her more since she had lost her job, in part due to depression and drinking, seven years before. Her alcohol use had subsequently increased to a minimum of three drinks a day, and often far more. She now had occasional blackouts, without seizures or clear medical complications from alcohol. She also self-medicated with diazepam.

Jenny's therapist suggested that her drinking might have started as a failed attempt at self-medication for her dysthymic mood and had now developed into a second psychiatric problem. He further suggested that there seemed to be a connection between exacerbations in Jenny's drinking and her marital frustrations. They focused on the role dispute between Jenny and Harry, in which she wanted greater intimacy and he sought to maintain distance. Indeed, a charting of her drinking revealed that she drank more after being frustrated or disappointed by Harry. Jenny refused to attend Alcoholics Anonymous meetings but did stop drinking and diazepam use in the early weeks of treatment. With role playing in sessions, she grew more assertive in confronting Harry and achieved some concessions: he did spend considerably more time with her, if not always enough for her needs. Her mood improved and dysthymic symptoms remitted. As termination approached, she began to take on the next challenge, the resumption of their dormant sex life.

EFFICACY

IPT has not demonstrated efficacy in two clinical trials with substance-abuse patients. In the first study, complicated by high attrition, Rounsaville et al. (1983) at Yale found no benefit for adjunctive weekly IPT for six months compared to low-contact treatment, a twenty-minute monthly meeting in which only the patients' depressive symptoms and social functioning were reviewed. All seventy-two patients were opiate abusers who had been maintained on methadone for at least three months prior to entering the trial. All patients received standard methadone maintenance treatment, which included weekly ninety-minute group counseling. Outcomes included illicit drug use, dropout, symptoms, and social functioning.

Recruitment for and retention in IPT was poor. Of twelve major outcome measures, only two differed significantly, one favoring IPT and one favoring the low-contact condition. Most patients in both treatments showed significant clinical improvement during the six months. No differences were found on follow-up after two and a half years (Rounsaville et al., 1986).

In a separate trial, the same research team found twelve weeks of IPT ineffective or marginally worse than Relapse Prevention, a behavioral treatment, for forty-two cocaine abusers attempting to achieve abstinence (Carroll, Rounsaville, and Gawin, 1992).

COMMENT

The investigators describe numerous reasons why the six-month study for opiate-addicted, methadone-maintained patients failed to show a treatment effect for IPT (Rounsaville et al., 1983). Most important was the fact that all patients were already receiving ninety minutes of weekly group counseling and were reluctant to spend more time in treatment. This was reflected in the difficulties the investigators had in recruiting patients for and retaining them in the study. Subjects had also had time to stabilize on methadone prior to entering the study, relieving cravings and dysphoria and lessening the motivation for psychotherapy. Other issues concerned administrative difficulties of the program.

The investigators did not question the assumption underlying the adaptation of IPT, namely, that drugs were used in a dysfunctional attempt to deal with interpersonal problems. An alternative hypothesis is that drug use had serious consequences for interpersonal relationships and that the addict's efforts to eliminate drug use through sustained methadone maintenance and the accompanying program participation may have obviated the need for additional services. However, a study of a similar drug-using population by Woody et al. (1983, 1985) in Philadelphia, comparing drug counseling alone versus its combination with either supportive-expressive psychotherapy or with CBT, found that both psychotherapy groups showed greater improvement than the drug program alone. On the other hand, the recent NIDA Collaborative Cocaine Study, presented at the American Psychiatric Association Annual Meeting in May 1998, found drug counseling more effective than either supportive-expressive psychotherapy or CBT. In the Philadelphia study, however, drug counseling was integrated into the drug treatment program, was less intensive and time-consuming than in the Yale program, and began at the same time as methadone maintenance, when depressive symptoms were highest. Finally, it is possible that the supportive-expressive psychotherapy used by Woody and colleagues was more effective than IPT.

We cannot conclude that IPT has any efficacy in treating patients with substance abuse or dependence. The two negative IPT studies suggest limits to the utility of IPT, but do not necessarily preclude its use for all substance-abuse patients. For example, IPT might be useful for newly abstinent recovering alcohol-dependent patients, who face numerous psychosocial stressors that have been shown to precipitate relapse (Cherry and Markowitz, 1996).

CHAPTER 21

Eating Disorders: Bulimia and Anorexia Nervosa

BULIMIA NERVOSA

Bulimia nervosa is defined in DSM-IV (American Psychiatric Association, 1994) by recurrent episodes of binge eating, accompanied by a perceived loss of control over eating during the episode, and followed by recurrent inappropriate compensatory behavior such as self-induced vomiting or misuse of laxatives, fasting, or excessive exercise.

IPT has been used in two acute clinical trials for bulimia. In the first, Fairburn at Oxford University used IPT as an individual treatment for bulimia without significant adaptation to the particularities of the disorder. Beyond some initial psychoeducation, eating problems were *not* addressed in the psychotherapy (Fairburn et al., 1991, 1993; Fairburn, 1998). The other study was the first attempt to use IPT as a group therapy for any psychiatric diagnosis (Wilfley et al., 1993).

RATIONALE

Bulimia is a prevalent and morbid condition, particularly among young women. Pharmacotherapy provides some but often limited benefit. Among psychotherapies, only cognitive behavioral therapy had received much outcome research prior to the Fairburn et al. study (1991). The rationale in the Fairburn et al. study seems to have been to use IPT as a control condition for CBT, although its performance then exceeded expectations. As IPT shares with CBT some of the nonspecific factors of psychotherapy, its presence was intended to highlight the specifically effective ingredients of CBT. In that study, IPT was minimally adapted for patients with bulimia, even though it was unclear how relevant some of the interpersonal problem areas (e.g., grief) might be to the treatment of bulimia. Fairburn and colleagues (1991, p. 464) did note that IPT might address the "often disturbed" interpersonal functioning of bulimic patients.

ADAPTATION

In individual psychotherapy of bulimia, the basic IPT principles remain essentially unchanged. First, bulimia is diagnosed as a medical illness and linked to an interpersonal problem area in a formulation. Once therapist and patient agree on a formulation, the symptoms of bulimia are related to the key interpersonal problem area—usually a role dispute or role transition—in the same manner as in major depression. In our experience, bingeing and purging often appear to be a behavioral response to an emotionally charged interpersonal encounter. Subjects benefit from exploring their interpersonal options, practicing them in therapeutic role playing, and then trying them out with significant others. As the interpersonal problem area is addressed, bulimic symptoms resolve.

Substituting bulimia for depression in IPT involves a paradigm shift. Although the general approach persists, the four interpersonal problem areas associated with depression may not apply equally to eating disorders. This requires further exploration. Fairburn and colleagues (1991) altered the scheduling of sessions, primarily to be compatible with the CBT to which it was being compared. Other than during the assessment phase, when a history of the eating problem is obtained, the content of the IPT approach is similar to that for depression. The first four sessions were devoted to determining the interpersonal context in which the eating disorder arose.

The design of the Fairburn et al. study allowed nineteen treatment sessions, lasting forty to fifty minutes, in the space of eighteen weeks. Sessions were scheduled twice weekly for a month, then weekly for two months, and biweekly for the final six weeks (Fairburn et al., 1991). In a significant shift from IPT for depression, after the initial sessions, Fairburn's therapists were instructed to let the talk of bulimia continue for no more than ten seconds. Unlike IPT for depression, which emphasizes the medical model of depression-as-illness, IPT for bulimia actively avoids the topic. This makes clinical sense: depressed patients are unlikely to focus on their depression as illness, often confusing the illness with their sense of who they are. In contrast, bulimic patients are all too symptomatically aware and tend to talk of nothing else. It may be helpful to shift the focus of bulimic patients from their symptoms to addressing their current life situation, stressors, and interpersonal interactions.

The therapist announces at the outset that he or she will be more active in the early sessions of the treatment, asking questions and providing psychoeducation, but that this will change as the therapy proceeds. The early sessions (roughly the first four) require the therapist to take histories of (1) the eating disorder, including periods of extreme weight gain, patterns of dieting and purging; (2) the patient's interpersonal functioning (the interpersonal inventory), past and present, including its relationship to the eating disorder; (3) significant life events; and 4) difficulties with self-esteem and depression. The therapist should particularly seek precipitants of bulimic episodes. The four histories can be combined to construct a life chart of the patient's history (Fairburn, 1998).

The therapist emphasizes that in order to break the pattern of bulimia, the patient must discover and address the interpersonal factors that perpetuate it (Fairburn, 1998). The therapist explains that interpersonal difficulties are common in bulimia nervosa, even if the patient's focus on weight, shape, and eating distracts her or him from those difficulties. Binges often follow a painful affect, such as those aroused by a dispute, by intimacy, or by feelings of loneliness. The therapist explains to the patient that treatment will focus on the interpersonal connections rather than on eating and weight. The formulation and the process of IPT for bulimia resembles those for depression. The therapist increasingly encourages the patient to take responsibility for trying to change the maladaptive interpersonal patterns. Therapists make the point—one that IPT therapists might well emphasize for all patients—that treatment "is an opportunity for change" (Fairburn, 1998). Therapist and patient together explore what the patient wants in interpersonal situations, the options for change, and the actual changes the patient then makes in his or her life.

CASE EXAMPLE

Elizabeth, a twenty-three-year-old single white businesswoman who had moved to New York from the South, presented with an eight-year history of bulimia as well as mild depressive symptoms. She reported having begun to grow concerned about her weight and appearance in junior high school, when she began to augment dieting with laxative use and induced vomiting in order to control her weight. She had initially resisted her parents' attempts to have her enter therapy. Eventually Elizabeth entered two courses of psychodynamic psychotherapy, lasting two and one and a half years, respectively, which she felt had done little good. An efficient worker who had earned two promotions at work, she felt that each step upward had increased her anxiety and sense of inadequacy. She described a series of superficial and brief relationships with men, which generally ended when she felt overwhelmed by intimacy and precipitated a rupture. Her symptoms persisted, with binges and purges occurring several times a week.

In eliciting Elizabeth's history, the therapist noted exacerbations of bingeing and vomiting at points of heightened anxiety associated with business and particularly with interpersonal relationships. Yet Elizabeth focused on her eating obsessively as an autonomous problem: it had to do with her weight, the way she looked in the mirror. She at first resisted her therapist's suggestion that her binges had an interpersonal context. When pressed, however, she agreed to try to work on this. The therapist made the formulation that Elizabeth had the illness called bulimia; that her discomfort with interpersonal situations, particularly in her relationships with men, triggered her overeating and purging; and that this treatable condition could be addressed by examining and changing these interpersonal patterns. They agreed to meet for sixteen sessions. Thereafter, the therapist interrupted Elizabeth whenever she began to focus on her eating, redirecting her to its interpersonal context.

Sessions began with the therapist asking, "How have things been since we last met?" Although Elizabeth responded in the early sessions with comments on her weight and eating, she quickly learned to see that bulimic symptoms could be related to social and occupational interpersonal stresses. Dating Jim, a new boyfriend, provided a role dispute and an opportunity to examine her discomfort with intimacy and the outlet that eating provided for such feelings. After returning home from dates, particularly dates that went well, she would feel anxious, then binge and purge. Patient and therapist explored alternative ways of dealing with her anxiety and risking intimacy with Jim. As Elizabeth became more comfortable asserting herself and expressing her feelings to Jim, her binges decreased and had essentially ceased by the time acute treatment terminated. At her one-year follow-up, she and Jim had become engaged, her job was going well, and she had not binged or purged in months: "Not even," she remarked, "when he proposed."

EFFICACY

The initial Fairburn study included twenty-four patients randomized to either CBT or an interpersonally focused treatment—not precisely IPT—for nineteen sessions over eighteen weeks. The treatments had comparable benefits (Fairburn et al., 1986). In a larger second study, seventy-five patients were randomly assigned to cognitive therapy (CBT), IPT, or behavioral treatment (BT) study for nineteen sessions over eighteen weeks, with a twelve-month follow-up. Patients carried the primary diagnosis of bulimia nervosa, although many had elevated scores on the Beck Depression Inventory (mean score=24). Few BT patients ceased binge eating and purging. Although CBT showed initial advantages (Fairburn et al., 1991), over time patients in CBT and IPT made equivalent and substantial changes across all symptom domains (Fairburn et al., 1993). At one-year follow-up, IPT and CBT showed equal efficacy, with each superior to BT.

A follow-up study assessed ninety-nine of the patients from both trials approximately six years after the completion of treatment. The major finding was that patients who received BT did poorly (86 percent still had an eating disorder), whereas those who received either IPT or CBT had a better prognosis: 28–37 percent had an eating disorder (Fairburn et al., 1995). The authors are now experimenting with using IPT supplemented by a CBT self-help program for bulimia (Fairburn, 1998).

A multi-site replication study comparing CBT and IPT for bulimia nervosa has been undertaken at Stanford and Columbia universities in collaboration with investigators at Oxford and Rutgers universities. It may help answer interesting questions of "mode specificity"; that is, whether the two treatments work by similar or different mechanisms. If such specific factors are found, therapists might use them to predict treatment outcome and thus to match particular patients to particular treatments.

A preliminary report from the multicenter study comparing IPT and CBT describes the outcome of CBT to be superior to that of IPT at the conclusion of treatment. However, at 8 to 12 month follow-up, there were no statistically significant differences in outcome. Because of CBT's more rapid effect, the investigators favor CBT as the first-choice treatment for bulimia nervosa (Agras et al., 1999).

GROUP FORMAT FOR BULIMIA (IPT-G)

Wilfley et al. (1993) have ingeniously adapted IPT as a group therapy for obese, nonpurging bulimic patients. One might wonder whether the mixture of different patients' interpersonal problem areas would confuse a group, disturbing the clarity of focus that is important to individual IPT. Wilfley et al. found that most of their bulimic subjects fit the problem category of interpersonal deficits, which simplified matters. Unlike depressed patients who fit the category of interpersonal deficits, these bulimic patients had sufficient social skills to tolerate a group setting. Their deficits evidently had to do with deeper issues of intimacy. Thus, whereas interpersonal deficits is an avoided category in IPT for depression, never used when other problem areas are present, in IPT-G it seems to serve as a catchall focus.

Groups met for sixteen weeks in ninety-minute sessions. Group discussions were augmented by individual write-ups the therapists sent home with each patient.

CASE EXAMPLE[1]

Karen, a fifty-three-year-old sales clerk, presented for treatment for binge eating disorder. At intake she reported three binge episodes a week, during which she consumed an unambiguously large amount of food (typically three to four fast-food sandwiches within a half hour) and felt a loss of control. She reported being most likely to binge eat when feeling uneasy, and stated that her overeating caused her marked distress.

Karen's binge eating began at age fifteen and had been followed by years of dieting and weight fluctuations. At 231 pounds, she was severely overweight, above the ninety-fifth percentile of weight for her age and height. She had an extreme fear of weight gain and great discomfort in allowing herself or others to see her body. She had no other Axis I psychopathology but met criteria for obsessive-compulsive personality disorder with a subthreshold diagnosis of self-defeating personality disorder.

Karen had never been in therapy before. Although she indicated a preference for CBT, she was randomly assigned to the interpersonal therapy group

---

as part of a binge-eating disorder psychotherapy treatment trial. Before the group sessions began, she met with her co-therapists for a two-hour pre-group meeting. In group IPT, this pregroup meeting parallels the first early sessions of individual IPT, eliciting a detailed inventory of the patient's interpersonal history and formulating problem areas and goals to guide the therapeutic work.

During this initial session, Karen was given her diagnosis and assigned the "sick role." She was also educated about binge eating disorder and reassured that it was the eating disorder, rather than a lack of motivation on her part, that was driving her incremental weight gain and out-of-control eating. After learning about her current symptoms by discussing a recent episode, Karen's therapists skipped back to her very first binge, using this as a frame through which to move forward chronologically. Together she and her therapists constructed a profile of relationship difficulties involved in the onset and maintenance of her binge eating.

Karen had a history of avoiding conflict and a fear of criticism. At the age of fifteen, she began a series of failed relationships that she had attempted to hide from her parents or to glorify (saying, for example, that she was married when she wasn't) in order to appear the "perfect" daughter and to not disappoint her parents. She binged when she was alone and used food to "numb out" in order to manage the feelings that she kept private. Her attempts at secrecy and use of food to disconnect from her feelings continued throughout Karen's subsequent marriage. Although her husband had been cruel and verbally abusive, Karen worked hard to "fool everyone for eighteen years" into believing that she had a fulfilling relationship because she didn't want anyone to think that she had failed in her marriage.

Since her divorce, Karen had been in a live-in relationship but remained emotionally disconnected from her boyfriend. She concealed her eating disorder from him, ate very little when they were together, and continued to binge eat when alone. At work, Karen reported that she put in fourteen-hour days because she felt uncomfortable "saying no" to customers' requests to see her before and after their business hours. Given the long periods of time she spent on her feet without breaks to eat or rest, Karen clearly disregarded her needs to an extreme degree. Consequently, she found herself binge eating at night, often on her way home from work, to avoid the conflictual feelings she had about experiencing resentment and frustration over her workload.

Karen and her therapists examined the use of binge eating as a primary coping strategy to manage her negative affective states and avoidance of conflict. Given her history of unfulfilling relationships and inability to manage her feelings interpersonally, Karen was assigned the problem area of interpersonal deficits.

To target her problem area, Karen was given three goals related to both her binge eating and her work resolving problems with interpersonal deficits. First, Karen was directed to become more aware of and to learn to identify her feelings when she began to binge eat or feel out of control with her eating. Many people who struggle with binge eating have difficulty identifying and labeling their affective states. Learning to do this would give Karen an extremely useful tool with which to begin to eliminate her binge episodes and, in a preliminary way, to help increase her connections with others. Second, she was encouraged to begin expressing her feelings with others—especially her boyfriend—rather than trying to avoid potential conflict. Years of lying to important people in her life and to herself to maintain an image of perfection had left Karen unable to communicate effectively or manage conflict. As a final goal, Karen was instructed to find ways to nurture herself rather then spending all of her energy caring for others. Consistent with her problem area, Karen had established a relationship pattern, common among binge eaters, of excessive caretaking for others.

Karen was encouraged to take better care of herself in order to break the vicious cycle of self-denial that she had established in her significant relationships. In addition, focusing on herself in relationships would also teach Karen about more effectively negotiating her interactions. Given the link between her problem area and binge eating, Karen's therapists explained that the exclusive focus on these goals would eliminate her binge eating.

Toward the end of the interview, the therapists helped prepare Karen for the work of the group and addressed her concerns about confidentiality. Her individual goals were linked to the group work by encouraging her to think of the group as an "interpersonal laboratory" where ties to others could develop, naturally occurring "impasses" in the formation of intimate relationships could be examined, and new approaches to handling interpersonal situations could be tried out. Karen was also instructed that the main focus of the group was to help her apply the skills learned in the group to her outside social life.

During the first phase of treatment, work with Karen centered on helping her connect her binge eating to difficulties in relationships. Consistent with a problem area of interpersonal deficits, Karen had difficulty initiating contact with other group members. In early sessions, she made comments that distanced herself from the group, such as stating that she was unlike the others because she had wonderful relationships, and had no problems to speak of other than her inability to diet effectively. A turning point came when group members began to explore their own unsustaining relationships. This group dialogue helped Karen realize that her relationships had not been as intimate or satisfying as she had first indicated.

Outside the group, Karen worked on the goal of caring for herself and expressing more feelings to her boyfriend. Having reduced her workload and become more physically active, Karen announced that she was feeling better about herself.

Throughout the second phase of treatment, Karen worked on goals in her outside life. Her therapists encouraged her to notice her style of glossing over problems, and Karen continued to receive helpful feedback about minimizing her feelings. As Karen spoke about her unhappiness during her first marriage, she began to understand that maintaining the facade of a perfect life prevented her from turning to others for assistance. Discounting her own feelings generally prevented her from experiencing her emotions or addressing them in adaptive ways. The progression of the group through the conflict phase of treatment further provided Karen with opportunities to observe that conflict could be worked through effectively. She was often surprised at the open discussions group members had with one another. Although discord made Karen very anxious at first, the successful resolution of a few instances of friction among group members helped her to see that disagreements could have positive outcomes and could even strengthen relationships. Outside of the group, Karen began discussing her feelings openly with her sisters, communicating with coworkers, and setting limits with customers by refusing some of their requests.

By the last phase of treatment, Karen was aware of the enormous energy she had spent concealing her problems. She was more open with her friends and family. She reported her relationships were more satisfying, and she and her boyfriend had become engaged. She continued to decrease her work hours and by the end of treatment had begun frank discussions with her daughters about their unresolved feelings about their father. Having learned to recognize her emotions and to make more time for herself, Karen was able to attend to negative feelings "without feeling as if the world was coming to an end." Karen had stopped binge eating by the time the final phase of treatment began. At post-treatment, she set the goal of giving more thought to conflict when it occurred rather than waiting for it to go away. At eight-month follow-up, Karen had lost seventy pounds from her initial assessment weight and remained binge-free.

EFFICACY

Drawing on the experience of Fairburn, a study by Wilfley et al. (1993) compared IPT in a sixteen-week group format to group CBT (CBT-G) and a waiting-list control (WL) for fifty-six women with nonpurging bulimia. At the end of treatment, both IPT-G and CBT-G significantly reduced binge eating, whereas WL did not. These results were sustained at one-year follow-up. Based on these results, a randomized clinical trial is under way for 162 women given either group IPT or CBT for twenty sessions over twenty weeks.

COMMENT

The application of IPT to eating disorders is still a new area. Final results of the initial studies are needed to confirm its efficacy. Further applications are possible: for example, to patients with anorexia nervosa.

ANOREXIA NERVOSA

Anorexia nervosa is an illness of high morbidity and mortality that principally affects young women.[2] Individuals suffering from anorexia may literally starve themselves to death. DSM-IV (American Psychiatric Association, 1994) characterizes this disorder as the refusal to maintain body weight at or above a minimally normal weight for age and height. Patients have an intense fear of gaining weight or becoming fat, even though often grossly underweight. They have a distorted sense of their weight and appearance and deny the dangers of their emaciated state. There is no definitive treatment (Hsu, 1986), and relatively little research has examined treatment outcomes. Psychodynamic psychotherapy (Bruch, 1978) and family therapy (Minuchin et al., 1978) have been among the psychotherapies proposed to treat the disorder.

McKenzie and colleagues in Christchurch, New Zealand, have adapted IPT for outpatients with anorexia nervosa, developing a manual (see Chapter 25) based on both the original IPT book (Klerman et al., 1984) and Fairburn's work on IPT for bulimia nervosa. The manual stresses the importance of building a treatment alliance and provides a rationale.

The premise of treatment, akin to that of IPT for bulimia, is that solving the patient's interpersonal difficulties, rather than focusing on the eating symptoms, will relieve the disorder. The four problem areas and general IPT strategies remain unchanged.

EFFICACY

There are as yet no efficacy data. In 1997, McKenzie and colleagues began a two-year, three-cell randomized treatment trial to compare twenty weeks of

IPT to CBT and Specialist Supportive Care. During an initial assessment phase of three sessions over the course of two weeks, all subjects are taught self-monitoring of food intake. Following randomization, the first four treatment sessions are scheduled twice weekly, followed by fourteen weekly sessions and two biweekly sessions. Follow-up assessments take place at three, six, nine, and twelve months.

The reader may find Chapter 23, describing IPT for Body Dysmorphic Disorder, of related interest.

NOTES

1. The authors thank Denise Wilfley, Ph.D., for background material and for the case reported in this section.

2. The authors thank Janice McKenzie, M.D., at the Department of Psychological Medicine, Christchurch School of Medicine, Christchurch, New Zealand, for providing the material for this section.

CHAPTER 22

Anxiety Disorders

Anxiety disorders may represent different territory from mood disorders, yet their symptoms frequently overlap and their relationship to life events may be similar. Unlike cognitive behavioral therapy, which has for some time been used to treat various anxiety disorders, IPT until recently had not been tested. Now, however, several research teams are exploring the utility of IPT to treat social phobia, panic disorder, and posttraumatic stress disorder (PTSD).

SOCIAL PHOBIA

Social phobia is, according to DSM-IV (American Psychiatric Association, 1994), the marked and persistent fear of social or performance situations in which one is exposed to possible scrutiny by unfamiliar people. The individual fears he or she will act in a way that will be humiliating or embarrassing, or that the appearance of anxiety symptoms will themselves have that effect. The resulting anxiety leads the person to avoid social situations, or causes marked distress if he or she attends them.

Social phobia is distinguished from simple shyness by its restriction of the sufferer's life to a small circle of friends or family, or to work with limited social interactions. Discrete symptoms of social phobia can occur in people who are otherwise outgoing and self-assured outside a specifically feared situation, such as public speaking or eating among strangers.

BACKGROUND[1]

Onset is usually in childhood or adolescence, and the condition is frequently chronic, although symptoms may remit if the feared situation can be avoided. The prevalence of social phobia in the general population is high, roughly 5–6 percent; it ranges still higher if the "impairment" criterion is loosened. Social phobia often occurs in conjunction with other anxiety disorders, major depression, dysthymic disorder, and substance abuse. Substance abuse may represent a failed attempt at self-medication to alleviate anxiety. Social and occupational impairment is high, and is associated with lower academic performance, income, and marriage rates, and difficulties in social relationships (Schneier et al., 1990; Sanderson et al., 1990).

Both pharmacotherapy and psychotherapy have been used as treatments. Phenelzine, a monoamine oxidase inhibitor, has the best established efficacy (Liebowitz et al., 1992), although the newer serotonin reuptake inhibitors are being tested as treatments. Cognitive behavioral therapy is the most widely tested psychotherapy and has established efficacy as well (Heimberg and Barlow, 1991).

RATIONALE

The interpersonal aspects of social phobia make it a natural starting place for testing IPT as a treatment of anxiety disorders.

ADAPTATION

Both individual and group adaptations of IPT for social phobia are being developed and tested. IPT has been modified for social phobia independently by Lipsitz at Columbia University and Stuart and O'Hara at the University of Iowa. Lipsitz has developed an extensive manual for social phobia (see Chapter 25).

Lipsitz reports that the common IPT ingredients—including the medical model, providing the "sick role," and the supportive therapeutic stance—seem to have a positive effect on most patients. The interpersonal formulation and linking of anxiety symptoms with interpersonal context has more appeal for some patients than for others. For example, a patient with prominent blushing insisted that her social anxiety was related to the blushing itself and had no connection to her relationships with other people or her ability to express emotion freely. IPT seemed to help her, nevertheless.

In general, the central principle is that excess social anxiety (the subjective experience of anxiety and the associated physical and cognitive symptoms) is reciprocally linked to impaired social functioning. Social anxiety interferes with the normal problem of mastering a new social situation. Avoiding social situations limits the patient's life. This social withdrawal further increases the sense that social situations are dangerous, compounding social anxiety.

CASE EXAMPLE

Leora, a thirty-seven-year-old divorced physical therapist, sought treatment for social phobia. She had difficulty at work because she "clammed up" every time a supervisor was near. She recalled that in high school she had felt intimidated by teachers and was reluctant to raise her hand in class. Although bright, she was afraid she would say something stupid and be laughed at by her classmates or rebuffed by her teachers. Leora's teachers had thought she was not interested and her grades suffered. A more outgoing and streetwise friend took Leora under her wing and initiated her into a local gang.

Leora dropped out of high school and hung out with the gang for the next two years. She used drugs when they did, although she denied liking them and said she did so only to fit in and gain approval. When she later left the gang and drugs behind and obtained her GED, her social anxiety persisted. In every work setting, Leora felt uncomfortable approaching her boss or supervisor. She could never view herself as advancing in her career and moved frequently from job to job.

DIFFERENCES BETWEEN IPT FOR DEPRESSION AND FOR SOCIAL PHOBIA

The distinction between IPT for depression and IPT for social phobia (IPT-SP) is largely semantic. In the former, the interpersonal problem area and the depressive syndrome are conceptually distinct. In social phobia, the definition of the disorder itself subsumes some aspect of role dysfunction (e.g., avoidance of social situations, expectation of humiliation). The goal of IPT-SP is the same as that of IPT: to decrease symptoms by decreasing social dysfunction. Yet the boundary between the disorder and the interpersonal anxiety is often less distinct than in depression. Thus the attempt made in some modifications of IPT to avoid discussion of symptoms (e.g., Fairburn et al., 1994) is not appropriate to IPT-SP.

The major interpersonal problem focus has been on role transition. Many social phobic patients have undergone or are in the process of major life changes, such as a move to a new location, career change or advancement, change in family constellation (e.g., separation from a significant other), or the onset of a major illness. Social anxiety may increase in intensity or may simply pose more of a problem for them in the context of these transitions.

Because social phobia often has an early onset and chronic course, and thus lacks an acute precipitant at the time of the patient's presentation for treatment, Lipsitz and colleagues have borrowed an approach from Markowitz's work (1993, 1998) on IPT for dysthymic disorder (see Chapter 12). By providing a medical model of social phobia, reassuring the patient that he or she has a disorder that is treatable, and instilling hope for change, the therapist induces a "therapeutic role transition." The patient recognizes that shyness, passivity, social awkwardness, and so forth, are symptoms or sequelae of a disorder and not the patient's true personality. This creates a positive "stressor," which serves as a dynamic frame for exploring current interpersonal experiences:

> It sounds like you can be quite assertive with your staff now that you're not let-ting the social phobia get in the way.
>
> You've dealt with this fear for so long that you've begun to think this is all you're capable of—that you're this low-key, passive person who belongs in the background. The reality is that social phobia has hindered you at every stage. Now that we've identified the social phobia and you're taking steps to over-come it, your *real* personality is beginning to show. You'll see that you have the ability to be more assertive, to take the lead, to be the center of attention and even enjoy it.

Lipsitz et al. have added an additional category of "role insecurity." This captures role difficulties subtler than those defined by interpersonal deficit. Role insecurity encompasses common concomitants of social phobia such as lack of assertiveness, conflict avoidance, difficulty expressing anger, and sensitivity to rejection—difficulties that social phobic and dysthymic pa-tients frequently share. These difficulties are less severe and less global than what were originally classified as interpersonal deficits in depressed patients. As with IPT for dysthymic patients, this formulation emphasizes the patient's natural potential for more competent behavior once the social phobia is resolved or mitigated. In most cases, social phobic patients have a fair idea of what to do in social situations but are held back by the symptoms of social phobia. In some cases, positive social skills are taught or reinforced using role playing as an adjunct technique.

Stuart and O'Hara, working independently, coined the term "interpersonal sensitivity" for patients with social phobia who have interpersonal deficits. They feel (S. Stuart, personal communication, 1997) that the label of "interpersonal deficits" has a derogatory connotation that may diminish the patient's optimism for recovery. "Role insecurity" and "interpersonal sensitivity" suggest a convergence in clinical approaches that makes sense for social phobia.

Stuart and O'Hara focus their IPT work on analyzing specific interactions between the patient and others, relying on communication analysis and role playing, and helping patients to set feasible goals for improvement. They discuss with patients the hypothesis that many of their problems derive from "hypersensitivity" to communication with others, particularly nonverbal communication. They suggest that because of patients' sensitivity, they are more prone than most people to overinterpret negative communications and ultimately develop a protective strategy that leads to social avoidance. This defensive reaction is cast as an understandable yet alterable means of dealing with interpersonal stress.

Patients with social phobia may have fewer relationships to address in therapy. Stuart and O'Hara report the utility of helping patients reconstruct in detail the interactions they have with others, particularly interactions that precipitate social avoidance. Both verbal and nonverbal communication are reviewed, with emphasis on how the patient may be misinterpreting communications of others, or not providing clear communications to others. The therapist helps the patient understand how he or she withdraws from interactions, nonverbally "pushing" others away. The therapist also discusses ways the patient can actively choose to continue an interaction or disengage without using nonverbal communications.

Their therapy also focuses on the patient's successful interactions. Positive reinforcement is crucial to the therapeutic process. At the same time, the therapist must set realistic goals. The therapist deems it unlikely that the patient will be able to function with minimal anxiety in social situations during the brief period of therapy. The patient can, however, "take steps in the right direction."

CASE EXAMPLES

Louise, a twenty-five-year-old woman, was bright and articulate but had chronic anxiety about speaking in public and attending parties and other social gatherings. She complained that she had "nothing to say" to people she met in these settings. The therapist suggested they role-play a conversation. "How are the potato chips?" she ventured. She then launched into a self-deprecating speech about how stupid a thing that was to say. The therapist challenged: "Not everyone who makes small talk at a party has a list of clever things to say. That's why they call it 'small talk.' You say something trivial and sometimes it leads to a conversation, sometimes it doesn't." The patient tried again and was happier with how the conversation progressed. "In your case," said the therapist, "social phobia has made it more difficult for you to get started. But once you do, you find as much to say as the next person." At the next party, Louise started a few brief conversations and was surprised at how easy it was.

Herb, a thirty-two-year-old man, presented for treatment of anxiety in social situations.[2] He reported difficulty in relating to others at work, and noted that his relationship with his wife of five years was deteriorating. He was also troubled by a fear of urinating in public restrooms. He felt that others were scrutinizing him in social situations and considered him inept and weak because of his inability to use public toilets.

Therapy initially focused on Herb's communication with others, which often consisted of avoidant, nonverbal messages. He discussed his feelings of inadequacy with the therapist and began revealing these feelings to his wife as well. As he began to make himself more vulnerable to others, he came to see himself in more realistic terms and came to grips with some of his fears. The therapist commented that he appreciated the risks that the patient was taking in self-disclosure, and noted that he was coming across as "more real" to the therapist.

At the conclusion of twelve sessions of therapy, Herb reported feeling much improved. Although he continued to feel anxious in public situations, he no longer practiced avoidant behavior. He also reported significant improvement in his marital relationship and his fear of using public restrooms was abating.

EFFICACY

An initial case series at each site has suggested the promise of IPT as a treatment for social phobia. Lipsitz has completed a fourteen-week open trial with nine patients with social phobia. At the end of the trial, seven (78 percent) were classified as responders by an independent evaluator and by self-report. Subjects showed significant improvement in social phobia on performance-fear and avoidance scales (Lipsitz et al., in press). Based on these results, Lipsitz is planning and has received funding for a fourteen-week controlled clinical trial, comparing IPT-SP to educational supportive psychotherapy, and incorporating six-month and one-year follow-ups. Stuart and O'Hara are conducting an open trial whose preliminary results suggest that IPT is highly effective as an acute treatment. Two-year post-treatment follow-up is planned to assess the enduring benefits of the intervention.

SOCIAL PHOBIA IN GROUP FORMAT

Weissman and Jacobson have adapted IPT in a group format for patients with extreme shyness. The patients had social phobia in unstructured interpersonal situations—e.g., parties, intimate discussions with significant others—but not in defined work situations. Most patients were successful in professional or business careers despite their phobias. All had been seen previously by Jacobson in individual psychotherapy (not IPT), in which some continued.

The main focus in a ten-session time-limited group was defining and describing the diagnosis, giving the patient the "sick role," and finding practical strategies for dealing with shyness in specific situations. Examples included developing a script to initiate a more personal conversation with an estranged father, and initiating a discussion with a spouse about having a child. Consonant with the report of Lipsitz, the chronic nature of the disorder led to a focus on therapeutic role transition from an impaired to a less-impaired state. The group format seemed to provide a safe haven for patients who could share their condition with others like themselves.

PANIC DISORDER

A panic attack is a discrete period of intense fear or discomfort, in which four (or more) of the following symptoms develop abruptly and reach a peak within ten minutes:

1. palpitations, pounding heart, or accelerated heart rate
2. sweating
3. trembling or shaking
4. sensations of shortness of breath or smothering
5. feeling of choking
6. chest pain or discomfort
7. nausea or abdominal distress
8. feeling dizzy, unsteady, lightheaded, or faint
9. derealization (feelings of unreality) or depersonalization (feeling detached from oneself)
10. fear of losing control or going crazy
11. fear of dying
12. paresthesia (numbness or tingling sensations)
13. chills or hot flashes

(Adapted from DSM-IV; APA, 1994)

A manual for IPT as an individual treatment for panic disorder is being developed by Arzt, van Rijsoort, and colleagues in Maastricht, the Netherlands.

RATIONALE

"Situational panic" occurs in interpersonal situations—for example, when patients are in public spaces or on public transportation. But even the more global diagnosis of panic disorder, whose attacks DSM-IV describes as "coming out of the blue" (American Psychiatric Association, 1994, p. 397), may have less obvious yet important interpersonal connections. Studies describe the occurrence of life events just prior to, hence potentially precipitating the onset of panic (Roy-Byrne et al., 1986; Last et al., 1984; Faravelli, 1985; Busch et al., 1991). Hence the connection between panic and life situations may be analogous to that of depression.

Panic onset has been associated, at least retrospectively, with physical or emotional separation or loss (Busch et al., 1991), or with changes in life expectation—i.e., role transitions.

ADAPTATION

Modification for IPT is under way, based on an assessment of the needs and clinical characteristics of panic patients. These have yet to be finalized.

CASE EXAMPLE

Peter, a thirty-one-year-old married actor, presented for treatment with a chief complaint of panic attacks in the past three months. His therapist initially treated him with pharmacotherapy, but in discussing the case with a supervisor several interesting points emerged. Peter had been married for eight years to a woman ten years his senior. A year before, while working abroad, he had a wild affair with a beautiful younger woman, which he then broke off upon returning to the United States. She, however, continued to write him, and he found her far more attractive than his wife. Peter and his wife began couples therapy for difficulties in their relationship, but he never mentioned the affair until his dog finally "uncovered" for his wife a love letter left in a pile of papers.

After this, Peter and his wife made a concerted effort to improve their marriage. About three months prior to Peter's presentation to the clinic, his wife urged that they have a baby. This seemed to reflect both an awareness of her "biological clock" and an attempt to cement the relationship. Peter felt ambivalent about having a child. It was in this context that his panic attacks—which were limited to nighttime, in his bedroom and in his wife's company—occurred. In discussing this obvious connection, the therapist pointed out that Peter had said he had no symptoms the previous last weekend when his wife was away.

Peter had no history of depression, no prior panic symptoms, and denied substance abuse.

Peter's panic could be treated as a role dispute with his wife over whether to have a baby (and whether to continue the marriage). As in treating a depressed patient, the therapy could focus on connecting the patient's interpersonal functioning, his ability to address and resolve his role dispute, to his panic symptoms. The interpersonal inventory would seek to define his handling of previous relationships, any difficulties with emotional intimacy he had there, his sexual interest and behavior with both his wife and his lover, and his patterns of coping. What does Peter want to happen? What keeps him in his marriage, and how much would he like to resume his affair abroad? How does he feel about having children? To the extent that Peter could first understand, and then act to resolve, his ambivalence about which relationship to be in, his panic would likely abate.

EFFICACY

There are as yet no efficacy data. A trial is planned in Maastricht.

POSTTRAUMATIC
STRESS DISORDER

Posttraumatic stress disorder (PTSD) is the consequence of exposure to an event that involved actual or threatened death or serious injury, and which evoked intense fear, helplessness, or horror. In the wake of this event, the patient suffers from a mixture of dissociative, anxious, and depressed symptoms (American Psychiatric Association, 1994).

RATIONALE

Like social phobia, PTSD is defined by a connection between symptoms and life situation, and hence lends itself to testing an IPT approach.

Krupnick at Georgetown University, Washington, D.C., is modifying IPT in a group format for low-income women with posttraumatic stress disorder (PTSD) subsequent to interpersonal trauma: sexual or physical molestation, assault, or abuse. A pilot group from a public-sector gynecology clinic consisted of women patients receiving family planning and gynecological services. These patients had been exposed to considerable interpersonal trauma, often from significant others, and had high rates of PTSD. Given that the patients' psychiatric diagnoses stemmed from relationship difficulties, Krupnick and colleagues felt that they could help them integrate prior traumas and maybe also avoid victimization in the future.

ADAPTATION

Many aspects of IPT for depression were retained. Group duration was sixteen sessions and focused on relationship disputes, role deficits, role transitions and losses. The here-and-now focus and connections between relationship difficulties and symptoms were retained. However, new emphasis was placed on relationship issues salient to interpersonal trauma histories: for example, issues of trust; learning whom it is safe to trust, how to identify interpersonal cues that might signal danger, and how to permit intimacy. The modification of IPT also provided therapist guidelines on cultural and social-class sensitivity for engaging low-income women, many of whom were ethnic minorities.

EFFICACY

The pilot group consisted of four women. All completed twenty sessions of ninety-minute group treatment. All met criteria for PTSD using a structured diagnostic interview and had histories of assault, abuse, or both. Pre- and post-treatment and four-month follow-up data on the women suggested the feasibility and potential effectiveness of IPT in this population. The model has subsequently been revised as a sixteen-session, two-hours-per-group model.

NOTES

1. The authors are grateful to Joshua Lipsitz, Ph.D., for contributing the material in this section and the case vignettes, which are used with permission.

2. The authors are grateful for the contribution by Scott Stuart, M.D., and Michael O'Hara, Ph.D., from the University to Iowa of this case and for a description of their use of IPT.

CHAPTER 23

Applications in Progress

Adaptation of IPT is flourishing, with researchers adapting it to address a variety of disorders. We do not know them all, nor can we vouch for their quality or appropriateness. These applications will eventually stand or fall on efficacy research. This chapter presents some of the promising new developments.

BODY DYSMORPHIC DISORDER

Body dysmorphic disorder (BDD) consists of a preoccupation with an imagined or minor defect in one's appearance (American Psychiatric Association, 1994).[1] A patient may obsess, for example, about devious-looking eyebrows, an excessively large nose or head, small genitals, or a stretched mouth. Their feelings of unbearable ugliness and pervasive preoccupation with appearance may lead to social withdrawal as well as repeated visits to dermatologists and plastic surgeons in an attempt to correct the imagined defect (Phillips, 1991). Common beliefs include: "If I am ugly or defective, then I am unlovable" and "My appearance has to be perfect" (Veale et al., 1996a, b).

The prevalence of BDD is unknown. Onset is usually in adolescence. Phillips (1991), in a clinical review, noted that symptoms tend to be unremitting, sometimes worsening over time. The body part of concern may shift over time and the preoccupation may progress to delusional thinking. The inordinate amount of time that patients spend on their preoccupation can lead them to neglect other aspects of life. There have been no published controlled efficacy trials of any treatment. Case reports of small numbers of patients have described the use of antidepressants or neuroleptics. Most of these reports have been negative, although some successes have been reported with serotonin uptake blockers. Some of these patients may have also been depressed (Phillips et al., 1994). In the domain of psychotherapy, Marks (1988) described successful results with exposure therapy in a small pilot study. Veale et al (1996b) found CBT superior to a waiting list for nineteen patients.

ADAPTATION

A group led by Veale in the United Kingdom has adapted IPT to treat BDD. The interpersonal inventory, problem areas, techniques, and time-limited framework of IPT were not changed. In the initial phase, patients were given the diagnosis of BDD, educated about its symptoms and prevalence, and told that BDD is often associated with problems in interpersonal relations. Patients were also taught to monitor the association between an increase in symptoms and current changes and disruption in their life. The therapist actively acknowledged the patient's distress and responded to this distress whenever expressed.

Symptoms of BDD were positively connoted as attempts on the part of the patient to cope with overwhelming feelings of personal distress. Dwelling on the symptoms of BDD was discouraged (compare IPT for bulimia, Chapter 21). Therapy focused on underlying feelings and relevant interpersonal circumstances. The patient was encouraged to develop more effective coping strategies to address his or her feelings and circumstances. The therapist also emphasized the need for change.

Since patients with BDD are often single or divorced, have high levels of social isolation, and typically have been ill since adolescence, interpersonal deficits were a frequent problem area. In such cases, therapists focused on interpersonal issues in relationships within the family of origin and their possible impact on current interpersonal functioning, and experiences within the treatment relationship could be used to help the patient understand current interpersonal functioning.

CASE EXAMPLE

Carla, a twenty-four-year-old woman, reported a twelve-year history of severe preoccupation with her appearance, particularly the size and shape of her nose, her breasts, and the appearance and texture of her skin. There was no objective evidence of deformity. One year before treatment, she had undergone what she considered an unsatisfactory rhinoplasty for her believed nasal deformity. In addition to the surgery, which failed to improve her symptoms, she had twice previously been treated with antidepressants by her general practitioner and had twice received general counseling in primary care. She was not clinically depressed on presentation.

Carla was the youngest of three children. At the time of assessment, she was unemployed and living with her parents. Despite previous counseling, she had difficulty describing her emotions and focused firmly on her perceived facial deformity. She initially made no criticisms of her father, but during the assessment period, which took four sessions, she revealed that he had physically and verbally abused her since childhood and that the abuse had continued to the present.

The case was formulated as an interpersonal role dispute, and symptoms were related to the dispute. For example, it emerged that, following abuse in childhood but also subsequently, Carla isolated herself in her room and persistently examined herself in the mirror. After it was established that she firmly wished to continue living with her parents, patient and therapist agreed that the dispute with her father had reached an impasse in which she was regularly the victim and he the perpetrator. Carla was encouraged to confront her father about his abuse and negotiate mutual expectations in their relationship.

The patient was surprised by the link between her abuse and her symptom. Initially, progress was patchy. Carla reported further episodes of abuse, and relatives left phone calls expressing concern about the degree of her depression. Carla considered and rejected an antidepressant medication prescription, residence in a women's refuge, and admission to a psychiatric ward. She remained preoccupied with her appearance, but to an apparently lesser degree, as treatment continued. She was able to link fluctuation in her symptoms to interpersonal circumstances. She became aware of her anger about her abuse and stopped blaming herself for her appearance and her "failed" operation. Although Carla never formally confronted her father, she did tell him that his assaults and criticisms were damaging to her. As her confidence grew, she sought training as an apprentice hairdresser. For the first time in years, she arranged holidays abroad with a female friend.

Termination was explored actively in the last three of her eighteen sessions. For two months prior to discharge, there had been no episodes of abuse. Carla felt confident that the abuse would not recur. She actively wished to terminate treatment and expected to maintain gains in the future. She attributed her improvement to increased insight into her circumstances and her reaction to them, which reduced her symptoms.

EFFICACY

There are no efficacy data for IPT with BDD. Veale and colleagues have begun a fifteen-week clinical trial in London comparing IPT to CBT.

COMMENT

The adaptation described here follows the IPT model. It is unclear whether comorbid depression is handled separately or as the consequence of BDD. Also, like dysthymic disorder, BDD is a chronic condition. More definitive focus on the transition to giving up the "sick role" may be useful. Further clinical experience and the results of the clinical trial will help to evaluate this approach.

SOMATIZATION DISORDER

Somatization disorder is characterized by nonspecific symptoms in multiple organ systems.[2] It begins before age thirty, extends over many years, and causes distress, disability, overutilization of medical resources, and often unnecessary medical procedures. It is essential to rule out medical conditions that cause multiple, vague symptoms. The course of somatization disorder is unpredictable and the exact prevalence unknown: estimates are between 0.2 to 2 percent among women, and 0.2 percent among men (American Psychiatric Association, 1994). Somatizing patients are intensely distressed by their symptoms and assume the "sick role" despite being in objective good health.

ADAPTATIONS

Scott Stuart, at the University of Iowa, notes that his experience with somatizing patients has led to several modifications of IPT specific to somatization disorder. The length of the treatment is sixteen weeks, a relatively long duration influenced by the patients' general mistrust of physicians. Such patients typically require six to seven sessions to establish a reasonable working alliance with their therapist. Stuart reports that, early in therapy, it is best to describe IPT as a treatment to help patients "cope" with their pain and physical ailments. Once an alliance is firmly established, the therapist introduces the concept that the patient's physical symptoms represent a means of meeting his or her interpersonal needs. The later work in IPT involves assisting the patient to develop new, more adaptive ways of satisfying those needs.

An additional modification is to invite the patient's primary care physician to accompany the patient to the first or second session. At this meeting, the therapist educates this physician about the therapist's conceptualization of the illness, and assists him or her in setting appropriate boundaries with the patient. This interaction occurs in the presence of the patient. Not surprisingly, primary care physicians have been eager to refer patients with somatization disorder for psychiatric treatment.

CASE EXAMPLE

Judy, a sixty-five-year-old woman, had seen numerous specialists for vague GI complaints. Numerous procedures had revealed no specific problems, but she persisted in her complaints, insisting that the doctors had not been diligent enough. At her first IPT appointment, she expressed great anger at her physicians, particularly several who had said that her problems were "all in her head." She angrily stated that she had come to the counseling appointment only because no one else had taken her problems seriously.

The first several sessions focused on framing the aim of the psychotherapy as helping Judy to cope with her physical problems, rather than invalidating her view of herself as ill. The therapist worked to establish a therapeutic alliance and to help Judy feel heard and understood. After five sessions, she began to disclose more personal information, including her feelings of being misunderstood by her physicians. She related that her problems had actually begun about two years before, when her husband had seen his doctor for stomach complaints. Within two weeks of this appointment, he had died of pancreatic cancer. She was able to relate this experience to her own fears that she, too, might be "really sick."

Judy also discussed interactions she had with her physicians. It became clear that she communicated her anger at being misunderstood and ignored by her doctors through demands and noncompliance. The therapist role-played some interactions with the patient, who practiced communicating her feelings more directly. The therapist disclosed to the patient that he had initially experienced her as hostile as well. She was able to accept this as a useful comment rather than as a criticism.

After sixteen weeks of therapy, Judy continued to complain of abdominal discomfort. She stated, however, that she now felt that she "would just have to learn to deal with it." She had agreed to see a single primary care physician for all her medical problems, and no longer demanded appointments with this doctor on a weekly basis.

Efficacy

Stuart is conducting an open trial of IPT for patients with somatization disorder. In addition to studying symptomatic improvement, he is assessing patient's utilization of health care resources prior to and following treatment—a key area for this patient population.

Scott and Ikkos (1996) in London have also modified IPT for patients with chronic somatization in primary care. Their adaptation adds a fifth problem area, the patient's relationship with health professionals and pursuit of medical care. Scott (personal communication, 1996) notes that the IPT medical model works readily with these patients because of their inappropriate use of the health care system. Treatment seeking is conceptualized as an interpersonal issue. Patients have been easy to recruit for IPT treatment.

A controlled trial is under way comparing IPT to a waiting-list control for thirty primary care patients in London, ages eighteen to sixty-five, with somatization disorder but without psychotic or depressive disorder.

Comment

We await the results of these studies, as well as more descriptive information so that the differences between these adaptations can be reconciled.

DEPRESSION FOLLOWING MYOCARDIAL INFARCTION

Numerous studies have shown an association between depression and adverse cardiac events (Musselman et al., 1998). The medical course of patients who have suffered myocardial infarction (MI) is complicated by major depressive disorder (MDD) (Stuart and Cole, 1996), which increases rates of morbidity and mortality. Stuart has adapted IPT for patients suffering from depression post-MI.

Stuart and Cole stress the need for careful initial evaluation of the patient's depressive symptoms, since post-MI patients who are not depressed often experience sleep disruption, decreased energy, and other vegetative symptoms frequently seen in depression. Moreover, many patients are referred while still hospitalized or in the early phase of recovering from their infarctions, further complicating the evaluation for depression. Medications require close review as well, as many cardiac medications have psychiatric side effects. In addition, the high morbidity and mortality rates associated with post-MI depression make speedy initiation of treatment for depression paramount.

ADAPTATION

Stuart and Cole modified IPT for treatment of depressed post-MI patients, reconceptualizing the problem area of grief to incorporate loss of health and loss of physical functioning as well as the actual death of a significant other. Patients often struggle with their own sense of mortality for the first time as a result of the MI, and often face real and permanent limitations to their functioning. Although post-MI depression could also be subsumed under the category of role transition, Stuart's experience has been that most patients describe the experience as a meaningful loss. Working with the metaphor that the patient uses to describe his or her problem enhances the therapist's ability to help the patient feel understood, fosters the development of a therapeutic alliance, and ultimately improves outcome.

Issues such as marital or interpersonal relationships, career or life goals, and new religious or spiritual beliefs may become treatment foci as well. Patients often feel compelled to make major changes in lifestyle: those who smoke, drink excessively, or are overweight may feel the need to radically change their health behavior. Many post-MI patients also have noted difficulty in communicating to others their need for help or support. Patients have consistently described difficulty in negotiating interpersonal relationships with significant others, especially if they have been forced into a passive, care-receiving role after a lifetime of independence.

CASE EXAMPLE[3]

Douglas, a fifty-eight-year-old man, was referred for treatment of depression of two months' duration six months following his first MI. His symptoms included constant fatigue, decreased motivation, anhedonia, and insomnia. He had a two-year history of angina. He also described a history of alcohol abuse: up to a fifth of alcohol a day during his twenties and thirties. This alcohol abuse had led to a difficult divorce, since which he had had no contact with his ex-wife or their children. He denied alcohol use over the last twenty years.

> The focus of therapy was conceptualized as grief over the loss of his family, his youth, and his physical health. Ways in which Douglas could resume contact with his children were explored. He also addressed unresolved anger, guilt, and sadness about his marriage and years of alcohol abuse for several sessions. By the conclusion of therapy, Douglas had returned to work and was no longer experiencing depressive symptoms. He had reinitiated contact with one of his children and had successfully completed his cardiac rehabilitation program.

Efficacy

Stuart is conducting an open trial of IPT in post-MI depressed patients. Reports of individual cases (Stuart and Cole, 1996) suggest the feasibility of the treatment and its potential effectiveness.

Comment

Grief in standard IPT is applied only to situations following a death (compare also bipolar disorder, Chapter 16). Since loss of health and physical functioning are paramount in post-MI patients, this might justify adding a fifth problem area such as "loss of health." Loss of health may cause interpersonal disputes in the family and could be handled in that focal area. Alternatively, the change in health status could be considered a role transition.

DEPRESSED PATIENTS WITH PHYSICAL DISABILITIES

People with physical disabilities have increased rates of depressive disorders, ranging from 9 percent to 25 percent in prevalence studies. Physical disability often disrupts the interpersonal network. Individuals undergo significant transitions in their interpersonal roles and relationships, and their disability may precipitate or worsen interpersonal disputes. McAnanama and Gillies in Toronto have offered IPT to patients with physical disabilities and comorbid depressive disorders.

Four patients have been treated thus far in an open trial. Two patients had congenital or childhood-onset disabling conditions, whereas the other two became disabled in adulthood. Role transitions and interpersonal deficits were salient foci for the latter group. In contrast, patients with childhood-onset disabilities tolerated severe nonreciprocal role relationships with nondisabled friends and lovers, often to the point of financial exploitation. They also had considerable difficulty in asserting their emotional needs in relationships with nondisabled individuals. Another dimension to relationship patterns was their interaction with personal-care attendants who provide intimate self-care functions on a daily basis. The negotiation of boundaries with self-care attendants proved a delicate balance when the disabled individual was also depressed. All patients showed clinical improvement in their mood status on the basis of changes on the Hamilton Depression Rating Scale (Hamilton, 1960).

PRIMARY INSOMNIA

Many patients suffer from sleep disturbance. Often this is related to a psychiatric or general medical condition, conditions that should be ruled out before the diagnosis of primary insomnia is made. Primary insomnia refers to difficulty in initiating or maintaining sleep, or having nonrestorative sleep, for at least a month (American Psychiatric Association, 1994). In conjunction with Schramm in Freiburg, Müller-Popkes and Hajak at the University of Kiel in Germany have begun the study of IPT as a treatment for this condition.

ADAPTATION

Schramm (unpublished, 1993) modified IPT for insomnia, incorporating some of the elements of social rhythm theory and treatment developed for the treatment of bipolar disorder at the University of Pittsburgh.

EFFICACY

Müller-Popkes and Hajak (1996) published a report of a pilot trial comparing random assignment of patients to twelve weeks of either IPT in fifty-minute sessions or progressive relaxation training (PRT) (Jacobson, 1929) in thirty-minute sessions. Twenty-five patients with primary insomnia were assessed on two occasions in a sleep laboratory: initially two weeks prior to treatment, and again after the last treatment session. IPT patients showed significant improvements in sleep efficiency, total sleep time, and nightly waking; sleep latency improved but the change did not reach statistical significance. In contrast, the PMR group showed no clinical or statistical improvement on sleep parameters.

COMMENT

These findings are preliminary, and it is conceivable that the lengthier treatment exposure of IPT accounted for differences in treatment outcome. Nonetheless, the results are interesting and this area bears further study.

BORDERLINE PERSONALITY DISORDER

Borderline personality disorder (BPD) is a disabling and costly disorder found mostly in young women. Personality disorder refers to a "deeply ingrained, inflexible, maladaptive pattern of relating, perceiving, and thinking of sufficient severity to cause either impairment in functioning or distress" (American Psychiatric Association, 1980, p. 103). The core features of BPD are affective instability and impulsivity and difficulty in interpersonal relations. The overlap with other disorders, particularly depression and anxiety disorder but also eating disorders, ADD, and substance abuse, and the associated 3–10 percent risk of suicide, raise questions about its specificity and epidemiology. Estimates of its prevalence vary widely (Merikangas and Weissman, 1986; Weissman, 1993). One long-term study suggests that patients with BPD, if they do not commit suicide, gradually achieve reasonable interpersonal stability (Stone, 1989).

Sometimes the diagnosis is used pejoratively to describe patients who have failed treatment, or who are demanding and difficult to treat. Difficulties in treating such patients arise from the strength and volatility of their affects: because of their expressed neediness and longings to be nurtured, their rage when these wishes and needs are inevitably not met, and their potential self-destructiveness. A variety of pharmacologic treatments have been used, with modest success and few controlled trials, including monoamine oxidase inhibitors, other antidepressants, carbamazepine, lithium, and low-dose neuroleptics. Their high rate of attrition from treatment makes these patients difficult to study.

Psychotherapy, especially long-term psychodynamic psychotherapy, has been the traditional treatment, and there is an extensive psychoanalytic literature describing approaches to patients with characteristics of BPD. There are no efficacy data, but clinical reports show a high attrition rate and poor response.

The most comprehensive clinical trial of patients with BPD was conducted by Linehan and colleagues (1991, 1994), who compared dialectical behavior therapy (DBT), a variant of cognitive behavioral therapy (Linehan, 1987, 1993), to treatment as usual. DBT uses problem-solving strategies, balancing change with validation of the patient's affect, and incorporates both individual and group modalities. Strategies include:

1. *Problem-solving strategies*: an active attempt to "reframe" suicidal and other dysfunctional behaviors as part of the patient's learned problem-solving repertoire.
2. *Contingency management strategies:* the use of interpersonal reinforcement to shape adaptive behaviors and extinguish those that are maladaptive.
3. *Irreverent communication strategies:* literal-minded attitude about current and previous parasuicidal and other dysfunctional patient behaviors (without being matter-of-fact about the patient's suffering).
4. *Capability enhancement strategies:* active teaching of the skills necessary to cope with oneself and with a sometimes invalidating environment.

The *dialectical* strategies include many techniques used by cognitive therapists but also add a focus on dialectical thinking, metaphor, paradox, comfort with ambiguity and inconsistency, and attention to the dialectical tensions in the therapeutic relationships. The role of the DBT therapist and treatment team is to consult with the patient about how to interact with others, not to consult with others about how to interact with the patient. Linehan et al. (1991) compared DBT to treatment as usual in forty-four women for one year and reported lower suicide attempt rates, improved social functioning, and reduced hospitalization for the DBT group.

ADAPTATION

Many psychopathological features of BPD might seem to lend themselves to IPT treatment: the interacting instability of mood and interpersonal relationships, the difficulties with anger and with separations. Gillies and colleagues in Toronto have adapted IPT for patients with BPD. This was a departure from the original IPT approach, inasmuch as IPT has explicitly not dealt with Axis II personality disorders. The adaptation maintains the time-limited format, the usual IPT techniques, and the four interpersonal problem areas, but adds a fifth potential focus, *self-image* (Gillies and Angus, 1994).

The early phase focuses on the assessment and exploration of symptom patterns of the disorder, such as anger and impulsivity in the context of interpersonal disputes. The therapist develops but does not articulate potential hypotheses about the patient's interpersonal problem areas. Often patients report that their past therapy experiences were difficult or unsuccessful because the therapist appeared uninvolved or distant. In contrast, IPT encourages an active and supportive approach.

Early sessions seek to imbue a sense of hope: the therapist must convey confidence. This is accomplished, in part, by stating that issues that have been raised initially will be addressed in detail in subsequent sessions. This is tied to a discussion of the importance of understanding how to handle difficult episodes so that they do not interfere with or interrupt relationships. Patients with BPD have a checkered and difficult story to tell. The therapist's goal in the first session is to obtain a broad overview, taking care not to be too assertive in pressing for detail or direction. If the patient identifies important interpersonal events spontaneously, he or she is told that they will be returned to in subsequent sessions. It is often useful to focus on the past six months when choosing a problem area. Since the course of the disorder can vary greatly over time, early history may differ remarkably from recent history of symptoms and difficulties.

The fifth interpersonal problem area, *self-image*, has been added because identity disturbance specifically related to uncertain self-image is a prototypical feature of BPD. While the five problem areas often overlap, one is chosen as the primary focus.

The intermediate phase focuses on the dysfunctional aspects of BPD in the context of the predominant interpersonal problem area. Relationship difficulties are viewed as being exacerbated by unstable affect—particularly with regard to anger regulation—and an uncertain and volatile sense of self. Therapists openly discuss with the patient the role that these dysfunctional characteristics play in the generation of interpersonal difficulties. The purpose of this discussion is to provide the patient with a cogent framework in which to develop an understanding of his or her own thoughts, behaviors, and feelings. Furthermore, it acknowledges the primary symptoms of the disorder.

Specific therapeutic tasks during the intermediate phase of the time-limited acute treatment include providing reassurance and support, clarifying cognitive/affective markers that precede and often obscure interpersonal difficulties, and active problem solving of interpersonal dilemmas. Identifying and clearly addressing components of the patient's maladaptive interpersonal style in sessions is an important task.

Unlike traditional psychodynamic approaches, in IPT the transference is not emphasized. If the patient's feelings about the therapist jeopardize the therapeutic relationship, the therapist openly acknowledges and explores the difficulties occurring in the sessions, using this dispute as a model for the resolution of interpersonal problems. The approach is interpersonal, not transferential, following the standard IPT model for depressed patients with interpersonal deficits. In practice this rarely arose.

One goal is to help the borderline patient both experience and understand ambivalent feelings within the context of the interpersonal problem area. Patients must learn to allow themselves to acknowledge the complex mix of changing feelings, judgments, and perceptions they experience in relationships with others. In what is often referred to as splitting, individuals with borderline personality disorder tend to view people dichotomously, as either all good or all bad. This tendency to polarize the actions and intentions of others is evident to therapists when they themselves are rapidly alternating between being idealized and denigrated, and is a normal aspect of work with BPD patients. Enactment of this pattern in the therapy affords the opportunity to carefully explore the generation and expression of these dysfunctional cognitive judgments and affective states. It is useful to assess patients' capacity to talk about problems as their own, rather than as occurring "out there" beyond the sphere of possible change. Another goal is to help patients reach an understanding of the role they play in generating and escalating interpersonal conflicts.

A major therapeutic challenge, particularly in the intermediate and late phases of treatment, is coping with multiple demands to respond immediately to urgent problems or crises. Frequent distressed phone calls from patients can become a common pattern during crises. The recognition and reflection of the affect of genuine distress, irrespective of its ostensible cause, is a critical precondition for the development of a safe and trusting relationship. Failure to initially acknowledge this acute distress can lead to therapeutic impasses in which further escalation of distress may develop.

The therapist must also recognize the stress that he or she experiences in response to these urgent demands for support and for immediate relief from long-standing problems. An important message to convey between sessions is that the therapist hears the patient's concerns but that a telephone conversation is not the most productive context for discussing them. This strategy assures patients that they are being heard between sessions, but that fuller exploration of the problems will take place during the scheduled sessions, not during emergency phone calls.

The final phase of the brief treatment program is characterized by an integration of major interpersonal themes discussed in earlier sessions and a focus on identifying and maintaining new interpersonal coping strategies. Termination is discussed throughout the therapy program, unlike traditional IPT but consonant with many brief treatment approaches. This discussion is important for borderline patients, who often have histories of attachment and separation difficulties. To address the often episodic crises of these patients, it is advisable that monthly or bimonthly continuation or support sessions be scheduled after the completion of the acute treatment. In the acute IPT program described here, therapy sessions are conducted once a week for four months, followed by monthly continuation sessions for another six months. The latter sessions provide ongoing opportunities to discuss termination and separation issues and provide a guided transition from intensive weekly work to establishing and maintaining relationships outside of therapy.

CASE EXAMPLE[4]

Suzanne was a twenty-seven-year-old assistant to a film producer. She had lived for two years with her thirty-four-year-old boyfriend, James, who also worked in the movie industry. Suzanne was referred by her primary care physician for evaluation of depression. She was a friendly, articulate young woman who easily established rapport during the assessment. She met DSM-IV criteria for both major depressive disorder and borderline personality disorder. She was treated with sixteen sessions of IPT: twelve consecutive weekly sessions followed by four monthly maintenance sessions. Her initial Beck Depression Inventory (BDI) score was 39, and her Diagnostic Interview for Borderline Personality Disorder (DIB) score was 10. She had had one prior psychotherapy at age nineteen. She felt that this open-ended psychodynamic treatment helped "somewhat," but found the therapist's silence daunting and dropped out after one month.

Terrified of being alone, Suzanne tolerated verbal abuse from her boss rather than risk abandonment. She also recounted becoming furious with her boyfriend during a discussion of their future together. At the time, she felt uncertain about whether or not she wished to continue the relationship and, indeed, about whether or not she was "the kind of person who could handle a relationship." During the argument, she jumped out of a moving car and skinned her knee and arm. This precipitated her entry to treatment. She identified her uncertainty about who she was as her primary concern and proceeded to work on self-image as her major interpersonal focus in IPT, although touching on interpersonal deficits and disputes.

Suzanne had a history of episodic relationships characterized by initial idealization, after which turmoil and dispute often swiftly followed. She tended to react impulsively when relationships fell apart, overspending on her credit cards and drinking heavily for brief periods. She had a history of cutting herself when she felt overwhelmed; she found the cutting relieving and calming. Suzanne identified herself as very reactive to the perceptions of others. She felt that she didn't know who she was, nor where her real interests were much of the time. She had made a number of career changes on the advice of friends or people whom she admired, and felt profoundly uncertain about herself and her talents.

Early sessions focused on identifying interactions with others that led Suzanne to doubt or to attack herself. She initially had little sense of what precipitated her mood instability and self-image difficulties, but worked with the therapist over the first few weeks of treatment to examine the effects of her communications with others. This was particularly important with regard to her cutting: she became able to identify the kinds of interpersonal interactions that precipitated cutting episodes. These experiences related to fear of loss or of inability to maintain her sense of identity when others were making demands on her.

For example, her boss was planning her future, encouraging her to become a film producer. Suzanne felt uncertain about whether this plan matched her interests and talents. Meanwhile, her parents felt she should return to school and pursue a law degree. She felt intense distress when faced with such competing expectations. After her mother sent her numerous law school applications, she cut herself. Able to see that her sense of her own identity felt fragile under such pressure, Suzanne worked with her therapist to examine communication patterns with her parents, boss, and boyfriend. In addition to giving her the "sick role," the therapist used other IPT strategies, including a weekly review of symptoms (both borderline and depressive), examining role reciprocity, and exploring gains and losses in the sense of self and in expectations about relationships.

In giving the sick role, IPT for borderline patients emphasizes helping the patient to understand his or her vulnerability to impulsivity, affective instability, and interpersonal difficulties. For Suzanne, part of taking the sick role involved establishing with her boyfriend that she might indeed misread situations at times and that she needed to take time out to gather her own thoughts and opinions. During the intermediate phase of treatment, she learned to delay decision making for brief periods rather than making impetuous and ultimately harmful decisions. This strategy helped her to sort out her own feelings and wishes. Suzanne also worked with her therapist to review her own nascent hopes for herself. She expressed an interest in visual arts and looked into a university fine arts program. This was a difficult transition, as it brought into conflict her own expectations for herself versus those of others. She had some stormy exchanges during the intermediate phase of treatment, particularly with her parents, but these seemed necessary for her learning to assert her own interests.

Suzanne found the end of treatment difficult. She had felt supported by her therapist and worried about being able to maintain her sense of self after treatment. Her depression had remitted (BDI=5) and she lost much of her borderline symptomatology (DIB=0). Her sense of emptiness and fear of abandonment persisted, and she was occasionally still impulsive. She recognized this and saw that it was important to pursue her own ambitions even in the face of real or perceived loss of relationships. She also had the experience of working through with her boyfriend a discussion of her own wishes. She was surprised that he could support her career decisions and also supported her evolving sense of herself in the relationship. They were able to disagree, and to agree to disagree, about minor issues. They also became more effective as a couple about communicating during arguments, making frequent use of "time out" strategies. Agreeing not to rush to solve arguments improved the tenor of their relationship.

Suzanne acknowledged a wish to continue in treatment with her therapist and noted that this was the first time she had felt understood and supported. They worked together to establish a sense that she could successfully engage in other relationships, and that learning to say a healthy good-bye was an important step. Suzanne contacted her therapist two years after treatment to let her know that she had enrolled in a graduate art history program and felt she had found an intellectual home. She and her boyfriend had become engaged and were looking forward to marriage. She had not experienced any serious depression in the interval and felt her borderline symptoms were well controlled.

EFFICACY

Gillies and colleagues undertook a pilot treatment trial with twenty-four borderline patients in Toronto, comparing IPT to Relationship Management Therapy (RMT) (Dawson, 1988; Marziali and Munroe-Blum, 1994) in twelve weekly sessions, then following patients monthly for six months. The randomized clinical trial used sequential treatment/therapist crossover design to control for therapist effects.

RMT focuses on helping the patient to deal with ambiguity and uncertainty. Unfortunately, the dropout rate for RMT was so high—more than 75 percent—that randomization was abandoned. Thirteen women aged eighteen and older, recruited through mental health professionals and general practitioners, were enrolled in IPT. Patients with criminal charges or current substance abuse were excluded. About a third were taking antidepressants or anxiolytics during the course of treatment, which were maintained at stable dosages throughout the trial. Eight percent of subjects met criteria for a current major depressive episode.

The attrition rate for IPT was less than 10 percent: twelve of the thirteen patients completed the full course. There was a decline in overall pathology and in self-reported symptoms. Patients identified the IPT therapist's high verbal activity as a helpful factor. The authors note (personal communication, 1998) that they had a liberal policy with regard to missed sessions and required three consecutive missed sessions as the criterion for dropping out. The permission to attend sporadically, the authors felt, may have helped patients to continue and complete the course. Patients absented themselves during periods of intense affect or anger.

COMMENT

The treatment of borderline personality disorder represents the first foray of IPT into personality disorder. It raises many questions: Can a time-limited psychotherapy treat a personality disorder? What are reasonable goals for such brief therapy with such difficult patients: simple containment of impulsive and self-destructive behaviors, rather than complete remission of symptoms? The exclusion criteria Gillies and colleagues used in their study may also have resulted in the selection of a less severely ill subset of patients meeting the diagnosis of borderline personality disorder. The concomitant use of pharmacotherapy is also a problematic confounding factor. Definitive statements about efficacy, particularly for a personality disorder, require a controlled clinical trial and long-term follow-up. In addition, on-going continuation or maintenance treatment may be indicated, like that used for recurrent major depression (Chapter 11), dysthymic disorder (Chapter 12), and other chronic disorders.

NOTES

1. This material on BDD is provided by Drs. M. D. Beary, London; A. Boocock, London; G. Ikkos and M. Morris, Southhall; and D. Veale, London.

2. The authors thank Drs. S. Stuart (University of Iowa), J. Scott, and G. Ikkos (London) for their contributions to this section.

3. Case provided by Scott Stuart, M.D. (University of Iowa).

4. Laurie Gillies, Ph.D., provided this case example as well as background material about her adaptation of IPT for borderline personality disorder.

PART FOUR
IPT RESOURCES

CHAPTER 24

IPT in New Formats: Group, Telephone, Patient Guide; Translation and Use in Other Languages and Cultures

GROUP IPT

Group psychotherapy is a popular modality. It costs less than individual therapy, and has traditionally been considered a setting in which patients can obtain social support and develop interpersonal skills. There are several ongoing efforts to modify IPT for a group format. The best-developed version, which also has the advantage of efficacy data, is the group treatment for bulimia described in Chapter 21 (Wilfley et al., 1993).

Wilfley's model involved relatively minor adaptations. As in much group therapy, sessions last ninety minutes, longer than most individual psychotherapy. There is a pregroup individual interview in which the therapist confirms the patient's diagnosis, completes the interpersonal inventory, explains the process of IPT and sets the treatment contract. Patients are told that the group provides an interpersonal laboratory to work on relationship problems and their social life. Patients with interpersonal deficits are encouraged to use the group as a social milieu to practice. After each session, the therapist summarizes the meeting, focusing on the interpersonal transactions, then mails this summary to participants.

Gillies in Toronto is testing group IPT for adolescent depressed mothers, and Mufson at Columbia University in New York is testing group IPT for depressed adolescents. Klier in Vienna is adapting IPT as a group treatment for postpartum depression, as have Gorman and O'Hara in Iowa. Krupnick and colleagues in Washington, D.C., are developing a group IPT approach for abused women with posttraumatic stress disorder. While the group format seems a natural adaptation of IPT, it requires further testing.

IPT BY TELEPHONE

Many people suffering from psychiatric disorders, particularly depression, receive no treatment. Barriers to treatment include stigma, familial prohibition, geographic distance, financial limitations, physical illness or disability, and the need to care for dependents at home. To make IPT more accessible, its administration by telephone is being assessed in two studies.

The telephone has been shown to be an effective and economical means of extending psychosocial services to medically ill patients (Frasure-Smith and Prince, 1985; Polinsky et al., 1991; Wasson et al., 1992). For example, telephone psychotherapy has been developed and tested for homebound cancer patients (Grumet, 1989; Mermelstein and Holland, 1991).

MEMORIAL SLOAN-KETTERING STUDY

Donnelly, Kornbluth, Holland, and others at Memorial Sloan-Kettering Cancer Center in New York City delivered a form of IPT by telephone to severely medically but not psychiatrically ill patients with metastatic breast cancer receiving a concomitant trial of high dose chemotherapy. The investigators note that the physical, psychological, and social stresses accompanying cancer and its treatment are well established (Holland and Rowland, 1989), as is the effectiveness of psychosocial interventions in facilitating adjustment to those stresses (e.g., Fawzy et al., 1995). As new cancer therapies develop, so does the need to maximize patients' psychological ability to tolerate and to adapt to these treatments. This pilot study was designed to test the feasibility and efficacy of telephone IPT.

Treatment was offered to patients ages eighteen and over and their partners in weekly thirty-minute sessions for approximately fifteen weeks. The patients and their partners faced severe stressors. All patients had metastatic breast cancer considered incurable by standard treatments. Their high-dose chemotherapy regimen was unusually disabling, requiring patients to live within minutes of the hospital for the first two to three months of treatment. This was a major disruption in the lives of most patients and their families. They took extended leaves from jobs, having to move and leave children and/or spouses at home. Role transitions were many and profound, both for patients and their families. They were expected to be too ill to attend office psychotherapy sessions.

The investigators' purpose was to adapt IPT to relieve cancer-related stress rather than depression. They developed a manual for telephone counseling that combined elements of IPT and IPC (see Chapter 17). Among the modifications was the routine offer of treatment to patients' partners. Therapists tended to focus on role transitions, and omitted mention of the "sick role," as patients did not necessarily have psychiatric diagnoses. Telephone counseling began with the onset of chemotherapy and continued in thirty-minute weekly sessions for its duration, about three months, and for four weeks beyond. Scheduling of sessions was flexible, based on the patient's medical status. Ratings were assessed at intake, end of chemotherapy (three months), and two weeks after the final telephone session (five months).

Fourteen women with breast cancer and ten of their partners (83 percent of eligible patients) entered the study. One dropped out early, shortly before withdrawing from chemotherapy. The other patients completed a mean sixteen sessions, while partners averaged eleven sessions. Based on Mental Health Inventory (Veit and Ware, 1983) Psychological Distress scores, five patients and three partners were rated improved; three patients and three partners remained essentially unchanged; and four patients and one partner worsened. Participants rated satisfaction with the therapy between "good" and "excellent," comparing it favorably to prior psychotherapy experiences. The major impediment to the therapy was the patient's physical health, which in six cases delayed outcome assessments.

COLUMBIA STUDY

Another pilot telephone trial is comparing IPT, delivered over the telephone, to no treatment in thirty depressed mothers who had been part of a ten- to fifteen-year naturalistic longitudinal study (Miller and Weissman, personal communication, 1998). These mothers have had recurrent depression but have not received regular treatment. No specific adaptation has been made other than the substitution of the telephone for face-to-face interviews. All patients had been assessed clinically as part of the longitudinal study, so that patients with a suicide history, psychotic disorder, or severe depression were excluded.

Patients were randomized to receive either IPT or no treatment in a controlled clinical trial. IPT subjects were offered twelve fifty-minute sessions. IPT was described as a brief psychological treatment for depression which had been shown to be helpful when delivered face-to-face, but which was only now being tested over the telephone. Patients were informed that should their level of depression pose a threat to themselves or to others, they would be encouraged to go to an emergency room, or else the psychotherapist would call to have an ambulance take them to the emergency room.

Therapists also arranged with patients to telephone at a mutually acceptable session time. Although patients were encouraged to maintain sessions at the same time each week, they were free to call ahead to reschedule when necessary. Patients were encouraged to find a time during the week when they were the only person at home, allowing them privacy and freedom from distraction.

CASE EXAMPLE

Patricia was a thirty-year-old married woman. At the age of twelve months, her now three-year-old daughter was diagnosed with a severe congenital disorder that precludes her walking, talking, or feeding herself. She also had behavioral problems that Patricia felt unable to control. Patricia has a history of recurrent major depressive disorder. At the time of initial telephone contact, she was mildly to moderately depressed, with a Hamilton Depression Rating Scale score of 18.

Patricia eagerly accepted the offer of IPT by telephone, stating that she "needed to talk to somebody," and answered the telephone promptly as scheduled for her initial session. In that session, she was forthcoming about her current life situation. Most of the session was devoted to her description of her role as full-time caretaker of her disabled daughter, whom she referred to as "my life." She felt isolated, embarrassed by the child's condition, and overwhelmed with guilt despite awareness of the genetic etiology of the illness and her certainty that she had fully complied with prenatal care.

A key interpersonal problem concerned her role as primary caretaker for her daughter. On the one hand, Patricia said she felt lonely and angry about having this role. On the other hand, she refused to include the school psychologist, teachers, nurses, or even her husband in decisions about her child's treatment for fear she would be "overpowered" or coerced into the wrong course of treatment. Patricia expressed concern that her dilemma in her caretaking role had recently precipitated significant medical problems. Several months prior to starting IPT, against the advice of the child's doctor, Patricia had adamantly refused the assistance of a live-in nurse (covered by her insurance) to assist with a home-based dietary treatment designed to ameliorate the symptoms of the girl's disease. When, due in part to her confusion in preparing the meals, the dietary treatment failed and the girl became quite ill, Patricia felt intense guilt and sank into an episode of depression.

Initial Phase

Patricia's interpersonal problem area was formulated as a role transition: her daughter's illness had pressed her into the narrow role of full-time caretaker. She now needed to expand her role to the broader one of mother and wife. Patricia readily acknowledged that her world had narrowed to exclude adult relationships and pleasant experiences outside the home. In collaborating on the formulation with the therapist, Patricia recalled that for more than a year she had neither seen a movie nor eaten at a restaurant with her husband. He felt that Patricia was being unreasonable and should make time for him. They often argued about her unavailability. Recognizing with the therapist the confinement of her role unleashed Patricia's frustration and her anger over her "not perfect life" and "not perfect" child.

When asked about her experience of the telephone as a medium for treatment, Patricia responded that she would only do therapy by telephone because the demands of her child's care left her no time to come to a clinic. She expressed appreciation of the opportunity to vent her frustration to a therapist in the familiar and private setting of her home.

Intermediate Phase

Patricia and the therapist now developed strategies to facilitate her role transition away from the sole role of caretaker. Interpersonal strategies included methods for building "partnerships" with other caretakers: the school psychologist, teachers, nurses, doctors, and, most important, her husband. In a relatively short time, Patricia became skilled at enlisting the help and concern of other caretakers by explaining her fears, posing treatment questions, and requesting help. As Patricia built partnerships, she became less overwhelmed and more interested in adult contacts, including those with her husband. She noticed that with these changes, her daughter began acting out less frequently in her presence.

When again asked to evaluate telephone treatment, Patricia replied that she looked forward to the weekly sessions as the only time designated specifically for her well-being. She emphasized that over the telephone she felt free to express herself.

Termination Phase

In the late phase of treatment, Patricia noted that building partnerships had somewhat eased the burden of her child's illness. She also remarked that as she made her husband a "partner" by asking him for help, they communicated better about their child. Improved marital communication produced both a stronger alliance and more arguments about issues in the child's care that had not been discussed. Patricia's handling of the role transition was thus creating a change in a complementary interpersonal problem area: a shift from impasse to conflict in the area of role dispute. This shift was discussed, and the treatment concluded with the development of strategies Patricia could use to maintain authentic communication with her husband.

In her transition beyond the role of sole caretaker, Patricia considered the possibility of having a second child. In the initial phase of treatment, she had expressed guilt that having a second child would "cheat my daughter." She also feared that she would give birth to another child with the same illness, despite having received reassurance to the contrary from a genetic counselor. Once she reformulated her role, she evaluated the prospect of pregnancy differently. In the last session, Patricia wondered whether "growing up with a sister like [her daughter] might make a sibling more sensitive than most kids." After a silence, she continued, "If the second child has the problem, then I just guess my calling in this life is to take care of disabled children."

Evaluation of Treatment

At Week 12, Patricia showed a decrease in scores on both the Hamilton Depression Rating Scale (a drop from 18 to 3) and on the Hamilton Anxiety Scale (a drop from 12 to 4). She claimed that she greatly valued her telephone treatment and would like to continue on a weekly basis, but would settle for a biweekly continuation treatment. She kept every scheduled session (two were rescheduled within the same week) and answered the telephone promptly when the therapist called. When asked at the end of treatment whether she would accept a face-to-face therapy, Patricia responded that she preferred the telephone. She was certain that she could not make the time to travel to a clinic, and she repeatedly mentioned that she felt "freed up" to talk in the privacy of her home without "having to deal with the reactions of still another hospital doctor." That Patricia expressed ambivalence about face-to-face treatment with a professional is consistent with her ongoing struggle to form partnerships with professionals. Given this interpersonal difficulty, the anonymity and leveling effect of the telephone may have allowed Patricia to engage in a brief treatment.

COMMENT

The therapists in both studies report the feasibility and patient acceptance of IPT over the telephone. Yet caution is in order. The cancer study excluded patients with psychiatric disorders, and the Columbia study excluded seriously mentally ill patients. Psychotherapy by telephone may be optimal for less symptomatic patients who do not require close monitoring. All patients were seen for an evaluation prior to starting treatment. We recommend that all patients receive a face-to-face evaluation before beginning treatment by telephone. The efficacy of this approach is pending.

PATIENT GUIDE

Weissman (1995) has developed a user-friendly patient guide to IPT with accompanying worksheets. This is designed for patients who want to learn about or who are receiving IPT. The idea is to help depressed individuals either to learn to cope with their depression or to understand some of the methods that trained therapists might use to help them.

We do not know whether reading a book about depression is helpful. This, too, deserves testing. We do believe that a clear understanding of the facts about depression and about the therapeutic strategy of IPT is useful to patients in treatment, and may be helpful generally. The patient guide is consonant with the psychoeducational component of IPT, and with its assumption that the more the patient knows about depression and the efficacy of antidepressant treatments, the better. The principle is that the educated patient is the best consumer of treatment.

The guide belongs to the current trend in the United States to destigmatize psychiatric problems and to demystify treatment so that people suffering from these disorders can get appropriate help early, before the symptoms have enduring consequences in their work and family life. We believe that patients with psychiatric symptoms should know what the available treatment options are, what to expect in treatment, and when to seek alternate treatments. We do not believe that there is only one treatment for depression or that IPT is best for all depressed patients.

An excerpt from the forms used to determine the problem areas follows:

During the intermediate session of IPT, you and your therapist will choose one or two problem areas to work on. These problems may change over the course of treatment. Do not be concerned if this happens. If you are not in IPT treatment, you may want to use these forms to help understand the problems associated with your depression.

1. When did your symptoms of depression *first* begin?
   _____(Month) _____(Year)

   Is this the first time you were depressed?
   ___Yes   ___No   ___Don't Know

   If this was not the first episode of depression, when did this episode begin?
   _____(Month) _____(Year)

2. Think about what was going on in your life when you started to feel depressed this time.

   Did someone you cared about die?
   ___Yes   ___No   ___Don't Know

   Was it the anniversary of someone's death?
   ___Yes   ___No   ___Don't Know

   Were you thinking about someone who died?
   ___Yes   ___No   ___Don't Know

   Were you having problems at home with your spouse or partner?
   ___Yes   ___No   ___Don't Know

   Were you having problems with your children?
   ___Yes   ___No   ___Don't Know

Worksheet questions are incorporated into the flow of the text for continuity. It is recommended that, prior to termination, patients redo all the forms to evaluate the progress of therapy and highlight any areas that may need further work. A separate booklet containing the worksheet or monitoring forms is also available. These forms can be used to continue to monitor problem areas after treatment ends. It is recommended that patients review their completed forms with the therapist.

The book is intended to facilitate treatment. Formal testing to determine whether the use of the patient book facilitates treatment has not been carried out. Informal reports by Gillies in Toronto, and by Markowitz in New York (personal communications, 1999), note that patient response has been positive and that some therapists have found it useful during training.

Weissman, in collaboration with Judd in Melbourne, Australia, is incorporating the monitoring forms into a study of IPC for depressed patients in primary care. Patients will be encouraged to complete the forms between sessions and return them to the therapist at the beginning of each session. This approach is designed to maximize the efficiency of patient/therapist contact. Feasibility and efficacy await testing. The patient guide (*Mastering Depression: A Patient's Guide to Interpersonal Psychotherapy*) can be obtained through The Psychological Corporation, Order Service Center, P.O. Box 839954, San Antonio, TX 78283–3954 (telephone: 1–800–211–8378).

TRANSLATION AND USE IN OTHER LANGUAGES AND CULTURES

Developed in the United States, IPT has attracted attention abroad. Some clinicians outside the United States have wondered whether the optimism and pragmatism of IPT represent an endogenously American, "Coca-Cola" approach untranslatable to other cultures or languages. Serious discussion has usually led to agreement that interpersonal problem areas are ubiquitous and that the IPT approach makes clinical sense regardless of geography. The ultimate answer to the question is taking the form of translation and controlled clinical trials to test the efficacy of IPT in different countries and languages (e.g., Blom et al., 1996; Rosello and Bernal, in press; see Chapters 10 and 13).

Cultural adjustments may prove necessary in certain situations. For example, it has been suggested that many Dutch women are taught that it is immodest to acknowledge wanting anything. Hence, it may be more difficult for them than for their American counterparts to verbalize their desires in certain interpersonal situations.

The transportation of IPT to other countries has occurred in several ways. There have been direct translations of the original manual (Klerman et al.,

1984). The English-language manual has been used to train bilingual therapists in the native language of their patients, e.g., in Holland, Spain, and Puerto Rico. IPT has also been used in English-speaking countries: the United Kingdom, Australia, New Zealand, and Canada.

The original IPT manual (Klerman et al., 1984) has been translated, in whole or in part, into Italian, Japanese, German, and Spanish. French and Thai translations are being planned. The translators are listed below. IPT has also been described in publications in other languages.

In 1997, a group of researchers and clinicians met at the Tenth World Congress of Psychiatry to launch a European IPT association (Solé-Puig, 1997).

Australia

Contact: Fiona Judd, M.D., The University of Melbourne, Department of Psychiatry, 7th Floor, Charles Connibere Building, c/o P.O. Royal Melbourne Hospital, Parkville 3050, Australia.

Dr. Judd is conducting a study in primary care.

Austria

Contact: Claudia Klier at the Universitätsklinik für Psychiatrie Wien (Allgemeines Krankenhaus, 1090 Wien, Währinger Gürtel 18–20, Austria) is conducting group IPT trials for depressed postpartum women.

Brazil

Contact: Marcelo Feijo De Mello (at Dr. Mario Ferraz 53, Apt. 51, São Paulo, Brazil 01453–010) is conducting a preliminary study of IPT for dysthymic patients.

Canada

Contacts: Laurie Gillies, Ph.D., Clarke Institute, 250 College Street, Toronto, Canada M5T 1R8; Gina Browne, Ph.D., Reg. N., Director, System-Linked Research Unit, McMaster University, Faculty of Health Sciences, 1200 Main Street West, HSC 3N47, Hamilton, Ontario, Canada L8N 3Z5.

Dr. Gillies heads an IPT clinic at the Clarke Institute in Toronto, has undertaken several adaptations of IPT (see Chapters 13 and 23), and has an IPT training program. Dr. Browne has completed a large study of IPT for dysthymic patients in primary care (see Chapter 12).

France

A French translation is planned by Professor Charles Pull, Centre Hospitalier de Luxembourg, 4 rue Barblé, L–1210 Luxembourg. (See also Switzerland.)

Germany

There is a German translation of part of the original book: Schramm, E. 1996. *Interpersonelle Psychotherapie bei Depressionen und anderen psychischen Störungen.* Stuttgart and New York: Schattauer.

Schramm has also conducted numerous workshops in Germany. Müller-Popkes in Hamburg is conducting research on IPT as a treatment for insomnia (Müller-Popkes and Hajak, 1996). Bauer and colleagues in Freiburg are developing an adaptation of IPT for patients with early Alzheimer's disease. Schramm is planning to test IPT as a treatment for inpatients in Freiburg, as hospital stays remain long in Germany.

Contact: E. Schramm, Ph.D., Klinikum der Albert-Ludwigs-Universität Freiburg, Universitätsklinik für Psychiatrie und Psychosomatik, Hauptstrasse 5 D–79104, Freiburg, Germany.

Iceland

Contacts: Högni Oskarsson, M.D., Sudurgata 12, 101 Reykjavík, Iceland; Halldóra Olafsdóttir, M.D., Nordurbrun 20, 104 Reykjavík, Iceland.

Italy

Translation: Klerman, G. L., M. M. Weissman, B. J. Rounsaville, and E. S. Chevron. 1989. *Psicoterapia Interpersonale della Depressione.* Translated by P. Galezzi; edited by G. Berti Ceroni. Torino: Bollati Boringhieri.

Contacts: Giuseppe Berti Ceroni, Servizio Sanitario Nazionale, Regione Emilia-Romagna, Unita Sanitaria Locale n. 27, Bologna Ovest, Italy; Giovanni de Girolamo, M.D., Azienda USL Città di Bologna Servizio di Salute Mentale, Viale Pepoli, 5–40123 Bologna, Italy; Luigi Grassi, M.D., Clinica Psichiatrica, Università di Ferrara, Corso Giovecca 203, 44100 Ferrara, Italy;

and Andrea Pergami, M.D., Psychiatric Unit, Azienda USSL 26, Ospedale Predabissi, 20077 Vizzolo, Milan, Italy.

Japan

Translation: Klerman, G. L., M. M. Weissman, B. J. Rounsaville, and E. S. Chevron. 1997. *Interpersonal Psychotherapy of Depression.* Translated into Japanese by Hiroko Mizushima, Makoto Shimada, and Yutaka Ono. Tokyo: Iwasaki Gakujyutsa.

Contact: Yutaka Ono, M.D., 5–22–8 Soshigaya, Setagaya-Ku, Tokyo 157, Japan. We are unaware of current research on IPT in Japan.

The Netherlands

IPT is flourishing in the Netherlands. A description of the general method of IPT and its adaptation has been published in Dutch (Blom, Kerver, and Nolen, 1997), although the manual has not been directly translated. IPT was listed as one of the proven efficacious treatments for depression without psychotic features in treatment guidelines developed at the 1994 Dutch Consensus Conference (Consensus-bijeenkomst Depressie bij Volwassenen, 1994).

Under the leadership of Hoencamp in The Hague, a pilot open trial of IPT was completed (Blom, Hoencamp, and Zwaan, 1996) demonstrating feasibility in ten depressed Dutch patients. A large, three-site clinical trial comparing IPT, nefazodone, their combination, and IPT plus placebo is under way. The goal, to recruit fifty depressed patients per cell, is more than half achieved. Other pilot trials are also under way: in Maastricht, a study of IPT for panic patients by Arzt and van Rijsoort; in Rotterdam, a study of adherence and outcome comparing IPT to treatment as usual for depression (Hoencamp and Jonker, personal communication, 1997); and in Leyden, a study comparing eight and sixteen sessions of IPT versus CBT (E. Hoencamp, personal communication, 1998).

Contacts: Marc Blom, M.D., Riagg Westhage, P.O. Box 17162, 2502 CD, Den Haag, Netherlands; Erik Hoencamp, M.D., Ph.D., Psychiatrisch Centrum Bloemendaal, Monsterweg 93, 2553 RJ, Den Haag Postbus 53002, Netherlands; Kosse Jonker, Ph.D., Psychiatrisch Centrum Bloemendaal, Monsterweg 93, 2553 RJ, Den Haag Postbus 53002, Netherlands; Herro F.

Kraan, M.D., Ph.D., Twents Psychiatrisch Ziekenhuis, Postbus 347, 7500 AH, Enschede, Netherlands; Pieternel Kölling, M.D., Twents Psychiatrisch Ziekenhuis, Postbus 347, 7500 AH, Enschede, Netherlands; Alex van Bemmel, M.D., Ph.D., Head, Academic Mood Disorders and Sleep Laboratory, University of Limburg, Maastricht, 6200 MD, Maastricht, Netherlands; Mirjam van Rijsoort, Department of Experimental Psychopathology, Dutch Institute for Research and Postgraduate Education, University of Limburg, Universiteitssingel 50, P.O. Box 616, ML–6200 MD, Maastricht, Netherlands.

New Zealand

Studies of eating disorders and depression are under way. *Contact:* Peter Joyce, M.D., The Christchurch School of Medicine, Department of Psychological Medicine, P. O. Box 4345, Christchurch, New Zealand.

Norway

Contacts: Martin Svartberg, M.D., and Aviva Mayers, M.S.W., University of Trondheim, The Medical Faculty, Department of Psychiatry and Behavioural Medicine, Ostmarka Hospital, P.O. Box 3008 Lade, N–7002 Trondheim, Norway.

Ms. Mayers conducts IPT training in Trondheim. There is a brief description on the use of IPT in Norwegian (Lorentzen, 1993).

Spain

IPT was introduced by Solé-Puig (Puig, 1995a, b), who has translated the IPT manual (Solé-Puig, 1998) and founded the Sociedad Española de Psicoterapia Interpersonal. IPT has also been used in Puerto Rico with Spanish-speaking patients (see Chapter 13, Rosello and Bernal, in press).

Contact: José Solé-Puig, M.D., Universitat de Barcelona, Department de Psiquiatría i Psicobiologia Clinica, Casanova 143, 08036 Barcelona, Spain.

Sweden

Contact: Roland Berg, M.D., Dalagatan 42, S–11324 Stockholm, Sweden.

Switzerland

Contact: Theodore Hovaguimian, M.D., 12 rue Verdaine, 1204 Geneva, Switzerland.

Thailand

Dr. Sughondhabirom in Bangkok plans to translate IPT into Thai.

United Kingdom

Contacts: Christopher Fairburn, M.D., Oxford University Department of Psychiatry, Warneford Hospital, Oxford OX3 7JX, United Kingdom; Steven Martin, M.D., and Elizabeth Martin, R.N., Sunderland Hospital, Sunderland, United Kingdom.

A U.K. report commissioned by the Department of Health on the efficacy of psychotherapies included IPT as a key treatment for mood disorders and bulimia. This report was subsequently published by Roth and Fonagy, 1996.

Studies include neuroimaging research by the Martins comparing response to IPT and pharmacotherapy for depression.

CHAPTER 25

Training and
Treatment Manuals

TRAINING IN IPT

IPT is designed for use by psychiatrists, psychologists, psychiatric social workers, nurses, internists, or other health professionals who have already achieved proficiency in some form of psychotherapy, have already learned the skills of listening and talking to patients, and have some clinical experience. Those who lack psychotherapeutic training can use interpersonal counseling (IPC; see Chapter 17). Table 25.1 summarizes requirements for IPT therapists.

The IPT therapist should have at least two years of clinical experience in psychotherapy for ambulatory depressed patients, or for patients with the diagnosis to which IPT is to be applied. For example, a therapist inexperienced in treating bulimia nervosa will need some exposure to and supervision for that diagnosis. Therapists are further evaluated by IPT training therapists to ensure that they meet an acceptable standard of clinical competence, including the ability to relate to patients with warmth, interest, and empathy; the ability to build a therapeutic alliance; and so forth. In addition, therapists should have a positive attitude about time-limited treatment and an open-minded approach to the use of interpersonal techniques. The IPT therapist should have no rigid attachment to an alternative therapeutic belief system. Finally, it is assumed that, on the basis of previous training and experience, the therapist recognizes his or her own strengths and weaknesses in relating to different kinds of patients.

TABLE 25.1   Training Requirements for IPT

Prerequisites
1. Advanced health care or mental health care degrees, e.g., M.D., Ph.D., M.S.W., R.N.
2. Experience as a psychotherapist (at least 2 years)
3. Experience in working with depressed (or other target diagnosis) patients

Training
1. Read IPT manual
2. Attend workshop or course
3. Supervision by a trained IPT therapist, using taped cases
   • ideally, supervision of 3 cases (for research certification)
4. Certification: supervisor's approval of competence

The IPT approach has been most readily learned by fully trained psychotherapists who are already experienced and proficient in psychotherapy. For therapists with a background in long-term psychodynamic therapy, adopting an IPT approach primarily involves refocusing and condensing the type of work they may already be doing with nonpsychotic outpatients. For such therapists, learning the IPT approach requires including a "medical model" approach to psychoeducation about depression; focusing interventions to follow the strategies for identifying and approaching the four types of interpersonal problem areas; and increasing the activity level in order to complete the work in a relatively limited number of sessions (twelve to sixteen) and a correspondingly brief time period. Adjusting to an IPT approach also means avoiding a focus on transference, the interpretation of dreams and relationships, a conflict-based approach to psychopathology, and a focus on personality. It means focusing on helping the patient to actively change aspects of his or her life rather than simply on understanding them. Thus, IPT bears a relationship to but still differs significantly from psychodynamic psychotherapy (Markowitz et al., 1998). Adherents of relatively "pure," long-term and open-ended forms of psychodynamic psychotherapy may conversely find IPT concepts differ from those they are accustomed to.

Psychotherapists who have been trained in a behavioral or cognitive approach need to adjust to different technical interventions. The focus of treatment shifts from affectively tinged ("hot") cognitions to the affects themselves as they arise in interpersonal situations. On the other hand, cognitive and behavioral approaches to depression often employ a similar time frame to IPT, and familiarity with a time-limited approach may make adjustment easier. Analogous to IPT, CBT therapists frequently treat specific disorders such as major depression, and some techniques, such as role playing, are common to both approaches.

The three components of IPT training are (1) the material assembled in this book; (2) a didactic seminar; and (3) supervised casework based on the supervisor's review of videotapes of psychotherapy sessions (Markowitz, 1999).

WRITTEN MATERIAL

The major instrument used to define, specify, and transmit the strategies and techniques of IPT is this book and its earlier version (Klerman et al., 1984). It discusses the theoretical background and general characteristics of the treatment. The current and earlier version of the IPT manual differ from most other books on psychotherapy by providing detailed instructions and guidelines for the actual conduct of the treatment. They demarcate both the external and the internal boundaries of IPT. The IPT approach comprises an operationalized list of techniques that may be drawn upon, a detailed outline of four general formulations (Markowitz and Swartz, 1997) and strategies for approaching the patient's interpersonal problems depending on the type of issues presented, a set of guidelines for handling specific problems (silence, lateness, and so on) that commonly arise in psychotherapy, instructions about the sequence of events to be followed in the different phases of therapy, and descriptions of the defining features of the relationship the IPT therapist attempts to form with the patient.

External boundaries of IPT are also delimited, and techniques that are not part of IPT are described. Also beyond the boundaries of IPT is the use of a therapeutic stance inconsistent with IPT, such as being overactive or directive, or insufficiently supportive or active. These manuals are designed to provide therapists with easily available guidelines by which to conduct IPT.

DIDACTIC SEMINAR

Original Seminars

In two- to five-day seminars, we attempted to help therapists in the early IPT studies to identify what they were already doing that was compatible with IPT, what they were doing that was not IPT, and the skills needed for the IPT approach. This teaching took the form of a review of the written material included in Part 1 of this book, intermixed with clinical illustrations using videotaped case material and role playing.

Our training experience is based on work with mental health professionals who had completed their highest professional degree and had a minimum of two years of psychotherapy experience using an insight-oriented, exploratory approach. These therapists were selected based on review of their credentials; on their having read IPT material and found it compatible with their work; and on a trainer's review of videotaped samples of their clinical work. Given this preselection, we found that IPT could be readily learned by most of those who attempted it. In three training courses involving twenty-seven therapists, twenty-three (85 percent) were certified as competent IPT therapists at the completion of training. However, there are several areas in which IPT trainees have had difficulty (Weissman, Rounsaville, and Chevron, 1982). These parallel the four areas of IPT emphasized in the training.

The first concerns the emphasis on depression as a psychiatric disorder. Psychotherapists who have not worked in a medical setting are sometimes reluctant to review depressive symptoms systematically, to define their onset as part of a medical syndrome, and to direct interventions toward mitigating and managing the symptoms. Instead, they tend to immediately focus on interpersonal issues without specifically addressing the patient's symptoms. This is a serious mistake, since patients usually seek treatment primarily because of their symptoms. Ignoring them may reduce a patient's sense of being heard and helped.

The second problem area concerns the emphasis on problems in current interpersonal functioning. Highly experienced psychodynamically trained psychotherapists may fall into lengthy discussions of childhood relationships or of transference rather than attempting to relate the uncovered interpersonal patterns to the immediate interpersonal problems. A short-term treatment lacks the time for lengthy explorations of all determinants of current behavior; nor is this an objective of IPT. If past determinants are discussed at all, they should be explicitly related to current interpersonal patterns in the "here and now."

The third problem concerns the exploratory aspect of IPT. Trainees may err in following the training manual in a rigid, "cookbook" fashion, failing to pay close attention to nuances of the therapeutic relationship or to subtle shifts in affect and emphasis by the patient. Whatever the structure and goals of a particular psychotherapy, the patient-therapist relationship is the central feature without which it cannot succeed. For example, although many tasks should be defined and accomplished in the initial sessions, it is unwise for the therapist to charge straight through them if the patient is severely symptomatic or manifests doubts and hesitations about the therapist or the treatment. The IPT therapist must recognize first and foremost the need to build a working alliance. For severely personality disordered patients, it may be necessary to spend additional time early in treatment establishing an alliance before proceeding with particular IPT techniques. Those who spend their energy going "by the book" miss this point.

The fourth problem relates to time-limited treatment. Many experienced psychotherapists with backgrounds in open-ended, long-term, psychoanalytically oriented treatment have difficulty adjusting to actively focusing the sessions and quickly offering interpretive feedback to the patient. Many IPT trainees have never explicitly attempted brief or time-limited treatment and tend to emphasize long-standing personality issues rather than more acute depressive symptoms. These trainees are often surprised and gratified to note the extent to which seemingly intransigent "personality traits" yield when depressive symptoms are relieved in the course of a brief treatment. Adjustment to the short-term nature of the treatment occurs most readily when the therapist comes to believe that meaningful work—i.e., symptom reduction and resolution of a specific interpersonal problem—can be accomplished in a limited time interval.

Subsequent Experience

In recent years we have continued to give one- and two-day seminars, workshops, and courses to mental health clinicians in various settings. These have corroborated earlier impressions. Scientific developments have familiarized many psychotherapists with the concept of time-limited treatments, and economic changes have increasingly coerced their use. Seminars help to reinforce the techniques described in the written material. Discussions often help seminar participants trained in other psychotherapies to resolve questions and to adopt the IPT mind-set.

We have been impressed that even relatively inexperienced psychotherapists, such as third-year psychiatric residents, can learn basic IPT techniques by reading the book, attending a course, and treating supervised cases (Markowitz, 1995; Markowitz, in press). Although residents lacked psychotherapeutic experience, they compensated for needed security in the therapeutic role with their enthusiasm, appearing to adjust relatively easily to the demands of conducting an active, time-limited approach. As relative novices, they also had fewer "bad habits" from other therapies to correct, and often enjoyed the relaxed, conversational stance of IPT. Some did need time to develop comfort in actively intervening with patients and focusing sessions. Videotaping of sessions for supervision and the availability of appropriately trained supervisors are important for training residents. The latter, especially, are not yet universally available.

SUPERVISED CASEWORK

After the didactic seminar, therapists are assigned two to four training cases, for each of which they receive weekly supervision on a session-by-session basis. Supervision may be done by telephone or in person and follows the review by the supervisor of the videotape or audiotape of the session. Both trainee and supervisor should have tape equipment and tapes available so that they can watch specific segments as they discuss the session. The primary purpose of supervision is boundary marking, or helping the therapists learn which techniques are included and which are excluded in IPT. It is also helpful if the supervisor reviews the ratings made by the patient during the session. Serial symptom ratings are helpful to therapist trainees, as they are to patients, in measuring progress toward remission.

Our first training program demonstrated the importance of basing supervision on review of videotapes. In this project, supervision was carried out in the traditional manner: reviewing therapy process notes. After each supervisory session, the supervisor rated the therapist's use of IPT techniques and strategies. Videotapes were also made of the supervisory sessions, and several months after the training, the two supervisors reviewed them, making ratings using the same format. What we found was that the two supervisors agreed with what they saw on the videotapes (Pearson's r = .88), but there was no significant relationship between the videotape ratings of the psychotherapists and those made on the basis of traditional supervision.

Two kinds of discrepancies between traditional supervision and viewing videotapes were noted. Several therapists who on videotape review were thought to be excellent had underrated their own work, whereas some who could talk IPT theory and technique and presented their cases well were rated poorly when actual sessions were viewed. This independence of impressions gained from process-note supervision and from viewing videotapes is a key issue that deserves consideration in other types of clinical training (Chevron and Rounsaville, 1983).

In recent years, IPT supervision has been conducted over great distances. Therapists in Europe and across the United States have taped treatment sessions (in English), shipped them by overnight mail to New York, reviewed them by telephone with their supervisors, and thus kept current in their training cases. This approach is expensive but effective, allowing therapists far from IPT research and training sites to learn the technique.

Evaluation Methods

In keeping with the research orientation of IPT training, we have been careful to evaluate the competence of trainees to perform IPT as defined in this book and to assess their progress systematically in the course of training. We believe that the best indicator that therapists have mastered this approach to treatment is their actual performance in psychotherapy sessions with depressed patients. For that reason, certification of psychotherapist competence is made on the basis of reviewing videotaped psychotherapy sessions. To evaluate the therapist's performance, a rating system has been devised that covers three levels of compliance with the IPT approach: (1) broadly defined use of appropriate IPT strategies; (2) appropriate use of specific IPT techniques; and (3) absence of use of techniques that are not part of IPT. In each area, the rater assesses both whether or not a strategy or technique has been utilized, and the quality of its use. Evaluators also rate general psychotherapeutic skills and patient cooperation.

Two evaluators assess trainee competence: (1) the supervisor, who also shares his or her impressions with the trainee; and (2) an evaluator independent of the training. The use of an independent rater who is not invested in the training process was thought necessary to determine whether the supervisory relationship might bias the rater in favor of his or her supervisees. In fact, the level of agreement between ratings of supervisors and independent evaluators has been high (Weissman, 1982).

Each evaluator bases ratings on review of entire psychotherapeutic sessions. The reason for reviewing the entire hour is that the domains being rated encompass more than the nature of the therapeutic relationship, which could be assessed in a shorter time. Evaluating the appropriate use of specific techniques and strategies requires knowledge of their context. Moreover, the IPT emphasis on the sequencing of strategies across sessions and focusing on targeted problems makes it desirable for evaluators to rate therapists with knowledge of what has occurred earlier in the treatment and what goals the therapist had in mind.

Effects of Supervised Casework

Because the therapist's competence to conduct IPT was rated on the basis of performance in psychotherapy sessions, the first ratings were made after trainees already had been carefully selected and the didactic seminar completed. Thus, ratings of change over time could reflect only the effects of supervised casework. In comparing ratings of therapists' first and final training cases, we found that degree of improvement was related to psychotherapists' experience.

In one training program, in which trainees had an average of fourteen years of experience, we noted a ceiling effect: ratings based on performance in the first supervised case had an average level of "excellent." Therapists had apparently been able to grasp IPT techniques simply by reading the manual and attending the seminar. In one to three additional training cases, experienced psychotherapists showed neither significant improvement nor significant deterioration in their performance of IPT. In a similar program where trainees had less than six years of experience, average performance in the first training case was rated "acceptable." Performance significantly improved in the second case, but ratings remained below the excellent mark. It is no surprise that more extensive supervised casework seems necessary for less experienced psychotherapists (Chevron, Rounsaville, and Weissman, 1983).

Even after training, less experienced therapists achieved significantly lower ratings of IPT performance than more experienced ones. Inexperienced therapists often became skillful at performing the more structured, best-defined aspects of treatment. For example, they scored highly on using a syndromal approach to depressive symptoms, completing tasks described for initial sessions and termination sessions, and focusing on a single, defined current interpersonal problem area. Yet they were more likely than experienced therapists to perform treatment in a stereotyped fashion, showing less ability to change direction in an exploratory fashion and to form working alliances with difficult or resistant patients (Chevron et al., 1983). Experienced psychotherapists were excellent at performing IPT in a subtle and flexible manner and at maintaining rapport with patients. They tended to have difficulty with the more structured aspects of treatment, such as reviewing depressive symptoms and keeping the work focused in order to complete it within the time limit.

IPT TRAINING TAPES

Two videotapes are available that present key features of IPT and may be useful for training purposes. Kingsley Communications (5307 Cherokee Street, Houston, TX 77005) produced "Interpersonal Psychotherapy of Depression," which features Drs. Weissman and Markowitz. The Lundbeck International Psychiatric Institute (Grevinde Danns Palae, Skodsborg Strandvej 113, DK–2942 Skodborg, Denmark) has produced complementary tapes about IPT and CBT.

USES OF THIS BOOK

IPT training involves adjusting and refocusing the type of work that many traditionally trained, experienced psychotherapists already do. Thus, highly experienced, selected psychotherapists who participated in a didactic training seminar and carefully reviewed the manual were able to perform IPT adequately in the first supervised training case. For less experienced therapists, more lengthy supervised casework was advisable.

Several research groups have essentially taught themselves IPT based on a reading of the 1984 book and, in one case, participation by some of the group's members in a brief didactic seminar. In two independent natural experiments, one group in Canada and another in the Netherlands began doing IPT in isolation from training centers in the United States. After some years, each requested a consultation to ascertain whether they were doing IPT correctly. It appeared that they were. Peer supervision by a nucleus of interested therapists, in conjunction with the use of a treatment manual (and perhaps the background of a didactic seminar), may suffice to learn IPT.

Our experience with training also suggests that psychotherapy practitioners not involved with research could well adopt elements of an IPT approach by carefully reviewing the strategies described in the book, especially Part 1, which is the core description of the method. Thus we hope that professional readers of this book will find its principles, strategies, and techniques useful in their own practice. We also appreciate that many of the adaptations of IPT for other disorders have involved minimal changes in IPT techniques, but do require experience and knowledge of the population under study. For example, a highly competent IPT therapist who has never treated adolescents may have difficulty in using IPT-A with this population.

CERTIFICATION

Certification was originally a research standard, important to ensure homogeneity of treatment techniques in outcome studies. Now clinicians are increasingly seeking certification in IPT, sometimes to satisfy managed care organizations that they can deliver effective therapy. There is increasing pressure for certification standards in other techniques, such as cognitive behavioral therapy, as well.

Certification has been provided by experts at research training centers. There is no parchment or paper certificate for IPT graduates, although some trainees have requested one. Nor is there an IPT bureaucracy invested with formal powers to certify therapeutic competence. The clinical spread of IPT may eventually lead to the development of a credentialing body, but the current system requires formal training within a somewhat informal framework.

How much training is enough to acquire competence in IPT? Any standard is to some degree arbitrary, but we feel that certification should require the successful completion of at least three taped cases, with hour-by-hour supervision of each by a certified IPT expert. This process ensures that certification carries meaning. For most psychotherapists, the first case will involve some hesitation as the therapist tries to recall the tasks for each session; the second case will proceed more smoothly; and the third will go smoothly indeed.

Although IPT is usually not that difficult to learn, some therapists simply may not grasp its concepts despite treating more than three cases. IPT training can impart strategies and techniques to good psychotherapists; it cannot necessarily make a weak psychotherapist into a strong one. Therapists who put in the initiative, hours, and effort to learn IPT without success have been relatively few, in part because they have been carefully selected for research trials. As the numbers of trainees grow, more are likely to have difficulty with the approach.

Informal Training

Some clinicians may wish to learn IPT for its clinical benefit but do not need the formal credentials necessary for a research trial. Such psychotherapists may benefit from reading the IPT manual, from attending IPT workshops at conferences, and from peer supervision, a less expensive alternative to individual supervision with an expert. Like the more formal training, peer supervision should use tapes of sessions (which require informed written consent from patients) to review content.

Training Centers in North America

A few centers have provided most of the recent training for researchers and clinicians, as of the publication of this book. We expect the number to grow and would like to hear from new groups so that we can update our lists. The centers as of 1999 are:

Cornell Psychotherapy Institute
   Cornell University Medical College
   525 East 68th Street, Room 1322
   New York, NY 10021
   Contact: John C. Markowitz, M.D. (212-746-3774)
   or Kathleen F. Clougherty, A.C.S.W. (212-721-2569)

Western Psychiatric Institute and Clinic
   3811 O'Hara Street
   Pittsburgh, PA 15213
   Contact: Cleon Cornes, M.D. (412-624-2211)

Interpersonal Therapy Clinic
   Clarke Institute
   250 College Street
   Toronto, Ontario
   M5T 1R8 Canada
   Contact: Laurie Gillies, Ph.D. (416-979-6925)

Department of Psychiatry
  University of Iowa
  200 Hawkins Drive
  Iowa City, IA 52242
  Contact: Scott Stuart, M.D., and Michael O'Hara, Ph.D. (319-353-6960)

Workshops and courses are also frequently given at the annual meeting of the American Psychiatric Association and similar conventions.

IPT TREATMENT MANUALS

At one time the very diversity of psychotherapists' approaches to patients discouraged research on psychotherapy. Each psychotherapist was unique, and in any case there was no way to know what he or she was doing in the office with a given patient. Psychotherapy was seen as an art that could not be addressed by science. Happily, that outlook has changed. Treatment manuals can teach psychotherapists to adapt their styles to a particular approach. Audiotaping or videotaping provides an objective record of how the therapists deliver that treatment, a record that evaluators can review and score for treatment adherence.

Treatment manuals currently represent the state of the art of psychotherapy research. By specifying and standardizing psychotherapy (and increasingly, also pharmacotherapy), manuals provide the basis for a relative homogeneity of approach and technique across therapists in a treatment study. If therapists can be trained to follow a manual, this controls to a degree the variations between therapists' techniques. A therapy manual thus makes psychotherapy a relatively uniform treatment that can be tested. It is a form of quality control analogous to packaging 20 mg. of fluoxetine in each treatment capsule.

Psychotherapy studies use treatment manuals together with adherence monitoring and diagnostic homogeneity in order to simplify clinical situations enough to make the results of trials interpretable. Adherence monitoring is performed by trained independent evaluators who listen to taped treatment sessions to determine whether therapists are actually following the manual. This validates the psychotherapy that occurs in a treatment study. The focus on patients who share a principal diagnosis, such as major depression, provides diagnostic homogeneity. Thus we can learn whether a particular approach works for a particular patient population.

Good psychotherapy manuals educate therapists about a technique without quashing their individuality. Manuals should not be "cookbooks" that stifle spontaneity. On the other hand, they must provide guidelines sufficient that different therapists tend to respond in similar ways to key therapeutic situations. A properly designed manual offers therapists reassurance that the therapy has been carefully thought out and defined, has coherence, and addresses problems that may arise for the patient and therapist. It should contribute to the therapist's confidence in the treatment, which can in turn be imbued in the patient.

IPT was defined in a manual for research therapists at the time of the initial Boston–New Haven studies of the 1970s. That manual became the 1984 book *Interpersonal Psychotherapy of Depression*, which the present volume updates. Its utility was documented by Rounsaville and colleagues (1988). While its basic principles apply to all IPT adaptations, the interpersonal situations of patient populations differ. Depressed adolescents face different life issues than depressed geriatric patients. Patients with medical illness face stressors not seen by the medically healthy. Patients with bulimia face somewhat different problems than do depressed patients. Hence IPT has been adapted to varying degrees in many of the research trials that have been done and are now being done.

This section lists the available manuals adapting IPT for particular treatment populations. It also explains how to develop a new adaptation in preparation for a research study.

Some manuals have been published, whereas others have been developed by researchers and restricted to the site of their study. In the latter case, the researchers may be contacted about their manuals. Several manualized adaptations are described in earlier chapters of this book.

Maintenance IPT for Recurrent Major Depression (IPT-M) (Chapter 11). Frank, E., D. J. Kupfer, C. Cornes, and S. M. Morris. Maintenance interpersonal psychotherapy for recurrent depression. In *New Applications of Interpersonal Psychotherapy*, ed. G. L. Klerman and M. M. Weissman, 75–102. Washington, D.C.: American Psychiatric Press, 1993.

IPT for Dysthymic Disorder (IPT-D) (Chapter 12). Markowitz, J. C. *Interpersonal Psychotherapy for Dysthymic Disorder*. Washington, D.C.: American Psychiatric Press, 1998.

IPT for Depressed Adolescents (IPT-A) (Chapter 13). Mufson, L., D. Moreau, M. M. Weissman, and G. L. Klerman. *Interpersonal Therapy for Depressed Adolescents*. New York: Guilford Press, 1993.

IPT for Late-Life Depression (Chapter 14). (a) Frank, E., N. Frank, C. Cornes, D. Imber, M. D. Miller, S. M. Morris, and C. F. Reynolds III. Interpersonal psychotherapy in the treatment of late-life depression. In *New Applications of Interpersonal Psychotherapy*, ed G. L. Klerman and M. M. Weissman, 167–98. Washington, D.C.: American Psychiatric Press, 1993.

(b) Frank, E., and N. Frank. *Manual for the Adaptation of Interpersonal Psychotherapy to Maintenance Treatment of Recurrent Depression in Late Life (IPT-LLM).* Unpublished. Contact: Ellen Frank, Ph.D., Professor of Psychiatry, Western Psychiatric Institute and Clinic, 3811 O'Hara Street, Pittsburgh, PA 15213.

Conjoint IPT for Depressed Patients with Marital Disputes (IPT-CM) (Chapter 15). Weissman, M. M., and G. L. Klerman. Conjoint IPT for depressed patients with marital disputes. In *New Applications of Interpersonal Psychotherapy*, ed. G. L. Klerman and M. M. Weissman, 103–28. Washington, D.C.: American Psychiatric Press, 1993.

IPT for Bipolar Disorder (Interpersonal/Social Rhythms Therapy) (Chapter 16). Contact: Ellen Frank, Ph.D., Professor of Psychiatry, Western Psychiatric Institute and Clinic, 3811 O'Hara Street, Pittsburgh, PA 15213.

IPT for Primary Care and Medically Ill Patients (Chapter 17). Schulberg, H. C., C. P. Scott, M. J. Madonia, and S. D. Imber. Applications of interpersonal psychotherapy in primary care practice. In *New Applications of Interpersonal Psychotherapy*, ed. G. L. Klerman and M. M. Weissman, 265–91. Washington, D.C.: American Psychiatric Press, 1993.

Interpersonal Counseling (IPC) (Chapter 17). Contact: Myrna M. Weissman, Ph.D., Columbia University College of Physicians and Surgeons, 1051 Riverside Drive, Unit #24, New York, NY 10032.

IPT for Depressed HIV-Positive Patients (IPT-HIV) (Chapter 18). (a) Markowitz, J. C., G. L. Klerman, K. F. Clougherty, and L. Josephs. *Manual for Interpersonal Therapy with HIV-Seropositive Subjects.* Cornell University Medical College, unpublished (1990). Contact: John C. Markowitz, M.D., 525 East 68th Street, New York, NY 10021.

(b) Pergami, A., L. Grassi, M. Gonevi, and J. C. Markowitz. *Il Trattamento Psicologico della Depressione nell'Infezione da HIV e nell'AIDS–La Psicoterapia Interpersonale.* Milan: Franco Angeli, s.r.l. (in press).

IPT for Depressed Antepartum Patients (Chapter 19). Contact: Margaret Spinelli, M.D., Columbia University College of Physicians and Surgeons, 722 West 168th Street, New York, NY 10032.

IPT for Depressed Postpartum Patients (Chapter 19). Contacts: Scott Stuart, M.D., University of Iowa, Department of Psychiatry, 200 Hawkins Drive, Iowa City, IA 52242; Michael O'Hara, Ph.D., Department of Psychology, 200 Hawkins Drive, Iowa City, IA 52242.

IPT for Substance Abuse (Chapter 20). Rounsaville, B. J., and K. Carroll. Interpersonal psychotherapy for patients who abuse drugs. In *New Applications of Interpersonal Psychotherapy*, ed. G. L. Klerman and M. M. Weissman, 319–52. Washington, D.C.: American Psychiatric Press, 1993.

IPT for Bulimia Nervosa (Chapter 21). *(a) Individual format:* Fairburn, C. G. Interpersonal psychotherapy for bulimia nervosa. In *New Applications of Interpersonal Psychotherapy*, ed. G. L. Klerman and M. M. Weissman, 353–78. Washington, D.C.: American Psychiatric Press, 1993. Contact: Christopher G. Fairburn, DM, MRCPsych, Department of Psychiatry, Oxford University, Warneford Hospital, Oxford OX3 7JX, United Kingdom.

(b) Group format (IPT-G). Wilfley, D. E. *Interpersonal Psychotherapy Adapted for Group (IPT-G) and for the Treatment of Binge Eating Disorder.* Yale Binge Eating Treatment Study, unpublished (1993). Contact: Denise E. Wilfley, Ph.D., San Diego State University-UCSD, Clinical Psychology Program, 6363 Alvarado Court, Suite 103, San Diego, CA 92120.

IPT for Social Phobia (IPT-SP) (Chapter 22). (a) Lipsitz, J., J. C. Markowitz, and S. Cherry. *Manual for Interpersonal Psychotherapy of Social Phobia.* Columbia University College of Physicians and Surgeons, unpublished (1997). Contact: Joshua Lipsitz, Ph.D., Columbia University College of Physicians and Surgeons, 722 West 168th Street, Unit #13, New York, NY 10032.

(b) Contacts. Scott Stuart, M.D., University of Iowa, Department of Psychiatry, 200 Hawkins Drive, Iowa City, IA 52242; Michael O'Hara, Ph.D., Department of Psychology, 200 Hawkins Drive, Iowa City, IA 52242.

IPT for Borderline Personality Disorder (Chapter 23). Angus, L., and L. A. Gillies. Counseling the borderline client: an interpersonal approach. *Canadian Journal of Counselling/Revue canadienne de counseling* 1994; 28:69–82. Contact: Laurie Gillies, Ph.D., Interpersonal Therapy Clinic, Clarke Institute of Psychiatry, 250 College Street, Toronto, Ontario M5T 1R8 Canada.

IPT Patient Guide (Chapter 24). Weissman, M. M. *Mastering Depression: A Patient Guide to Interpersonal Psychotherapy.* San Antonio, Tex.: The Psychological Corporation, 1995. (Copies can be ordered directly through The Psychological Corporation, Order Service Center, P.O. Box 839954, San Antonio, Texas 78283–3954.)

HOW TO DEVELOP A TREATMENT MANUAL

To know whether IPT will work for a particular diagnosis or subpopulation within a diagnosis requires testing its efficacy. The development of IPT has followed this empirical approach: first, an open trial to show whether the treatment has promise; then, if it does, a controlled clinical trial comparing IPT to alternative treatment conditions. IPT has worked without significant adaptation as a therapy for several populations (e.g., primary care patients), but has been modified for others. There has been no hard rule to determine when to modify IPT and when to leave it unchanged. Our guess is that the decision has depended upon clinical experience and the researcher's idiosyncratic approach to the problem.

Several steps precede the actual treatment studies.

1. Clinical experience, with both IPT and with the treatment population in question, is prerequisite to developing a manual. The researcher should be certified in IPT and familiar with the target illness and its treatment approaches.

2. A preliminary step is often to undertake a needs assessment of the population under study. A survey of patients in a specialty clinic (bulimia, alcohol abuse, infertility, general medicine, etc.) might bring to light particular psychosocial and interpersonal problems these patients face. If these problems suggest a meaningful modification of the standard IPT approach, then a new manual might be warranted. An example is the development of a fifth interpersonal problem area, the single-parent family, for depressed adolescent patients.

3. Modifications of IPT deriving from the needs assessment can be addressed in the manual through the development of case vignettes and scripts. Case vignettes familiarize therapists with the problems of a particular patient population and the therapeutic approach used to address them. Scripts provide guidelines for how to intervene. For example, in IPT for HIV-positive patients, the developers decided it would be useful to link depression and HIV infection as dual, treatable medical illnesses (Markowitz et al., 1992). The treatment manual provided a script for therapists to work from in explaining this variation of the "sick role" to patients.

Modifications should not distort IPT beyond recognition. Radical changes may raise questions about whether the treatment is really IPT or a different treatment altogether. An interesting example of an amalgam of IPT and a more behavioral therapeutic approach is the IPT/social rhythms treatment developed by Frank and colleagues for the adjunctive treatment of bipolar disorder.

Practical decisions about treatment need to be incorporated into the manual. These guidelines reflect the nuts and bolts of a research project. How long and how frequent will psychotherapy be? IPT has been variously dosed as a twelve-week, fourteen-week, and sixteen-week treatment, in addition to being used as a monthly maintenance treatment. How should the therapist tell subjects to avoid unblinding independent raters by mentioning which treatment they are receiving?

4. Once a new manual has been developed, it deserves a test-drive before being used in a treatment trial. Pilot cases may bring to light problems with the manual, or raise new issues that should be added to it. Manuals may evolve as a study progresses and new situations arise. In order to ensure a uniform approach, it is best to have as polished a document as possible at the time the treatment trial begins.

5. Once complete, the manual may be used to train therapists. Therapists themselves often raise questions that may lead to updates of the manual. The goal, however, is to have a manual sufficiently comprehensive that it influences the therapists more than the reverse.

This chapter does not attempt to describe the full complexity of psychotherapy treatment trials. They require careful planning and training, and they are not easy to do. Treatment manuals, while central to the testing of psychotherapy, are only one element in the training, design, and other decisions important to such research (Bergin and Garfield, 1994).

NOTES

1. Advanced health care or mental health care degree: e.g., M.D., Ph.D., M.S.W., R.N.
2. Experience as a psychotherapist (at least two years).

3. Experience in working with depressed (or other target diagnosis) patients.

Training:
1. Read IPT manual.
2. Attend workshop or course.
3. Supervision by a trained IPT therapist, using taped cases (and, for research studies, ideally, supervision of three cases).
4. Certification: Supervisor's approval of competence.

PART FIVE
THE FUTURE OF IPT

The Future of IPT

In the past twenty years IPT has built a solid foundation in research. Its clinical range and number of practitioners are growing. Where will it be twenty years hence?

FIGHTING THE DECLINE
OF PSYCHOTHERAPY

Statistics indicate that the use of psychotherapy in the United States is declining. Under the pressure of managed care, which considers pharmacotherapy a less expensive option, fewer patients are being treated with talking therapies. Yet populations with psychiatric disorders need alternatives and adjuncts to pharmacotherapy.

PREDICTIONS

The psychotherapy pendulum has swung and will likely rebound. As managed care itself changes, and as access to psychotherapy is choked, there is likely to be a resurgence of psychotherapy in the United States. Those psychotherapies that survive and grow are likely to be those with empirical support. There is already a shaking out of psychotherapy candidates. Books such as Fonagy and Roth's *What Works for Whom?* (1996) illustrate the evidence-based approach that should increasingly separate therapies of tested efficacy from those reliant solely on belief. IPT and CBT will probably be joined by other therapies of demonstrated utility, while others will fade away.

THE STRENGTHS OF PSYCHOTHERAPY

Despite the adverse economic environment, some psychotherapies have been gaining ground, at least from a scientific standpoint. We know more about when psychotherapy works, and to some degree about how it works, than ever before. There have been gains in standardization of treatments and increasing numbers of efficacy studies. Ironically, reimbursement has been decreasing at the same time that these gains have been occurring.

Economic studies of psychotherapy, albeit few, have not demonstrated a cost offset (Klerman et al., 1987; Schulberg et al., 1996). Yet cost offset studies have only looked at whether treatment affects overall costs for individuals *within* the health care system (see Chapter 17), ignoring other, "outside" costs such as those for social services, which the Hamilton, Ontario, study (Browne et al., 1997) found that IPT reduced. Health care systems also pay for *families*, not individuals, and costs of depressive and other disorders to the family can be expensive. Children of depressed patients are at risk for depression themselves, and have higher health care costs than other children (Weissman et al., 1997; Kramer et al., 1998). None of this is captured in cost offset studies, which might show added economic as well as health benefits for psychotherapies if they took a broader scope.

PREDICTIONS

Studies of wider scope may demonstrate the economic benefits of efficacious psychotherapies. We look forward to more such studies involving IPT. Whether or not IPT proves to have a cost offset, we expect that it will be shown to be cost-effective.

THE PSYCHOTHERAPISTS
OF THE FUTURE

Who will future psychotherapists be? The current emphasis on health care costs has limited patients' access not only to psychotherapy but also to particular therapists ("providers"). Managed care organizations that do reimburse psychotherapy have tended to authorize only the least expensive providers. Thus psychiatrists and psychologists have been displaced by less highly paid therapists; psychiatric social workers and nurses and master's-level psychologists are in turn being squeezed by bachelor's-level providers. Will the psychotherapist of the future be a psychiatrist? A social worker? A health professional? Or a nonprofessional?

And who will train these psychotherapists? IPT is not "basic training" in psychotherapy, but a specialized, advanced course for therapists who already have fundamental skills. If less trained therapists become the standard, how well will they learn IPT, and how well will they deliver it in treating patients? It is also unclear who will pay for that training.

PREDICTIONS

Effectiveness studies may answer these questions. It might be worth comparing highly trained therapists to those with minimal background to test for differences. We expect that psychiatrists will be pressed into the position of doing less psychotherapy, but it may prove cost-effective as well as clinically sensible for them to provide combined psychotherapy and pharmacotherapy to certain patients (Dewan, 1999). This, too, deserves research. We also believe that IPT should become a standard part of the training curriculum for psychiatric residents, psychology and social work graduate students, and other mental health professionals.

CERTIFICATION AND
QUALITY CONTROL

Certification and quality control follow from the previous issue. There is already great interest among clinicians about certification in IPT. High quality of IPT therapists has been maintained to date in part because there have been so few therapists, highly trained for research studies. What will happen to IPT as it spreads among clinicians?

Among the most pressing issues for IPT is its translation from a purely research therapy to a clinical treatment. For IPT to survive and develop as a psychotherapy, it must ultimately become a widespread clinical treatment. How this process occurs may importantly influence the nature of training programs, the certification of IPT therapists, and other ramifications. Research should determine clinical indications for IPT, but what should be the standards for training and certifying clinicians? (See Chapter 25.)

CBT, another time-limited, research-tested psychotherapy of similar age, established clinical training institutes early in its existence. There are meetings and journals devoted to CBT, and an organizational body is being formed to set standards for formally certifying CBT psychotherapists (*Cognitive Therapy Today*, 1997). In contrast, Klerman and colleagues declined to train therapists in IPT before the treatment had been repeatedly tested. His death further delayed the dissemination of training. As a result, a relative handful of clinicians were trained in IPT, and almost solely for research protocols. Increasingly, however, there have been workshops at academic institutions and hospital clinics, courses at mental health meetings, and requests for training. Therapists and institutions seek to learn IPT in order to ensure managed care reimbursement for a "proven" therapy.

Because IPT has *not* yet spread widely in clinical circles, it may have preserved a relative purity in comparison to psychodynamic psychotherapy and CBT, which have developed variants over geography and time. The opportunity exists to maintain IPT quality earlier in the dissemination process, to provide quality control at the outset, setting standards for training, certification, and credentialing. We know that IPT works in the hands of well-trained psychotherapeutic clinicians who get research-level IPT training (typically, three audio- or videotaped cases, supervised hour-by-hour). There is presumably a decrement in efficacy as training rigor and clinical talent fall. We need to determine thresholds and requirements for training for clinicians at large.

The risks and benefits of setting standards are apparent. Without guidelines and standards, IPT is likely to become a catchphrase without much actual value: therapists can take a brief course and then tell patients, "Oh, yes, I do IPT." On the other hand, we have concerns about creating a bureaucratic monster to oversee the clinical spread of IPT. Its inventors, Klerman and Weissman, have kept matters informal, an approach that was feasible when IPT was small and research-centered. As IPT grows, some more formal—but ideally not too formal—organizational approach will be needed. Sessions at meetings of the American Psychiatric Association and elsewhere now provide opportunities to discuss clinical credentialing for IPT both in the United States and abroad. A newsletter may be useful to keep IPT therapists abreast of developments in the field.

Other educational issues require the participation of mental health leaders who may not themselves know IPT. For example, should IPT be taught in residency training programs? Unlike psychodynamic psychotherapy and cognitive behavioral therapy, training in IPT is not currently mandated by the Program Requirements for Residency Education in Psychiatry (American Medical Association, 1995). Some foresighted training directors have incorporated IPT into time-limited therapy curricula, but these programs as yet constitute a small minority. It is noteworthy, however, that the programs that do teach IPT include, but are not limited to, those with strong traditions of psychotherapy training. Some residency programs that once disdained and provided the bare minimum of psychotherapy instruction have come around to time-limited treatments, in large part because of the empirical evidence supporting the efficacy of IPT and CBT.

PREDICTIONS

There will be some need for a bureaucracy, ideally not too cumbersome, to certify IPT therapists and ensure quality control in training (Markowitz, 1997). This does not address the question of *ongoing* training or assessment to prevent diminished adherence over time.

THE RANGE OF IPT

As this book documents, IPT has been the subject of a great deal of research. This has established both its efficacy for some populations (especially mood disorders; also bulimic patients) and its limitations for others (negative studies for opioid- and cocaine-abusing patients). Yet much more research must be done to fully determine its therapeutic limits for a range of disorders, as well as its optimal dosing and duration, its sequencing and combination with pharmacotherapy, and its translation from efficacy studies to effectiveness in general practice.

We anticipate that IPT will prove efficacious for patients with many of the anxiety disorders now under study. Similarly, we anticipate that IPT would be a good treatment for depressed or anxious patients who face clear psychosocial stresses: for example, caregivers of Alzheimer's patients, patients in early recovery from alcohol dependence, and patients with major medical illnesses. We doubt that it will help patients with obsessive-compulsive disorder or schizophrenia.

The medical model of IPT fits neatly with that of pharmacotherapy, and research has suggested acute (DiMascio et al., 1979) although not chronic (Frank et al., 1990) synergy of IPT and antidepressant medication. Far more needs to be known about the indications and the timing of combined treatments: i.e., for which patients, and with what timing, should IPT and medication be combined? We also need more than the scarce current data on serial treatment: i.e., if psychotherapy fails, when should one try pharmacotherapy, and vice versa?

IPT as an acute treatment has been generally set at twelve to sixteen sessions for somewhat arbitrary reasons related to comparison with pharmacotherapy in outcome research. We do not know the optimal length or dosage of IPT for particular disorders. And, although IPT is the only therapy whose maintenance efficacy has been demonstrated in the treatment of major depression, there are only two studies, sharing a single dosage, currently in the literature (see Chapter 11). We also know little about adapting IPT to other modalities: e.g., group IPT or IPT by telephone.

Future research must study the translation of *efficacy* in research trials to *effectiveness* in standard clinical settings. There has been little research attention to effectiveness for most psychiatric treatments, including most psychotherapies. Because IPT has been almost entirely a research intervention, the need to study its clinical effectiveness is the more pressing.

We also know relatively little about the process of IPT. Whereas, historically, psychotherapy process research overwhelmed outcome research, the late Gerald L. Klerman felt that process research was superfluous until one had determined that the treatment worked. If it lacked efficacy, why would the ingredients of the therapy matter? Now that the efficacy of IPT has been demonstrated for some disorders, exploration of its active ingredients deserves greater attention. What makes IPT work? Its focus on life events seems to make it a credible approach for patients who have experienced significant life changes. But that premise deserves careful assessment.

No psychotherapy should aim to provide all things to all patients or to all therapists. From its inception, IPT has been driven by research, targeted to diagnosis, and has staked out one diagnostic area after another based upon empirical outcome findings. This approach should continue. We should determine treatment based on outcome findings rather than on ideology (Klerman, 1991). Psychotherapies should learn to coexist in the future, even within the same psychotherapist. The best-prepared psychotherapist will be one who can choose among psychotherapies in his or her treatment armamentarium, applying the optimal strategy to a given diagnosis or difficulty.

Predictions

How will IPT survive the role transitions of clinical expansion, further research, and the shifting economics and practice of psychiatry and other mental health professions? We think it is likely to come through well; it should be a growth industry. With appropriate preparation, its clinical expansion can maintain a high quality of training without unduly burdensome bureaucratization. The research accomplishments of the past provide a template and a direction for future studies. And because of IPT's limited treatment aims (limited, that is, by diagnosis) and empirical testing, it should adjust well to the economic future of psychotherapy.

An Integrative Case Example

A case of grief and loss illustrates both the strategies and techniques of IPT and offers a good way to compare them with those used in other psychotherapies. It also illustrates the use of IPT at the levels of chronology, problem areas, techniques, and therapist stance. This detailed presentation includes a description of strategies and sequence of events; a comparison of the IPT approach with that of other approaches in psychotherapy; a discussion of the levels of intervention; and a review of the techniques used.

STRATEGIES AND SEQUENCE OF EVENTS

INITIAL PHASE (SESSIONS 1–2)

Ruth, a sixty-two-year-old woman, came for treatment of a depression that had lasted a year and that she "became aware of" after her husband's death from a progressively debilitating illness caused by diabetes associated with vascular disease.

She had no previous history of depression. Her symptoms included unshakable sadness, with little change in mood regardless of events around her; preoccupation with memories of her husband's death and guilt about her feelings of inadequacy at being unable to get her affairs in order since he died; a tendency to oversleep; retardation and severe difficulty concentrating; social withdrawal so acute that she had restricted her outside contacts to her two grown children and felt that she was a burden on them. The depressive symptoms represented a continuation of her grief reaction, and she had thought these feelings were normal. Later, as the symptoms persisted, she became progressively more desperate and hopeless about being able to overcome them, though she denied suicidal feelings.

Ruth had sought treatment at another clinic two months before this first meeting with the psychotherapist. At that time, she had been treated with antidepressant medication and had begun to experience some improvement in mood. However, the treatment was discontinued when she was hospitalized for treatment of psoriasis. While in the hospital, she remained somewhat asymptomatic, but she became as depressed as ever when she returned home. She met the DSM criteria for major depression.

Interpersonal Context

Ruth clearly associated her depression with the illness and death of her husband, who had been progressively debilitated from the time they both retired four years ago. Although they had planned to travel during their retirement and held off taking vacations in anticipation of this, she accepted a restricted, isolated lifestyle centered on caring for her husband. She seldom left the house without him and cut off contacts with friends and acquaintances. Most disturbing about her husband's illness was his mental deterioration. Shortly before his death, he had to be hospitalized at a state mental hospital, where he developed more severe vascular disease that necessitated a transfer to another hospital and amputation of one leg. From that point until his death, Ruth's husband was completely incoherent.

Review of the past family life led to Ruth's assertion that the relationship had been fine and completely satisfying before her husband's illness. They had been married for thirty-five years. Her relationships with the two children, a son of thirty-one and a daughter of twenty-eight, had been characterized by her difficulty giving up control over them. The son was an alcoholic who had been abstinent for more than a year and was living at a halfway house. Apparently his progress toward rehabilitation was linked to Ruth's being able to reduce her attempts to help him with this problem. The relationship with the daughter was less troubled, probably because the daughter was described as more "self-sufficient" and independent of Ruth.

They had quarreled somewhat in the past because of Ruth's intrusiveness into her daughter's affairs, but the relationship had improved in recent years.

Although Ruth recognized that she needed to develop new activities and social contacts, she felt pessimistic about ever being able to do so. She described having a "dual personality" about this because there was a marked contrast between what she experienced with other people and her anticipation of it. She had done well in her job as a secretary for many years and had a number of friends from work. She felt that she had no difficulty making friends or meeting them, although she had tended to center her activities in her family. Her husband's illness had led her to cut off contact with friends more or less completely, especially during the last year of his life. Ruth felt she would be unwelcome with her old friends because they would be offended at her neglect of them. Thus she anticipated rejection if she were to attempt to get involved with people once again.

Her anticipation of rejection and her feeling that she would not enjoy other people's company contrasted sharply with what actually occurred when others asked her to join them in social activities. She reported that she did enjoy herself and that others seemed to appreciate her company. For example, when she was leaving the hospital, her roommates had told her they were sad to see her go because they had enjoyed her company. She recognized that she would probably be able to perform adequately in social relations if only she could get over anticipating a bad time and having to force herself to plan activities. But she also brought out long-standing fears of being taken over and exploited by others if she allowed friendships to reach more than a superficial level of interaction.

Comment on Strategy

The therapist conducted the initial information-gathering sessions with the aim of obtaining two general kinds of information: (1) an assessment of the type and severity of the depressive symptoms; and (2) a determination of the interpersonal issues associated with the onset of the current depressive episode. The initial part of the session began with general inquiries ("What brought you to the clinic?"), which were followed by a relatively systematic symptom review. This in turn was followed by an assessment of the current social situation (review of social supports and important activities such as work and friends) and of the events preceding and succeeding the onset of the depressive symptoms.

Initial Symptom Management.   From the review of the depressive symptoms, the therapist determined that they were of moderate severity, not requiring hospitalization, and that they had been somewhat responsive to medication in the past. Given the situational nature of Ruth's depression, it was decided to hold off initiating pharmacotherapy until there was further evaluation. The thought was that she might have some remission of symptoms as a result of entering psychotherapy. The issue of symptoms was handled in the first session with education and reassurance such as:

> The different ways that you have felt bad—the sadness and crying, being unable to get yourself going, trouble concentrating, not wanting to face other people—are all part of a picture of a depression that seems to have hit you as a result of losing many things over the past several years. As you pointed out, the way you are now is clearly different from the way you were: you've lost your husband; you lost his companionship even before that; you lost the plans you had for a happy retirement. It's very hard to get over these losses. Part of what we will be doing is trying to help you do this . . . confront what you've lost and help you manage it. As we do this, I expect that your symptoms will improve.

Initial Formulation of Therapeutic Strategy.   From the review of the context of the current depression, the therapist tried to determine what it was about and to begin to develop an understanding of how changes could be made. Part of the plan was also to develop an alliance with the patient by beginning to work on problems even in the first session; to provide the patient with feedback so that she felt she was being heard and to let her know what to expect from psychotherapy. Ruth clearly associated the depression with the death of her husband but was at a loss to determine why she was unable to get it out of her mind. From the review of her husband's last years, it became apparent that many aspects of the death were important in preventing Ruth from successfully mourning the loss.

She had responded to his long illness and gradual deterioration with denial, which had led her to expect him to act more responsibly than he was able. Thus his mental deterioration and helplessness led her to become angry with him (and probably to wish for his death). These feelings would be the source of severe guilt after his death. In particular, she felt bad about participating in his hospitalization, from which he did not return. Although his illness was out of his control, Ruth also felt angry that her husband's debility had caused them both to give up their plans for a happy retirement.

The first major goal of treatment was defined as helping Ruth overcome her guilt surrounding her handling of the illness and death and to develop a more realistic understanding of what had happened. The strategy was to review the relationship with the husband, the circumstances surrounding the death, and the ways she continued to think about him. While reviewing this material, the therapist kept in mind typical feelings associated with pathological grief, including shame over helplessness at not being able to prevent the event; rage and guilt about the lost person; survivor guilt, for feeling relieved that the other person died and not oneself; and sadness over the loss.

When material related to these themes was discussed, the therapist attempted to clarify the feelings to Ruth and to point out, where appropriate, their unrealistic nature. This kind of work was begun in the initial session, even while taking the history. For example, when Ruth discussed how guilty she felt about committing her husband to a state psychiatric hospital during the last few months of his life and expressed sadness at not having been able to talk to him about it, the therapist responded by eliciting information about her husband's condition and found out that he had become unmanageable—wandering around at night; incoherent; violent and threatening. On the basis of this information, as well as her account of what she would have liked to say to her husband, the therapist acknowledged Ruth's feelings of guilt and sadness at not being able to care for her husband by herself toward the end, but pointed out that she had no choice.

A second major goal of treatment, helping the patient to resume meaningful activities, was also defined on the basis of initial information gathering. At the onset of treatment, Ruth's social functioning was restricted to contact with her children and managing household chores. She hesitated to look up old friends, not only because she felt guilty about neglecting them but also because she was afraid she would not be able to control her depressed mood with them. She was aware of an active senior citizens' center in her neighborhood but was hesitant to become involved in it alone. She had started taking a course at a local community college but was considering dropping it. In addition, her mode of dealing with others often took the form of caretaking and self-sacrifice that was accompanied by fears of being exploited. Despite her current social deficiencies, the patient had had relatively active relationships with friends before she retired. Moreover, she acknowledged that once she got involved with other people she tended to enjoy the contact in spite of severe anticipatory anxiety about it.

To help her begin reusing her evident social skills, the therapist began a process of reviewing Ruth's options for getting involved with others and encouraging her to act on them. In this process, there was an emphasis on eliciting negative expectations about how various options would turn out and on confronting her about their unrealistic nature. For example, in the first session Ruth discussed how her relationship with her former best friend had lapsed when she couldn't visit the friend and leave her husband unattended, and had been too embarrassed at her husband's condition to invite the friend to see her. She felt now that she could not bring herself to call the friend because she would be insulted at being neglected. The therapist wondered if the friend would understand her explanation if she offered it, and the patient acknowledged that she might.

In reviewing Ruth's loss of her husband and her current social functioning, the therapist was not only taking the history but helping Ruth clarify these situations and beginning to help her develop alternative ways of thinking about them. At the end of the first session, after saying that the depression seemed to be related to the loss of her husband, the therapist gave Ruth this introduction to IPT treatment:

> One of the reasons people sometimes have difficulty starting up again after losing a loved one is because it's been hard to really look the loss straight in the face, and to really think about what it means, and allow yourself to feel the painful feeling. I think one of the things we can do in therapy is try to look at what's happened with you and your husband, to look at what he meant to you. We will go through that in a way that may be painful, but I think it's very necessary to do that if you are going to go back to an active life. The other side of trying to look at what's happened with the loss of your husband is for us to look into the ways you can start enjoying life again. And it seems that in fact you've made a start as far as that is concerned. However, it also seems that you

have a number of attitudes that to some extent you realize aren't realistic, such as the difference between the way things turn out and the way you anticipate them. Also, you have a lot of fears: that somehow people won't like you, that they're avoiding you or perhaps going to exploit you. We will spend some time trying to look at just what makes these things seem so powerful and likely to happen. Also, we'll look at ways you can overcome these hesitations. We'll be meeting for twelve sessions and I'd like you to bring in concerns that you have, ways you've been feeling or thinking that you would like to talk over, as well as taking the approach that we will be surveying the important relationships that you've had in the past and in the present.

Evaluation continued in the second session, as Ruth discussed two major topics related to the treatment goals: (1) her experience of her husband's life and death, and (2) her attempts at reestablishing a life of her own without him. Discussion of her family of origin revealed a highly disorganized or disrupted childhood. Her mother had died when she was five and the state split up the family, taking the children away from her alcoholic father when she was seven. From that time until the age of eighteen, she lived for relatively brief periods in a series of foster homes. She described this experience as painful and frustrating because the foster parents tended to look at the foster children as unpaid household help. At eighteen she moved in with an older sister, and she married her husband five years later, after a lengthy courtship. He had been her only serious suitor. Throughout the session, Ruth discussed progressively disturbing memories of her husband's final years, particularly his painful inability to care for himself. Toward the end, he had become psychotic, and verbally abusive to her. She again described her guilty relief when he was institutionalized and when he died. The therapist tried to be accepting and sympathetic as he drew out details of her memories of this time.

Interwoven with this theme was the topic of Ruth's getting involved with new activities. She discussed senior citizens organizations, future college courses, volunteer work, and seeing friends, mostly in terms of her fears about these things. She felt particularly apprehensive because she was single now and could no longer be as selective of others as she had been when her husband was there to fall back on. She also felt that married former friends would no longer be interested in her because she was no longer part of a couple. And she thought her depression so obvious that no one could possibly be interested in seeing her. The therapist was gently confrontational around these points, inducing her to give counterexamples and pointing out unrealistic aspects. Toward the end of this session, the therapist decided to start Ruth on an antidepressant medication. This decision was based on her continued high level of depression, which was noticeable throughout the session, and her history of positive response to medication in the past.

INTERMEDIATE PHASE (SESSIONS 3–8)

In Session 3, Ruth reported feeling better, and she had passed several minor milestones on the way to a more active life. She had driven at night for the first time (she said her husband had instilled a fear of night driving in her), she had had friends in to dinner for the first time since her husband's death, and she had started to go out more frequently, having made contact with a local senior citizens' center.

Ruth had also begun to think about how much she had restricted herself over the years in response to her husband's inhibited personality. She realized that she was still acting as if her husband were alive, and feeling guilty if she did things he would not have approved of. Moreover, she felt guilty if she spent money both of them had earned, or if she made changes around the house. Discussion of her day-to-day living revealed that she continued to keep space for him around the house, sleeping only on her side of the bed and using only her side of the closet. The session ended with a new realization that she, not he, could choose either to restrict herself or to allow herself to act. Moreover, coupled with the loss of a valued loved one was a level of freedom that she had not experienced for forty years.

In Session 4, the material from previous sessions was repeated and enlarged on. Ruth discussed her increased social life and her plans for future courses at college and volunteer work. As she talked, she realized that she was not merely regaining her old level of performance but was acting and thinking of herself in entirely new ways. She said she realized that most of her life had been spent in controlling, restricted environments—in foster homes and then with a cautious, controlling husband. She had taken these restrictions and limitations for granted, and was just now starting to sort out how much she wanted to change these things. For example, she followed a household routine in which each day of the week was spent on a specific task: for instance, Monday was wash day. When a desirable activity came up on a Monday, she was embarrassed at the degree of conflict she felt if she switched her wash day. However, she felt that the level to which she had routinized her life was excessive.

Session 5 marked a turning point. Two weeks had passed since the previous session, during which time Ruth received the results of her research ratings (various checklists and inventories that provide the patients with ratings on their degree of improvement). She felt that these ratings showed that she had improved considerably. She felt she had nothing more to talk about and was wasting the therapist's time. The therapist took these statements at face value and began to discuss the possibility of terminating after another session or two, encouraging her to review the course of treatment and discuss problems that might remain. In response to this, she discussed her fears that her health would deteriorate as she grew older. She was also concerned at not having closed the file of bills from her husband's treatment, and she feared that her improvement had been due entirely to medication and that she would relapse if it was discontinued. Despite these pessimistic themes, she also discussed her feeling that she had begun to learn new rules to live by. The therapist suggested that therapy did not have to consist simply of discussions of symptoms, which had now been reduced, but could focus on her experience of learning to live differently. Relieved and grateful, she indicated that she would like to remain in treatment after all.

Session 6 focused on the meanings behind a peculiar, persistent "frenzied" feeling she had begun to have, "as if I had to get everything done" before something dreadful happened. She had been feeling better and better, and was becoming more and more involved in new activities, especially in preparation for the Christmas holidays, the first to be celebrated without her husband. In this session, she reviewed aspects surrounding her husband's death and was able to relate her frenzied feeling to the fear that she would die, too, as a punishment, just when life looked promising again. She also revealed that her two cats had disappeared shortly after her husband's death, and this loss had greatly increased her despair. Discussing the fact that she had not yet gotten a stone for her husband's grave, she realized that in some ways she still could not bring herself to leave her husband in his place, the grave, while she went on to enjoy her life.

Ruth began Session 7 with a review of the progress she had made. She said she was feeling better than she had ever felt, that she was experiencing a kind of rebirth, making up for time lost to depression and preoccupation with her husband. She had become acutely aware of how depressed she had been through talking to another widowed woman who was still depressed.

She also expressed some embarrassment about how she must have appeared to others when she was depressed. She went on to say that she missed her husband as the holidays approached but these feelings were manageable and even pleasant in a bittersweet way. She said that he had been the only person with whom she could discuss much of her past life and only he had really understood her. Following this was a discussion of how she would continue to manage without him. Asked how she liked her involvement with the senior citizens' center, she replied that her enjoyment of it involved admitting that she was an "old lady" herself. She was somewhat concerned about becoming depressed again after treatment, and this called for a review of different treatment options and of circumstances that might make her depressed again. She had begun to take new things into her life, including listening to new songs, developing confidence in driving, and getting two cats to replace the two she had lost shortly after her husband's death.

In Session 8, Ruth brought Christmas cookies, which the therapist accepted and thanked her for without further discussion. Early in this session, Ruth was reminded that there were only four more visits left after this one. Ruth described her successful holidays, which included a Christmas dinner she had prepared for her family, and other social activities. She professed to be "happy, or at least as happy as I get." After a short silence, she said that one thought did continue to concern her and came repeatedly to mind. This was her memory of trying to strangle her husband shortly before he was placed in a hospital. The rest of the session was spent in a detailed review of just how bad the last year of her husband's life had been. The incident she recalled had occurred after he had agitatedly accused her of having imaginary lovers. Around this time, he had become not merely incompetent and incoherent but also paranoid. He slept at odd hours, and had to be watched lest he damage the house or hurt himself trying to repair something. What made the situation worse was the doctor's refusal to recognize her husband's mental deterioration, so that she felt she must be exaggerating things. The scene she remembered was a breaking point for her, and her husband was hospitalized shortly afterward.

Comment on Therapist's Stance in Intermediate Sessions

Having identified the probable cause of the depression and the two main interpersonal goals of the treatment during early sessions, the therapist approached each succeeding session with the general plan of listening for material related to the treatment goals and looking for opportunities to make incremental progress toward these goals. In the typical session, the topics discussed were those brought in by the patient, who, as her depression improved, was highly articulate and motivated for treatment. The therapist listened to the Ruth's discussions with the intention of focusing and expanding material related, first, to thoughts and feelings about her husband and his death, and about life without him. In particular the therapist was alert to discussions of the ways she continued to restrict her life based on memories of him and on angry feelings about him, with the plan of helping her to recognize that she was free to run her own life and to accept the angry feelings.

Second, the therapist listened for discussion of plans for new or expanded activities. In these discussions, the therapist was alert for statements that indicated hesitations based on unrealistic assumptions and took opportunities to help the patient expand her thinking about options open to her.

Thus the therapist entered each session with general strategies in mind and tried to lead the discussion in specific directions. However, the specific topics discussed and the flow of the discussion followed from material the patient brought in.

Allowed to take the initiative in choosing topics, Ruth indicated in varied and surprising ways the extent to which her life revolved around continuing to grieve for her husband and refusing to give this up enough to allow new things in. The therapy sessions nearly always contained material on the two major themes of the therapy, mourning her husband and taking on new activities. However, as these issues were discussed in each session, new issues arose and progressively deeper revelations were made, culminating in Ruth's statement that part of her guilt centered on her having attempted to strangle her husband in a fit of rage. Ruth was able to reveal this secret only after developing a trusting relationship with the therapist and after accepting less difficult aspects of her dealing with her husband's illness and death. This repetition of the original version of the current picture with progressively greater revelation of guarded material is typical of a successful therapy and is often arrived at only after a seemingly meandering sequence of sessions in which the patient seems to progress only to move back to a level of discussion that characterized earlier sessions. An aspect of this repetition is the importance of significant detail, represented in this case by the discussion in Session 6 of her lost cats that had disappeared shortly after the husband's death and the follow-up in Session 7 of having acquired two new cats.

TERMINATION PHASE (SESSIONS 9–12)

In Session 9, Ruth again reviewed her progress at school (she had gotten an A+ in her first-semester English course) and her activities with the senior citizens' center and friends. She described accepting the companionship of old people, which she had hesitated to seek at first because she could not accept the fact that she herself was really getting old. She was pleasantly surprised that an anticipated post-holiday slump had not occurred. She then discussed her concern that all this involvement with friends would hamper her independence, which she felt she must always guard fiercely. She recounted how, in foster homes as a teenager, she had received sexual advances from the men of many households. She felt that since that time she had always been cautious about trusting others. Discussion of termination was begun but was limited to her indication that she felt ready to stop and did not anticipate problems.

In Session 10, Ruth mainly ran through a list of the areas in which she had made progress. She felt confident that her improvement would continue, although she was still concerned that medications were solely responsible for this. Twenty to thirty minutes into the session, and after a long silence, Ruth asked if she could end the session early and the therapist consented.

Session 11 was focused on reviewing the depression and the therapy, and on discussing termination. The husband's decline and Ruth's reaction to it were again briefly reviewed, as well as the progress she had made, which included an improved mood, increased comfort and freedom in day-to-day life on her own, improved relationships with her children, a wider range of activities and interests, and many new friends. She discussed her reactions to the therapy: she had been apprehensive at first but had become increasingly positive. She also said she had gotten better too quickly, and could not understand how things could change so much.

The therapist explained that *the therapy had not really made her different, but had only allowed her to use the strengths and resources she already possessed.* She had gotten depressed largely because she was socially isolated during her husband's long illness. What therapy had done was help her put this loss and her feelings about him in perspective. This had been sufficient to allow her to grow in the direction of her own interests and abilities.

No new material was discussed in Session 12. Ruth's progress was reviewed and plans were made for the transfer of her pharmacotherapy to her internist. The patient expressed her confidence in the future and her gratitude to the therapist.

Comment on Termination Sessions

In this case, termination represented a winding down of therapy. The patient had experienced complete symptomatic improvement and had made much progress toward resuming an active life. In addition, in Session 8 she had revealed an important secret about the degree of rage she had felt toward her husband. After that, there were no more detailed reviews of the husband's final years and death and the intensity of the sessions was much reduced. Discussion of termination began and was part of each session after that. The therapist took care to make the ending date explicit and to elicit the patient's reactions to this. The patient was aware of primarily positive feelings about the therapy and the therapist. The patient's progress was frequently reviewed, and the therapist emphasized to the patient how much she had contributed to this progress by active participation in the therapy and by overcoming many obstacles in order to take on new activities. There was also explicit discussion of treatment options should depression recur, with a review of the kinds of symptoms that might indicate that she was becoming depressed again.

CASE SUMMARY

Ruth's case is an example of a straightforward treatment of pathological grief. The patient had been unable to give up the grieving process because of excessive guilt associated with her anger toward her husband before and after his death. She had responded to his illness with self-denial but secret resentment. As he became progressively debilitated, she was at once horrified at the deterioration of a man on whom she had depended and angry with him for becoming such a burden on her. Her desire for him to die was conscious and even acted upon during a fit of anger. Moreover, she saw her decision to hospitalize him as signing his death warrant. After he died, she felt continued resentment at being deprived of his company and his help in handling affairs, including the bills for his illness. Given her anger and her guilt in reaction to it, the patient could not allow herself to pleasurably pursue a life alone. Although she had many personal and social resources, she could not bring herself to take advantage of them.

The focus of the treatment was to help Ruth relieve her guilt while prodding her in her efforts to develop new interests. To help her complete the mourning process, Ruth's relationship with her husband, as well as his death and her reactions to it, were exhaustively reviewed, with special attention to painful affects such as sadness and guilty fear that she would be punished for her anger. Her personal resources were such that resolution of the mourning allowed her to improve dramatically.

IPT COMPARED WITH OTHER APPROACHES

INTERFACE WITH OTHER TYPES OF PSYCHOTHERAPY

The therapist's handling of the case of Ruth illustrates several of IPT's similarities to and differences from other short-term psychotherapies.

The types of psychotherapy most like IPT are psychoanalytically oriented psychodynamic therapies such as those described by Malan (1963); Sifneos (1979); and Davanloo (1982). In these therapies, the principal hypothesized curative feature is interpretation, which entails the linking of current conflicts, conflicts in childhood, and the transference relationship with the psychotherapist. The IPT conceptualization of the nature of the patient's problem is similar to that of psychodynamic therapists: that the patient was unable to complete the mourning process because of excessive guilt about her rage at her husband before and after his death. Much of Ruth's behavior can be explained by this guilt. Fearing massive retaliation for her angry thoughts, she needed to deny that her husband was dead to prevent a feeling that she had contributed to his death and needed to punish herself to expiate her imagined transgressions against him. Thus she kept her house the way it was when he was alive and continued to feel miserable and deprive herself of opportunities for happiness.

The handling of this issue in IPT was, however, quite different from that of the other types of therapies (cf. Markowitz, Svartberg, and Swartz, 1998). The IPT therapist concentrated exclusively on a review of the patient's experience of life with her husband and his death, attempting to elicit the affects related to this. There was no attempt to explore childhood events in any detail or to link these with the patient's reactions to her husband's illness and death. Moreover, there was no attempt to explore the relationship with the therapist, despite many opportunities for this. For example, in Session 5 the patient expressed the desire to end the therapy early because she had experienced a symptomatic improvement and felt she was wasting the therapist's time. In response, the therapist discussed the possibility matter-of-factly, focusing on what lay ahead of the patient rather than on what had gone on between patient and therapist. As the patient revealed many apprehensions about what might happen next, she realized that she was not ready to stop. Faced with a patient who wants to terminate prematurely, the IPT therapist may choose to discuss aspects of the therapeutic relationship, but discussion of transference issues and "resistance" are avoided.

Similarly, when the patient brought Christmas cookies to the therapist in Session 8, there was no discussion of the meaning of this because productive work was being done in the discussion of topics more centrally related to the short-term treatment. The acceptance of small gifts simply reflects the strength of the therapeutic alliance. And in the termination sessions, the therapist did not challenge Ruth's discussion of having only positive feelings about the therapy and handled her apprehensions regarding a possible relapse with a realistic discussion of options rather than an attempt to elicit a discussion of her ambivalent feelings about dependence on others. She had reason to have such positive feelings about the therapy. It was important, however, for the therapist to credit Ruth for the gains that she had made, in part because she had in fact made so many helpful life changes, and also so that she could leave therapy feeling competent and capable following a major loss and a year of depression.

Thus, one key difference between IPT and other types of psychodynamic short-term psychotherapies is what is *not* focused on, which in this case was the transference and childhood antecedents to current problems.

The way Ruth's depressive symptoms were addressed illustrates a second difference between IPT and other psychodynamic therapies. Here the patient was explicitly reassured about the positive prognosis and treatment with medications began after the second session, at which point it had become apparent that reassurance alone had not resulted in symptomatic improvement.

A third difference is the degree to which the IPT therapist engaged in repeated discussion of specific changes the patient could make to get involved with life again by finding new and more satisfactory roles. In these discussions, the therapist was careful not to advocate any specific course of action to the exclusion of others. Rather, there was an attempt to discuss options, with the implication that trying these out would be useful.

Fourthly, IPT also differs from psychodynamic therapies in the handling of personality issues. Throughout her life, Ruth's handling of interpersonal relationships showed that she had unresolved feelings of dependency, which she managed through denying the importance of others to her, keeping her distance from others, and taking care of others even when this was an intrusion into their lives, as in her relationship with her alcoholic son. Her surprise at the extent to which the death of her husband affected her is an indication of the counterdependent attitudes she had adopted.

The IPT therapist tried to help the patient formulate treatment goals consistent with her personality style. Since she needed others but had trouble acknowledging it, the therapist encouraged her to think about options for getting involved with others that included offering assistance to them. Hence, many of the options included volunteer jobs and friendships in which she offered something, such as transportation, to the other person. Although in the past this type of functioning had sometimes led to resentful feelings about being "used," these feelings had not usually led to disruption of the relationship. Thus the goal of IPT was to restore the patient to a previous level of functioning that she had considered adequate even though it might not be ideal. In contrast, the goal sought in the other psychodynamic therapies is resolution of key intrapsychic conflicts, which is supposed to lead to personality change.

IPT Versus Behavioral and Cognitive Therapies

The IPT therapist's emphasis on unresolved guilt differentiates this approach from a behavioral one, which might focus on the patient's failure to avail herself of reinforcing life experiences, and the cognitive therapist's emphasis on dysfunctional attitudes toward herself and her future. However, in Ruth's case the most striking differences between IPT and more behavioral treatments are technical. The IPT therapist was far less directive than a behavioral or cognitive therapist would have been. Although therapist and patient defined general areas in which work would be done, there was no explicit discussion of specifically targeted goals. Sessions were loosely structured around key issues, in contrast to the setting of an agenda that is part of cognitive therapy. Attempts to help the patient develop new activities took the form of discussions of options in which the therapist implicitly encouraged the patient to attempt new behaviors. No homework was assigned, progress was assessed in an informal manner, and specific suggestions were given sparingly. In contrast, behaviorist and cognitive therapies frequently involve repeated, explicit discussion of progress made, assignment of homework, and specific planning of actions the patient might take. In IPT, homework is implicit in the goal of resolving an interpersonal problem area, but no specific weekly tasks are assigned. The goal and the time limit of the therapy suffice to induce the patient to confront the task at hand.

Unlike social skills therapy, the treatment focused on an interpersonal problem area rather than on skills building per se.

LEVELS OF
INTERVENTION

The IPT therapist may try to bring about change through interventions at four different levels. In this case, three of the levels of change were attempted and effected.

COMBATING DEMORALIZATION AND
MANAGING DEPRESSIVE SYMPTOMS

In this case, the patient's depressive symptoms were elicited, summarized to her, and drawn together by the therapist as indications of a depressive episode in which her functioning was clearly different from what preceded it. She was reassured about prognosis. And in view of her good previous history of treatment response, she was treated with antidepressant medication.

INCREASING ACCEPTANCE OF SELF AND OTHERS

This was a key to the therapy. The patient had had the opportunity neither to evaluate the impact of her husband's death nor to get a realistic perspective on her handling of it. She had an exaggerated sense of having been excessively angry and inadequately caring. The therapy focused on helping her acknowledge and accept her angry feelings as natural and normal under the circumstances, and to give up her need to continue punishing herself for them.

TEACHING INTERPERSONAL
COPING STRATEGIES

The patient had an adequate repertoire of methods for making friends, getting involved in activities, and keeping occupied with meaningful activities. However, she had temporarily lost her social contact through her exclusive involvement with her husband and she was now prevented from getting involved with others by excessive guilt and the need to deny her husband's death and her own independence. Hence, as her symptoms decreased and her guilt abated, she was able to use her interpersonal skills more effectively. The therapist's interventions in this area were focused on countering unrealistic or excessive fears of rejection from others through a thorough discussion of options for new activities.

HANDLING OF PSYCHODYNAMICS

As noted in the discussion of the interface between IPT and psychodynamic therapies, the importance of excessive guilt was recognized by the therapist and focused on in the treatment. However, explicit interpretation of this material with reference to parallels in past and present relationships was not attempted.

TECHNIQUES

EXPLORATORY TECHNIQUES

Most of the therapist's activity in this case involved using exploratory techniques. The aim in their use was to formulate a goal that would help the therapist determine what areas of discussion to expand upon. For example, in intermediate sessions the therapist was likely to elicit further information about the patient's reluctance to visit her husband's grave rather than a discussion of a visit from her son.

The general goal of nondirective exploration is to help the patient and therapist pinpoint what actually goes on in the patient's life, in an attempt to begin assessing where changes need to be made. Thus, there is an interplay between exploration and clarification and feeding back small formulations to the patient. An example of this pattern occurred in Session 1, when the therapist tried to develop an understanding of the things that kept the patient from seeing old friends. In this discussion, it became clear that there was a distinction between anticipation of the event and the patient's actual ability to enjoy herself once in it.

PATIENT: I think I have a fear of . . . rejection so much that I don't institute any kind of a plan for anything. If anybody calls me and says do you want to do so-and-so, I'm glad to go, but I will not . . . initiate any type of activity . . . with anybody.

THERAPIST: How do you mean, fear of rejection?

PATIENT: Well, if they say no, I can't do it today, even though they give me a good excuse, it sort of throws me, you know, down into a hole, it's . . . almost like my fault that they can't do it, you know.

THERAPIST: Um-hm. Or that they're just making it up?

PATIENT: Yeah.

THERAPIST: I mean, is that really something that has happened to you a lot, that people have sort of found you hard to be with or . . . ?

PATIENT: I don't think . . . I don't think so. I think that's . . . in my mind.

THERAPIST: Hm. You've . . . tended to feel like that for some time, or just more recently?

PATIENT: I probably . . . just . . . maybe more recently. . . . Before, I, I think I always [sighs] probably had this feeling that, well, so what if anybody did reject me? Whatever . . . I initiated, I always had my husband to fall back on, you know, to, well, so that . . .

THERAPIST: Um-hm.

PATIENT: But now it's a little bit different. You just sort of, you hang up the phone, and you can't . . . [unclear] you know, other plans, or something. It's sort—you sort of say, well, what do I do now?

THERAPIST: Um-hm. When you make plans, it's hard to . . . you don't like to make plans very far in advance, or . . . ?

PATIENT: No.

THERAPIST: How come?

PATIENT: I don't know.

THERAPIST: So it's like you'll call up someone and want to do something today or tomorrow, that kind of thing?

PATIENT: Well, if I make a plan for, you know, an event, I can do that all right. But when the time comes, I sort of beat myself for having made that particular plan, because I really don't want to do it, you know, or at least I think I don't want to do it, I . . .

THERAPIST: And then when you do it?

PATIENT: Very opposite person or something . . . when I do it, I find I enjoyed it.

THERAPIST: Um-hm. So it really is, then a marked contrast between that antici . . .

PATIENT: I have sort of a conflict of some sort.

THERAPIST: Um-hm, it's like the anticipation of the event is really different from . . . the way it actually turns out.

PATIENT: Very.

THERAPIST: Just like . . . your anticipation that people won't or don't like you, and the way it turned out for instance when you were in the hospital, and people didn't want you to leave, that there is somehow . . . those things don't jibe.

PATIENT: Well . . . I don't have trouble getting along with people, I mean people generally like me. I'm not, you know, I'm not a pushy person, I don't . . . I . . . I'm pleasant enough, when I'm with people. . . . I, uh . . . I'm nervous inside, because I feel like I should be always chattering. And sometimes I come away from a group and think, you know? why, why do I always feel that I have to be always, my mouth always has to be going, and. . . . It's just that I can't stand silence, it's . . .

THERAPIST: Hm . . .

PATIENT: I can't stand silence in my house, my radio's going all the time.

THERAPIST: Um-hm. Do you get the message from people that you . . . talk too much, or that you . . .

PATIENT: No . . .

THERAPIST: So, once again, I mean it seems . . . that . . . you kind of have a sense . . .

PATIENT: Like I'm a dual person, you know?

THERAPIST: How do you mean, a dual person?

PATIENT: Like part of me can do . . . do things that, uh, you know, I should be doing, and the other part of me just fights against doing them.

MANAGEMENT AND
ENCOURAGEMENT OF AFFECT

Elicitation of affect was a key aspect of Ruth's treatment. In reviewing her relationship with her husband, there was an explicit attempt to help her experience sadness over the loss, with the plan of helping her realize that she could bear it; to feel her anger at her husband, with the plan of helping her realize that it is an acceptable and normal feeling; and to experience loving feelings about her husband, with the plan of helping her see that she need not give these up even if she began to allow new people and experiences into her life. Encouragement of affect took three primary forms: discussion of significant details in the patient's current and past life; naming her feelings; and encouraging her to accept the feelings as manageable and understandable.

Significant details were elicited throughout the therapy. These included the discussion of how the patient acted as though her husband were still in the house by sleeping on one side of the bed and keeping half of the closet open for him; discussion of what it was like when she attempted to visit the grave; discussion of her reactions to the loss of her cats; and many other significant details.

The following segment from Session 4 illustrates the exploration of significant details.

PATIENT: The holidays are . . . sort of . . . a sad time for me because [unclear] isn't going to keep me from doing . . . from, you know, decorating a little bit. I like Christmas. I like decorating the house. So . . . I-I just, when my husband isn't there, I still will . . . decorate.

THERAPIST: Mm-hm, mm-hm.

PATIENT: Because they're, they're pretty, the red, green—pretty colors.

THERAPIST: Mm-hm, mm-hm. It's still hard to think about doing things for yourself.

PATIENT: Well, I think that's where the guilt comes in, that he isn't here, you know. I don't . . . do that much for myself. I—well, no, I'm picking up, I'm doing quite a bit—but every once in a while . . .

THERAPIST: Mm-hm.

PATIENT: I get this pang of guilt, thinking, well, gee, you shouldn't be, you shouldn't be so happy about things.

THERAPIST: Hm, mm-hm. Because if you're enjoying things, that means you can't be thinking about him?

PATIENT: I think about him less and less, but I don't . . . suddenly, all of a sudden, when I'm doing something that I'm enjoying, the thought intrudes that, you know, you shouldn't be so happy [chuckles].

THERAPIST: Hm, hm. I guess.

PATIENT: I'm sure he wouldn't want me to be—sad . . .

THERAPIST: But in a way, hanging on to those sad thoughts . . . is a little like hanging on to him?

PATIENT: Probably. Something yesterday that I've been wanting to do for a long time, but yet not being able to, not . . . I guess maybe I didn't admit to myself that—that it had to be done . . . I called about a stone, for the, the grave.

THERAPIST: Hm.

PATIENT: And . . . probably will go out next week and pick it out. And maybe that'll help . . . lay things to rest a little bit. I have not been able to do it before.

THERAPIST: Hm. What, what had happened before, when you . . . tried to do it, or . . . think about it?

PATIENT: [sighs] I just couldn't think about it, I couldn't deal with it at all. When, in fact, I have been . . . I went to the cemetery once . . .

THERAPIST: Hm.

PATIENT: And . . . I was appalled, because . . . I went there, and I couldn't find . . . his grave, because there's no marker, or anything, and I had not . . . looked to see what was on either side of course, so I was . . . Maybe four or five graves there, with nothing on them. I didn't know which one . . . was, was his, which one was ours. And I was so appalled to think that . . . I'm not a cemetery person, I do not go every weekend, I wouldn't, because that doesn't, I—I, I just—does nothing for me.

THERAPIST: Mm-hm.

PATIENT: But occasionally, it doesn't hurt, you know. I wasn't so appalled that I couldn't find him . . . where they are, and everything, where I'm getting the stone is . . . that I got the locks.

THERAPIST: Mm-hm.

PATIENT: So I've never been back there again, because there's just no need to go. But I'm not a—I am not one of these people that just goes out and . . . cries, and . . . which would . . .

THERAPIST: Mm-hm.

PATIENT: Which would probably make me too sad for a while.

THERAPIST: What's too sad?

PATIENT: That he's down there and I'm up here, I guess [laughing].

THERAPIST: How would you be if you're too sad?

PATIENT: I would, I . . . probably would have a crying fit. Really, probably take me a couple days to get over it, you know . . . that's so—you know feeling like that is very immobilizing, I don't do anything. I wouldn't do anything. Where now I'm at least accomplishing something.

THERAPIST: Mm-hm.

PATIENT: May not sound like much to somebody else, but to me, it's . . . I have been. I'm—I feel like I've sort of . . . grown a little bit.

THERAPIST: Hm.

PATIENT: I don't have any fears about my mind going, at all, not at this point.

THERAPIST: Hm. Mm-hm.

PATIENT: And I'm not that old yet, either.

THERAPIST: So if you found a stone for him, though, he would have a place?

PATIENT: Probably that's the feeling I have, yeah.

THERAPIST: And that there would be . . .

PATIENT: And if I went there, it would be sort of . . . that would be sort of comforting, to know that I did, you know, get the things that—the right thing, probably.

THERAPIST: Mm-hm.

PATIENT: If there's a right and wrong, you know.

THERAPIST: Mm-hm.

PATIENT: I feel that would be the right thing to do.

THERAPIST: Mm-hm. But in a way, if he . . . doesn't really have a place, then . . . ?

PATIENT: He's just not laid to rest, you know, sort of.

THERAPIST: Mm-hm.

PATIENT: It's not, it's not finished, and I, I'd like it, at this point, like everything finished . . .

THERAPIST: Mm-hm, like with the bills, too.

PATIENT: Right. I've just got about a couple more things, as far as the bills go.

THERAPIST: Mm-hm.

PATIENT: And [sighs] that will be settled. And I think that's, I just—I—I mean it'll be a big relief, when I can just put everything aside, and just go on.

THERAPIST: Mm-hm. But I guess there are two sides to the relief. I mean, one is that you really have settled them, and he's in a place, and, you know, the place is definitely not with you, and he is dead.

PATIENT: Yeah.

THERAPIST: But, on the other hand, I guess, having these things still to do, in a way, keeps him around longer. You don't have to give him up.

CLARIFICATION

Naming the patient's feelings—clarifications—were done frequently. For example, when Ruth discussed having been so angry that she tried to strangle her husband, the therapist commented: "He did things to you that make anyone enraged—his threats, his suspiciousness, his helplessness were enraging, and you got so angry you temporarily lost control."

In Ruth's therapy, clarifications usually took the form of tying together the different ways the patient discussed feelings, in an attempt to show her how they related to guilt thoughts and feelings regarding her husband. The intention was to help her recognize that the guilty fantasies were unrealistic and to help her develop an appropriate level of distance from the event. One example of this type of clarification comes from Session 4. The patient had discussed her happy anticipation of Christmas as well as the worrisome fact that her doctor had found a spot on her lung. Her immediate thought was that she had cancer and was going to die quickly, just as she was beginning to enjoy life.

THERAPIST: Mm-hm, I wonder if through the . . . guilty pang, and the . . . feeling that you're, you know, going to really get sick and die, if those really aren't kind of related in a way, you know, like, almost like you feel . . . that . . .

PATIENT: I should have died?

THERAPIST: Yeah . . . or that, you know, that it just, it's fitting that you would get sick, now he's gone.

PATIENT: I hope not.

THERAPIST: Mm-hm. But I think that maybe it's thoughts, you know.

PATIENT: Yeah, yeah . . .

THERAPIST: I mean, they're not realities. But . . . you know, I wonder . . .

PATIENT: I had them a while ago, I, I had that type of fear maybe a while ago but not . . . in the last couple of months.

THERAPIST: Mm-hm. Mm-hm.

PATIENT: I mean where, after, after he died, maybe two, three, a couple of months afterward.

THERAPIST: Mm-hm, Mm-hm.

PATIENT: I had those . . . types of thinking, but I haven't now.

THERAPIST: Well, but, you know, I guess the thing is, that as you're enjoying things, you know, and feeling . . .

PATIENT: Mm-hm.

THERAPIST: I don't, I don't think that those thoughts, I think you can think other things, you know.

PATIENT: Yeah . . .

THERAPIST: It's just that it seems to me that, uh . . .

PATIENT: They go together.

THERAPIST: Yeah, that, you know, that as you are starting to enjoy things, and feeling guilty, you know, it would sort of seem like . . . you know . . .

PATIENT: Just my luck.

THERAPIST: Yeah, right. I mean that this would be kind of a retribution for . . .

PATIENT: Yeah . . .

THERAPIST: For starting to enjoy yourself.

PATIENT: Well, the mind does a lot of crazy things, I guess.

THERAPIST: Hm, mm-hum, mm-hum. Well, I guess it's hard, because it—you know, if you do enjoy things, then you really are giving him up.

PATIENT: Yeah.

THERAPIST: You know, and you really are . . .

PATIENT: Maybe I'm not ready, quite ready to let go.

THERAPIST: Yeah. Entirely, that . . . and I think that, you know, the fact that you sort of stay away from . . . the grave, you know, because it scares you still, how sad you can get.

PATIENT: Yeah.

THERAPIST: You know, I, think that uh . . . I think that it's really . . . impressive that you are making the kind of progress that you are, but on the other hand, I guess the thing is that, you know, I think you . . . you don't have to . . . forget about him. You know, you don't have to be . . . entirely without the memories.

PATIENT: Yeah . . . well, outside of that little guilty pang, thinking about him doesn't hurt quite as much as it had, but . . .

THERAPIST: Hm, mm-hm.

PATIENT: The hurt and the guilt—are, I don't know, are they related, sort of? I find that I'm not . . . uh, as lonely in the house at all. In fact, I enjoy being alone now, more . . .

THERAPIST: Hm.

PATIENT: And, uh . . . if I, when my daughter asks me to come over, just to sit, or, you know, I don't mean to baby-sit, but to come over, I don't feel the need that I have to run right over. If I'm tired, I say, I don't think I will tonight, you know.

THERAPIST: Mm-hm.

PATIENT: So [sighs] at one point, I just couldn't wait to get out of that house, but now it's beginning to take . . . shape . . . for me. My things are beginning to be . . . displayed. And, you know . . . little by little, his things are disappearing.

THERAPIST: Mm-hm.

PATIENT: Outside of a picture or two, you know.

THERAPIST: Mm-hm.

PATIENT: But . . . I have not been able to wholly . . . get rid of all of his clothes, for instance. . . . I don't know why I'm waiting, I have a couple of bathrobes that are hanging there, and I thought, why did I leave these here? I don't know why I left them here.

THERAPIST: Mm-hm.

PATIENT: But I know that I'll get rid of them, you know . . . as soon as I start.

THERAPIST: Mm-hm. You'll get rid of them when you . . .

PATIENT: When it's time, yeah . . .

THERAPIST: When it's time. Mm-hm, mm-hm. And it's a little-by-little process.

PATIENT: Yeah, yeah. . . . Sometimes, after I've gotten . . . think of that, of something like that, I feel real good about it, I don't feel sad at all.

THERAPIST: Mm-hm.

PATIENT: In fact, I . . . most of these things, I took off to the thrift shop, where, you know, they're sold to the, for the poor people . . . wearable. My son didn't want anything, so I just thought, well, I would— rather than put, dump them in the Salvation Army, they have a thrift shop where nice . . . you know, the churches have it. . . .

THERAPIST: Hm.

PATIENT: And I find my going down to the cellar doesn't bother me quite as much as it did. And that's something else I have to get straightened out, but I'll do that after the holidays. . . .

THERAPIST: Mm-hm. So you can put some things off.

PATIENT: I can?

THERAPIST: You can.

PATIENT: Yes.

THERAPIST: Mm-hm.

PATIENT: My mind gets, my mind gets very . . . [chuckles] mixed up when I think of leaving. If anything happened to me, I think, oh, what a job it's going to be for somebody.

Another clarification occurred in Session 5:

PATIENT: I deserve staying in bed.

THERAPIST: Mm-hm. You mentioned, before, feeling guilty about going out, that you can go out now without feeling guilty . . .

PATIENT: Well, it's just . . . I don't know what it is, feeling that—I shouldn't be enjoying myself. I don't know why.

THERAPIST: Hm.

PATIENT: But it's . . . I've sort of gotten . . . gotten over that, I think . . . or . . . this past week I didn't allow myself to think about it. I just have this feeling that all . . . [sighs] this is not happening to me, that . . . my house isn't mine, that I, you know . . . It's really—I always felt it, that, you know, the money that was made in that house was always his anyway, and that he never . . . showed that or anything. It was, it was just me that, you know, that way, so that I never spent money freely, or . . . unless it was my own money.

THERAPIST: Mm-hm.

PATIENT: Uh . . . because . . . you know, we would talk things over, before we bought anything, so it was a ha—a long, long habit, so it's still sort of ingrained in me that I shouldn't be doing this, without finding out [chuckles] if I can or not.

THERAPIST: Hm. Mm-hm. Feeling like you ought to discuss it with him?

PATIENT: Right.

THERAPIST: Mm-hm, mm-hum.

PATIENT: But gradually it's dawning on me that I'm my own person, and I've got to just, you know, stand on my own two feet, do what I want to do.

THERAPIST: Mm-hm. So, in other words, if you want to go out to lunch or . . .

PATIENT: Just what I did this past week, right.

Therapist: If you want to go to a movie.

Patient: Or if I want to stay in bed, see.

Therapist: Mm-hm, mm-hum. But it's like you sort of anticipate . . . that something bad will happen if you—

Patient: Not necessarily. I don't think I went that far. It was just . . . something . . . that's just left over from when, from living with another person so long, and always . . . thinking, before I made any plans, whether, you know, he would like to go, or whether he would rather I didn't go. I, I really wasn't . . . as free when we were married as I am now. I do have a lot of freedom now, but—that was of my own making, too. I think that . . .

Therapist: Hm. He probably would have thought it was OK if you were more independent?

Patient: Yeah. Right. Yeah, I'm sure he would have. I think a lot of my problems were made . . . in my mind.

Behavior Change Techniques

As the therapist initiated discussions of different possibilities for developing a more active life, these took the form of reality-oriented considerations of options. Affordability and transportation were discussed, as well as what needs Ruth might satisfy with activities of various sorts. Techniques such as direct advice and role playing were not necessary, since the patient herself took a great deal of initiative. This illustration of a discussion of options comes from Session 3:

Therapist: You know, last week we had discussed, we had talked about the fact that, you know, it seems like . . . getting back to what we talked about a little earlier . . . that really, this is one of the first times in your life that you've really been as free as you are.

Patient: Yeah, in all my life, I think it's my . . .

Therapist: Mm-hm.

Patient: This is the freest I've ever been. And I really sometimes get very annoyed with myself, that I don't put my time to better use.

Therapist: Like . . . ?

Patient: Well, like doing something for somebody else, you know, I still have . . . perhaps doing some, doing some volunteer work somewhere . . .

THERAPIST: Hm.

PATIENT: I've been talking to a couple . . . people that I know who are doing some, one of the women . . . working in the convalescent home . . . goes in a couple of times a week and she loves it.

THERAPIST: Hm.

PATIENT: And it gives her a feeling of, you know, usefulness.

THERAPIST: Mm-hm. That seems like a big step to take?

PATIENT: Yes . . . it's a big step for me to take to call up. I'm . . . not a telephone person. I hate telephones, I've got to be . . . really desperate to pick up a telephone and call somebody . . . or something.

THERAPIST: Mm-hm. What about dropping by?

PATIENT: I never thought of that [chuckles]. That to me would be easier than telephoning.

THERAPIST: Mm-hm, mm-hum. Well, I mean, I . . . I suppose most places where you would volunteer, there must be someone there, you could . . . just go by and see. Or maybe you could go with a friend, or something like that.

PATIENT: Yeah . . . mm-hm. . . . Well, I-I-I'm still busy trying to get myself . . . in order, that, I'll . . . sort of let that rest a little while.

THERAPIST: Mm-hm. Well, I guess the thing about, though, having a lot of freedom is that it really, always brings up . . . issues like—you know, what are the things that are satisfying to you? You know, what is it that you want out of life?

PATIENT: Well, see. I always wanted to go, I'd always—I grew up thinking that I never was able to go to college. . . .

THERAPIST: Hm.

PATIENT: So . . . now I've got this freedom, and my son said, "Why don't you take a course? That'll keep you occupied and interested."

THERAPIST: Mm-hm.

PATIENT: So [sighs] he said, "Why don't you go down to . . ." you know . . . the one down on . . . Anyway, I took South Central, because I thought it was easier for me to get there than it was to go to Southern.

THERAPIST: Mm-hm, mm-hum. I think South Central also generally does have more . . . community people.

PATIENT: Yeah . . .

THERAPIST: Instead of, you know, Southern tends to be more eighteen-year-olds.

PATIENT: Yeah . . .

THERAPIST: That kind of thing. Mm-hm.

PATIENT: Of course, as a senior citizen, there are a lot of things that are open to you, like I don't have to pay for the courses that I take.

THERAPIST: Hm.

PATIENT: I pay for my books, but I don't have to pay.

THERAPIST: Mm-hm, mm-hm. Well, have you thought of taking more than one course? Or are you really trying to get a degree?

PATIENT: Well, I have, I have . . . well, I thought I would like to get an associate degree. I don't know in what, but I always like that, because South Central . . . South Central is . . . a two-year course anyway. So I have to talk to, I have to go down, to get to talk to a counselor there, see what's open for me.

THERAPIST: Mm-hm, mm-hum.

PATIENT: Well, this course that I'm taking now, English course, is . . . a lot of writing, I . . . think, my goodness, if I took two courses I'd go crazy.

THERAPIST: Mm-hm. Well. I guess that's the thing about freedom, is that you have to—decide on what you're . . .

PATIENT: Yeah.

THERAPIST: What it is that you want.

PATIENT: Because I still want some freedom. For myself.

THERAPIST: Mm-hm.

PATIENT: To do . . . other things that I like to do.

THERAPIST: Well, so, so one of the things then, that you want to have in your—as part of your life—picture—the way that you would be organizing your life—would be . . . at least a minimum amount of time at home, or, you know, taking care of the house and I guess being in the house that you like.

PATIENT: Yeah . . .

THERAPIST: And . . . you know, just having a sense that it's yours, and relaxation, that sort of thing. And, you know, another aspect of it I guess would be that you'd want to make sure that you had time to . . . you know, do some socializing.

PATIENT: Mm-hm.

THERAPIST: To, maybe . . . after all, one of the advantages of being retired is that you can . . . spend time doing recreation.

PATIENT: That's right.

THERAPIST: That kind of thing.

PATIENT: As long as you're healthy enough to do that.

THERAPIST: Mm-hm. But . . . on the other hand, it seems like . . . there are other things . . . that you want to be able to have a sense of building, or of accomplishment.

PATIENT: Yeah, I've got to, I've got to really sort of pinpoint what I really want to do, because my mind whirls around . . . doing this, this, this, this, and . . . uh . . .

THERAPIST: Well, what . . . ?

PATIENT: And I don't think that you can . . .

THERAPIST: Mm-hm.

PATIENT: . . . you can [sighs] do a good job at everything that you want to do, you know.

THERAPIST: Mm-hm, mm-hum. Well, what are the things that you've been considering?

PATIENT: Nothing specific, it's just that my mind is just whirling around.

THERAPIST: Well, where does it whirl?

PATIENT: Well, first the volunteer stuff, that, that part . . .

THERAPIST: Mm-hm. Any particular kind of volunteer?

PATIENT: No, I hadn't really thought about any kind of volunteer work, and I've been sort of . . . I don't know, I don't know whether I want to work with the elderly or the children . . .

THERAPIST: Mm-hm.

PATIENT: Sometimes I think I'd like to work with the elderly, and, you know, then I think maybe I'd rather work with children, so I have to make up my own mind about that.

THERAPIST: Mm-hm.

PATIENT: And I think that . . . I haven't really . . . gone into it, I think the senior citizens do have a program . . . for volunteer work too, so that . . .

THERAPIST: Hm.

PATIENT: I might be into something there.

THERAPIST: Mm-hm.

PATIENT: As I get better acquainted.

THERAPIST: Mm-hm. So one possibility would be to do some . . . volunteer work, which I guess would be satisfying in the sense that . . .

PATIENT: Yeah, if it's just one day a week, I think it would sort of satisfy me . . .

THERAPIST: Mm-hm, mm-hm.

PATIENT: I think this woman I was talking about, I think she started with one day and decided she had to go two days, because she enjoyed it, and they . . . really looked forward to having her come.

THERAPIST: Mm-hm.

PATIENT: So it sort of gives her a sense of being needed, and accomplishing something too.

THERAPIST: Mm-hm. Then another whole area, though, is the idea of—I guess learning more: I'm going to still be curious about things, and . . .

PATIENT: Yeah.

THERAPIST: Wanting to . . . ?

PATIENT: Yeah, I certainly don't want to just sit in a chair and watch television. I don't . . . watch that much television, anyway. Nothing much on, you know?

COMMUNICATION ANALYSIS

In this case, communication analysis was not used at all. If, for example, the patient had had difficulty in engaging others in discussion as she tried to get involved in the senior citizens' group, this might have been used.

USE OF THE THERAPEUTIC RELATIONSHIP

If the patient had been more resistant to the work of the psychotherapy, the therapist might well have tried to draw parallels between the patient's interpersonal problems outside of therapy and her behavior in the therapy sessions. As it turned out, this was not necessary.

Literature References

Agras, W. S., B. T. Walsh, G. T. Wilson, and C. G. Fairburn. 1999. A multisite comparison of cognitive behaviour therapy (CBT) and interpersonal psychotherapy (IPT) in the treatment of bulimia nervosa. Presented at Eating Disorders '99, London, April 20–22, 1999.

Alter, C. L., S. Fleishman, A. Kornbluth, J. C. Holland, D. Baiano, R. Levenson, V. Vinciguerra, and K. R. Rai. In press. Supportive telephone intervention for patients receiving chemotherapy: A pilot study. *Psychosomatics*.

American Academy of Pediatrics, Committee on Drugs. 1994. Transfer of drugs and other chemicals into human milk. *Pediatrics* 93:137–50.

American Medical Association: Graduate Medical Education Directory 1998–1999. Chicago: American Medical Association, 1998, 828.

American Psychiatric Association. 1980. *Diagnostic and Statistical Manual of Mental Disorders*, 3d ed. Washington, D.C.: American Psychiatric Association.

———. 1987. *Diagnostic and Statistical Manual of Mental Disorders*, 3d ed., rev. Washington, D.C.: American Psychiatric Association.

———. 1994. *Diagnostic and Statistical Manual of Mental Disorders*, 4th ed. [DSM-IV]. Washington, D.C.: American Psychiatric Association.

———. 1994. Practice guidelines for the treatment of patients with bipolar disorders. *Supplement to the American Journal of Psychiatry*. 151(12):1–36.

American Psychiatric Press. In press, 2000. *Handbook of Psychiatric Measures*. Washington, D.C.: American Psychiatric Press.

Angold, A., M. M. Weissman, K. John, K. R. Merikangas, B. A. Prusoff, P. Wickramaratne, G. D. Gammon, and V. Warner. 1987. Parent and child reports of depressive symptoms in children at low and high risk for depression. *J. Child Psychol. Psychiatry* 28:901.

Angst, J. 1986. The course of major depression, atypical bipolar disorder, and bipolar disorder. In *New results in depression research*, ed. H. Hippius, G. L. Klerman, and N. Matussek, 26–35. New York: Springer-Verlag.

Angst, J., K. Merikangas, P. Scheidegger, and W. Wicki. 1990. Recurrent brief depression: A new subtype of affective disorder. *Journal of Affective Disorders* 19:87–98.

Angus, L., and L. A. Gillies. 1994. Counseling the borderline client: An interpersonal approach. *Can. J. Counseling/Rev. Can. de Counsel* 28:69–82.

Arieti, S., and J. Bemporad. 1978. *Severe and Mild Depression*. New York: Basic Books.

Bakish, D., Y. D. Lapierre, R. Weinstein, J. Klein, A. Wiens, B. Jones, E. Horn, M. Browne, D. Bourget, A. Blanchard, C. Thibaudeau, C. Waddell, and D. Raine. 1993.

Ritanserin, imipramine and placebo in the treatment of dysthymic disorder. *J. Clin. Psychopharmacol.* 13:409–14.

Barber, J. P., and L. R. Muenz. 1996. The role of avoidance and obsessiveness in matching patients to cognitive and interpersonal psychotherapy: Empirical findings from the Treatment for Depression Collaborative Research Program. *J. Consult. Clin. Psychol.* 64:951–58.

Barrett, J. E., J. A. Barrett, T. E. Oxman, and P. D. Gerber. 1988. The prevalence of psychiatric disorders in a primary care practice. *Arch. Gen. Psychiatry* 45:1100–1106.

Basco M. R., and A. J. Rush. 1996. *Cognitive-Behavioral Therapy for Bipolar Disorder.* New York: Guilford.

Bauserman, S.A.K., I. Arias, and W. E. Craighead. 1995. Marital attributions in spouses of depressed patients. *Journal of Psychopathology & Behavioral Assessment* 17(3):231–49.

Beardslee, W. R., M. B. Keller, P. W. Lavori, and G. L. Klerman. 1988. Psychiatric disorder in adolescent offspring of parents with affective disorder in a nonreferred sample. *Journal of Affective Disorders* 15:313–22.

Beck, A. T. 1978. *Depression inventory.* Philadelphia: Center for Cognitive Therapy.

Beck, A. T., A. J. Rush, B. F. Shaw, and G. Emery. 1979. *Cognitive Therapy of Depression.* New York: Guilford.

Becker, J. 1974. *Depression: Theory and Research.* New York: Wiley.

Becker, R. E., R. G. Heimber, and A. S. Bellack. 1987. *Social Skills Training Treatment for Depression.* New York: Pergamon.

Beckham, E. E., and W. R. Leber, eds. 1995. *Handbook of Depression,* 2d ed. New York: Guilford.

Bemporad, J. R. 1988. Psychodynamic treatment of depressed adolescents. *J. Clin. Psychiatry* 49:26–31.

Bergin, A. E., and S. L. Garfield, eds. 1994. *Handbook of Psychotherapy and Behavior Change.* 4th ed. New York: John Wiley and Sons.

Bersani, G., F. Pozzi, S. Marini, A. Grispini, A. Pasini, and N. Ciani. 1991. 5-HT$_2$ receptor antagonism in dysthymic disorder: A double-blind placebo controlled study with ritanserin. *Acta Psychiatric Scand.* 83:244–48.

Bibring, E. 1953. Mechanism of depression. In *Affective Disorders,* ed. P. Greenacre. New York: International Universities Press.

Bigelow, G. E., and K. L. Preston. 1995. Opioids. In *Psychopharmacology: The Fourth Generation of Progress,* ed. F. Bloom and J. Kupfer, 1731–74. New York: Raven Press.

Blatt, S. J., D. M. Quinlan, P. A. Pilokonis, and M. T. Shea. 1995. Impact of perfectionism and need for approval on the brief treatment of depression: The National Institute of Mental Health Treatment of Depression Collaborative Research Program revisited. *J. Consult. Clin. Psychol.* 63:125–32.

Blazer, D. G., and C. D. Williams. 1980. Epidemiology of dysphoria and depression in an elderly population. *Am J Psychiatry* 137:439–44.

Blom, M.B.J., E. Hoencamp, and T. Zwaan. 1996. Interpersoonlijke Psychotherapie voor depressie: Een pilot-onderzoek. *Tijdschrift voor Psychiatr.* 38:398–402.

Blom, M.B.J., M. J. Kerver, and W. A. Nolen, eds. 1997. *Inleiding in de interpersoonlijke psychotherapie.* Houten: Bohn Stafleu Van Loghum.

Bronisch, T., and G. L. Klerman. 1991. Personality functioning: Change and stability in relationship to symptoms and psychopathology. *J. Personality Disorders* 5:307–17.

Brent, D. A., D. Holder, D. Kolko, B. Birmaher, M. Baugher, C. Roth, and B. Johnson. 1997. A clinical psychotherapy trial for adolescent depression comparing cognitive, family, and supportive treatments. *Arch. Gen. Psychiatry* 54:877–85.

Brent, D. A., D. J. Kolko, M. J. Allen, and R. V. Brown. July 1990. Suicidality in affectively disordered adolescent inpatients. *J. Am. Acad. Child Adolesc. Psychiatry* 29(4):586–93.

Brent, D. A., C. Roth, D. Holder, D. Kolko, B. Birmaher, B. Johnson, and J. Scweers. 1996. Adolescent depression: A comparison of three psychosocial interventions. In *Psychosocial treatment for child and adolescent disorders: Empirically based strategies for clinical practice*, ed. D. Hibbs and P. S. Jensen, 187–206. Washington, D.C.: American Psychological Association.

Brown, A., and D. Finkelhor. 1986. Impact of child sexual abuse: A review of the research. *Psychol. Bull.* 99:66–77.

Brown, C., H. C. Schulberg, M. J. Madonia, M. K. Shear, and P. R. Houck. 1996. Treatment outcomes for primary care patients with major depression and lifetime anxiety disorders. *Am. J. Psychiatry* 153(10):1293–99.

Brown, G. W., and T. O. Harris. 1978. *Social Origins of Depression: A Study of Psychiatric Disorder in Women.* London: Tavistock.

Brown, G. W., T. Harris, and J. R. Copeland. 1977. Depression and loss. *British Journal of Psychiatry* 130:1–18.

Browne, G., M. Steiner, J. Roberts, A. Gafni, C. Burne, E. Dunn, E. Jamieson, M. Webb, B. Bell, M. Mills, L. Chalklin, D. Wallik, and J. Kraemer. 1997. A randomized trial of the effects and expense of Zoloft (sertraline) vs. interpersonal psychotherapy, alone or in combination for people with dysthymia in primary care. Health and Social Service Utilization Unit, McMaster University. Unpublished report.

Burch, H. 1978. *The Golden Cage.* Cambridge, Mass.: Harvard University Press.

Burgess, J. W. 1993. The psychotherapy of giving medications: Therapeutic techniques for interpersonal interventions. *Am. J. Psychother.* 47(3).

Busch, F. N., A. M. Cooper, G. L. Klerman, R. J. Penzer, T. Shapiro, and M. K. Shear. 1991. Neurophysiological, cognitive-behavioral, and psychoanalytic approaches to panic disorder: Toward an integration. *Psychoanalytic Inquiry* 11:316–22.

Campbell, M., and E. K. Spencer. 1988. Psychopharmacology in child and adolescent psychiatry: A review of the past five years. *J. Am. Acad. Child Adolesc. Psychiatry* 27:269–79.

Carroll, K. M., B. J. Rounsaville, and F. H. Gawin. 1991. A comparative trial of psychotherapies for ambulatory cocaine abusers: Relapse prevention and interpersonal psychotherapy. *Am. J. Drug Alcohol Abuse* 17:229–47.

Cassano, G. B., G. Perugi, I. Maremmani, and H. S. Akiskal. 1990. Social adjustment in dysthymia. In *Dysthymic Disorder*, ed. S. W. Burton and H. S. Akiskal. London: Gaskell.

Centers for Disease Control. 1987. Revision of the CDC surveillance case definition for acquired immunodeficiency syndrome. *Morbidity and Mortality Weekly Report* 36:3S–15S.

_____. 1990. HIV prevalence estimates and AIDS case projections for the United States: Report based upon a workshop. *Morbidity and Mortality Weekly Report* 39:1–31.

Chambers, C. D., K. A. Johnson, L. M. Dick, R. J. Felix, and K. L. Jones. 1996. Birth outcomes in pregnant women taking fluoxetine. *N. Engl. J. Med.* 335:1010–15.

Cherry, S., and J. C. Markowitz. 1996. Interpersonal psychotherapy. In *Clinical Depression During Addiction Recovery: Process, Diagnosis, and Treatment,* ed. J. S. Kantor, 165–85. New York: Marcel Dekker.

Chevron, E. S., B. J. Rounsaville, E. D. Rothblum, and M. M. Weissman. 1983. Selecting psychotherapists to participate in psychotherapy outcome studies: Relationship between psychotherapist characteristics and assessment of clinical skills. *J. Nerv. Ment. Dis.* 171:348–53.

Chodoff, P. 1970. The core problem in depression. In *Science and Psychoanalysis,* ed. J. Masserman, vol. 17. New York: Grune and Stratton.

Christie, K. A., J. D. Burke, D. A. Regier, D. S. Rae, J. H. Boyd, and B. Z. Locke. 1988. Epidemiologic evidence for early onset of mental disorders and higher risk of drug abuse in young adults. *Am. J. Psychiatry* 145:971–75.

Clarke, G., and P. M. Lewinsohn. 1989. The Coping with Depression Course: A group of psychoeducational interventions for unipolar depression. *Behavior Change* 6:554–69.

Clarke, G. N., W. Hawkins, M. Murphy, L. B. Sheeber, P. M. Lewisohn, and J. R. Seeley. 1995. Targeted prevention of unipolar depressive disorder in an at-risk sample of high school adolescents: A randomized trial of a group cognitive intervention. *J. Am. Acad. Child Adolesc. Psychiatry* 34(3):312–21.

Clum, G. A., G. A. Clum, and R. Surls. 1993. A meta-analysis of treatments for panic disorder. *J. Consult. Clin. Psychol.* 61:317–26.

Cochran, S. D. 1984. Preventing medical noncompliance in the outpatient treatment of bipolar affective disorders. *J Consult Clin Psychol.* 52(5):873–78.

Cohen, M. B., G. Blake, R. Cohen, F. Fromm-Reichmann, and E. Weigert. 1954. An intensive study of twelve cases of manic depressive psychosis. *Psychiatry* 17:103–37.

Cohen-Cole, S. A., and K. G. Kaufman. 1993. Major depression in physical illness: Diagnosis, prevalence, and antidepressant treatment (A ten-year review: 1982–1992). *Depression* 1:181–204.

Conte, J. R., R. Plutchik, K. V. Wild, and T. B. Karasu. 1986. Combined psychotherapy and pharmacotherapy for depression: A systematic analysis of the evidence. *Archives of General Psychiatry* 43(5): 471–79.

Coryell, W., and G. Winokur. 1994. Course and outcome. In *Handbook of affective disorders,* 2d ed., ed. E. S. Paykel. New York: Churchill Livingstone.

Coyne, J. C. 1976. Depression and the response of others. *Journal of Abnormal Psychology* 85:186–93.

Cross-National Collaborative Group. 1992. The changing rate of major depression: Cross-national comparisons. *JAMA* 268(21):3098–105.

Cytrn, L., and D. H. McKnew. 1985. Treatment issues in childhood depression. *Psychiatric Annals* 15:401.

Dalton, K., and W. Holton. 1996. *Depression after childbirth: How to recognize, treat, and prevent postnatal depression.* New York: Oxford University Press.

Davanloo, H. 1982. *Short-Term Dynamic Psychotherapy.* New York: Jason Aronson.

Dawson, D. F. 1988. Treatment of the borderline patient, relationship management. *Can. J. Psychiatry* 33:370–74.

De Groot, P. A. 1995. Consensus depressie bij volwassenen. Nederlands Tijdschrift voor Geneeskunde 139:1237.

Depression Guideline Panel. 1993a. *Clinical Practice Guideline: Depression in Primary Care: Detection and Diagnosis.* Rockville, Md.: U.S. Dept. of Health and Human Services, Agency for Health Care Policy and Research. AHCPR Publication 93-0550, 1.

———. 1993b. *Clinical Practice Guideline: Depression in Primary Care: Treatment of Major Depression.* Rockville, Md.: U.S. Dept. of Health and Human Services, Agency for Health Care Policy and Research. AHCPR Publication 93-0551, 2.

———. 1993c. *Clinical Practice Guideline: Quick Reference Guide for Clinicians: Depression in Primary Care: Detection, Diagnosis, and Treatment.* Rockville, Md.: U.S. Dept. of Health and Human Services, Agency for Health Care Policy and Research. AHCPR Publication 93-0552.

———. 1993d. *Clinical Practice Guideline: Depression Is a Treatable Illness: A Patient's Guide.* Rockville, Md.: U.S. Dept. of Health and Human Services, Agency for Health Care Policy and Research. AHCPR Publication 93-0553.

———. 1993e. *Clinical Practice Guideline: Depression in Primary Care.* Vols. 1–4. Rockville, Md.: U.S. Dept. of Health and Human Services, Agency for Health Care Policy and Research. AHCPR Publication 93-0550-0553.

Dewan, M. 1999. Are psychiatrists cost-effective? An analysis of integrated versus split treatment. *Am. J. Psychiatry* 156:324–26.

DiMascio, A., M. M. Weissman, B. A. Prusoff, C. Neu, M. Zwilling, and G. L. Klerman. 1979. Differential symptom reduction by drugs and psychotherapy in acute depression. *Arch. Gen. Psychiatry* 36:1450–56.

Dobson, K. 1989. A meta-analysis of the efficacy of cognitive therapy of depression. *J. Consult. Clin. Psychol.* 57:414–19.

Dujorne, V. F., M. U. Barnard, and M. A. Rapoff. 1995. Pharmacological and cognitive behavioral approaches in the treatment of childhood depression: A review and critique. *Clinical Psychology Review* 15:589–611.

Dutch Consensus Conference: Consensus-bijeenkomst Depressie bij Volwassenen. C.B.I.T/N.v.P. 1994. ISBN 90-6910-170-X.

Earls, F. 1980. Prevalence of behavior problems in three-year-old children: A cross-national replication. *Arch. Gen. Psychiatry* 37:1153–57.

Ehlers, C. L., E. Frank, and D. J. Kupfer. 1988. Social zeitgebers and biological rhythms. A unified approach to understanding the etiology of depression. *Arch. Gen. Psychiatry* 45:948–52.

Elkin, I., M. T. Shea, J. T. Watkins, S. D. Imber, S. M. Sotsky, J. F. Collins, D. R. Glass, P. A. Pilkonis, W. R. Leber, J. P. Docherty, S. J. Fiester, and M. B. Parloff. 1989. National Institute of Mental Health treatment of depression collaborative research program: General effectiveness of treatments. *Arch. Gen. Psychiatry* 46:971–82.

Emslie, G., A. J. Rush, W. A. Weinberg, R. Kowatch, T. Carmody, and T. L. Mayer. 1998. Fluoxetine in child and adolescent depression: Acute and maintenance treatment. *Depression* 7:32–39.

Emslie, G. J., A. J. Rush, W. A. Weinberg, R. A. Kowatch, C. W. Hughes, T. Carmody, and J. Rintelmann. 1997. A double-blind randomized placebo-controlled trial of fluoxetine in depressed children and adolescents. *Arch. Gen. Psychiatry* 54:1031–37.

Emslie, G. J., J. T. Walkup, S. R. Piszka, and M. Ernst. 1999. Nontricyclic antidepressants: Current trends in children and adolescents. *J. Am. Acad. Child Adolesc. Psychiatry* 38(5):517–28.

Endicott, J., and R. Spitzer. 1978. A diagnostic interview: The schedule for affective disorders and schizophrenia. *Arch. Gen. Psychiatry* 35:837–44.

Erikson, E. H. 1968. *Identity, youth, and crisis.* New York: W. W. Norton.

Eysenck, H. J. 1952. The effects of psychotherapy: An evaluation. *J. Consult. Clin. Psychol.* 16:319–24.

Fairburn, C. G. 1998. Interpersonal psychotherapy for bulimia nervosa. In *Interpersonal psychotherapy,* ed. J. C. Markowitz. Washington, D.C.: American Psychiatric Press.

Fairburn, C. G., R. Jones, R. C. Peveler, S. J. Carr, R. A. Solomon, M. E. O'Connor, J. Burton, and R. A. Hope. 1991. Three psychological treatments for bulimia nervosa: A comparative trial. *Arch Gen Psychiatry* 48:463–69.

Fairburn, C. G., R. Jones, R. C. Peveler, R. A. Hope, and M. O'Connor. 1993. Psychotherapy and bulimia nervosa: Longer-term effects of interpersonal psychotherapy, behavior therapy, and cognitive behavior therapy. *Archives of General Psychiatry* 50:419–28.

Fairburn, C. G., J. Kirk, M. O'Connor, and P. J. Cooper. 1986. A comparison of two psychological treatments for bulimia nervosa. *Behav. Res. Ther.* 24:629–43.

Fairburn, C. G., P. A. Norman, S. L. Welch, M. E. O'Connor, H. A. Doll, and R. C. Peveler. 1995. A prospective study of outcome in bulimia nervosa and the long-term effects of three psychological treatments. *Arch. Gen. Psychiatry* 52:304–12.

Faravelli, C. 1985. Life events preceding the onset of panic disorder. *J. Affect. Disorders* 9:103–5.

Fawcett, J., P. Epstein, S. J. Fiester, et al. 1987. Clinical management—imipramine/placebo administration manual. NIMH Treatment of Depression Collaborative Research Program. *Psychopharm. Bull.* 23:309–24.

Fawzy, F. I., N. W. Fawzy, L. A. Arndt, and R. O. Pasnau. 1995. Critical review of psychosocial interventions in cancer care. *Arch. Gen. Psychiatry* 52:100–113.

Fendrich, M., V. Warner, and M. M. Weissman. 1990. Family risk factors, parental depression and psychopathology in offspring. *Developmental Psychology* 26:40–50.

First, M. B., R. L. Spitzer, M. Gibbon, and J.B.W. Williams. 1995. *Structured clinical interview for DSM-IV Axis I disorders: Patient edition* (SCID-I/P, version 12.0). Biometrics Research Department, New York State Psychiatric Institute.

Fitts, S. N., P. Gibson, C. A. Redding, and P. J. Deiter. 1989. Body dysmorphic disorder: Implications for its validation as a DSM-III-R. *Clin. Syndrom. Psychol. Rep.* 64:655–58.

Fleming, J. E., and D. R. Offord. 1990. Epidemiology of childhood depressive disorders: A critical review. *J. Am. Acad. Child Adolesc. Psychiatry* 29:571–80.

Fleming, J. E., D. R. Offord, and M. H. Boyle. 1989. The Ontario Child Health Study: Prevalence of childhood and adolescent depression in the community. *Br. J. Psychiatry* 155:647–54.

Foley, S. H., S. O'Malley, B. Rounsaville, B. A. Prusoff, and M. M. Weissman. 1987. The relationship of patient difficulty to therapist performance in interpersonal psychotherapy of depression. *J. Affect. Dis.* 12:207–17.

Foley, S. H., B. J. Rounsaville, M. M. Weissman, D. Sholomskas, and E. Chevron. 1989. Individual versus conjoint interpersonal psychotherapy for depressed patients with marital disputes. *Int. J. Fam. Psychiatry* 10:29–42.

Folstein, M. F., S. E. Folstein, and P. R. McHugh. 1975. "Mini-mental state": A practical method for grading the cognitive state of patients for the clinician. *J. Psychiatr. Res.* 12:189–98.

Frances, A., J. F. Clarkin, and S. Perry. 1984. *Differential Therapeutics in Psychiatry: The Art and Science of Treatment Selection.* New York: Brunner/Mazel.

Frank, E. 1991. Interpersonal psychotherapy as a maintenance treatment for patients with recurrent depression. *Psychotherapy* 28:259–66.

Frank, E., and N. Frank. May 1988. Manual for the adaptation of interpersonal psychotherapy to maintenance treatment of recurrent depression in late life (IPT-LLM). Unpublished manuscript. Pittsburgh, Pa.

Frank, E., N. Frank, C. Cornes, S. D. Imber, M. D. Miller, S. M. Morris, and C. F. Reynolds III. 1993. Interpersonal psychotherapy in the treatment of late-life depression. In *New applications of interpersonal psychotherapy,* ed. G. L. Klerman and M. M. Weissman, 167–98. Washington, D.C.: American Psychiatric Press.

Frank, E., S. Hlastala, A. Ritenour, P. Houck, X. M. Tu, T. H. Monk, A. G. Mallinger, and D. J. Kupfer. 1997. Inducing lifestyle regularity in recovering bipolar disorder patients: Results from the maintenance therapies in bipolar disorder protocol. *Biol Psychiatry* 41:1165–73.

Frank, E., D. Kupfer, C. L. Ehlers, T. H. Monk, C. Comes, S. Carter, and D. Frankel. 1994. Interpersonal and social rhythm therapy for bipolar disorder: Integrating interpersonal and behavioral approaches. *Behav. Therapist* 17(7):143–46.

Frank, E., D. J. Kupfer, and J. M. Perel. 1989. Early recurrence in unipolar depression. *Arch. Gen. Psychiatry* 46:397–400.

Frank, E., D. J. Kupfer, J. M. Perel, C. Cornes, D. B. Jarrett, A. G. Mallinger, M. E. Thase, A. B. McEachran, and V. J. Grochocinski. 1990. Three-year outcomes for maintenance therapies in recurrent depression. *Arch. Gen. Psychiatry* 47:1093–99.

Frank, E., D. J. Kupfer, E. F. Wagner, A. B. McEachran, and C. Cornes. 1991. Efficacy of interpersonal psychotherapy as a maintenance treatment of recurrent depression. *Arch. Gen. Psychiatry* 48:1053–59.

Frank, E., R. F. Prien, R. B. Jarrett, M. B. Keller, D. J. Kupfer, P. W. Lavori, A. J. Rush, and M. M. Weissman. 1991. Conceptualization and rationale for consensus definitions of terms in major depressive disorder. *Arch. Gen. Psychiatry* 48:851–55.

Frank, J. D. 1973. *Persuasion and Healing: A Comparative Study of Psychotherapy.* Baltimore: Johns Hopkins University Press.

Frasure-Smith, N., F. Lesperance, R. H. Prince, P. Verrier, R. A. Garber, M. Juneau, C. Wolfson, and M. G. Bourassa. 1997. Randomised trial of home-based psychosocial nursing intervention for patients recovering from myocardial infarction. *Lancet* 350:473–79.

Frasure-Smith, N., F. Lesperance, and J. Talajic. 1993. Depression following myocardial infarction: Impact on six-month survival. *JAMA* 270:1819–61.

Frasure-Smith, N., and R. Price. 1985. The ischemic heart disease life stress monitoring program: Impact on mortality. *Psychosomatic Medicine* 47:431–44.

Fromm-Reichmann, F. 1960. *Principles of Intensive Psychotherapy.* Chicago: Phoenix Books.

Garber, J., M. R. Kriss, M. Koch, and L. Lindholm. 1988. Recurrent depression in adolescents: A follow-up study. *J. Am. Acad. Child Adolesc. Psychiatry* 27:49–54.

Garrison, C. Z., M. D. Schluchter, V. J. Schoenbach, and B. K. Kaplan. 1989. Epidemiology of depressive symptoms in young adolescents. *J. Am. Acad. Child Adolesc. Psychiatry* 28:343–51.

Geller, B., E. C. Chestnut, M. D. Miller, D. T. Price, and E. Yates. 1985. Preliminary data on DSM-III associated features of major depression disorder in children and adolescents. *Am. J. Psychiatry* 142:643–45.

Geller, B., T. B. Cooper, D. L. Graham, F. A. Marsteller, and D. M. Bryant. 1990. Double-blind placebo-controlled study of nortriptyline in depressed adolescents using a "fixed plasma level" design. *Psychopharmacol. Bull.* 26:85–91.

Geller, B., D. Reising, H. L. Leonard, M. A. Riddle, and B. T. Walsh. 1999. Critical review of tricyclic antidepressant use in children and adolescents. *J. Am. Acad. Child Adolesc. Psychiatry* 38(5):513–16.

Gershon, S., and J. C. Soares. 1997. Current therapeutic profile of lithium. *Arch. Gen. Psychiatry* 54:16–20.

Gitlin, M. J., and L. L. Altshuler. 1997. Unanswered questions, unknown future for one of our oldest medications. *Arch. Gen. Psychiatry* 54:21–23.

Glick, I. D., J. F. Clarkin, J. H. Spencer, G. L. Haas, A. B. Lewis, J. Peyser, N. DeMane, M. Good-Ellis, E. Harris, and V. Lestelle. 1985. A controlled evaluation of inpatient family intervention: I. Preliminary results of the six-month follow-up. *Arch. Gen. Psychiatry* 42:882–86.

Glover, V. 1997. Maternal stress or anxiety in pregnancy and emotional development of the child. *Br. J. Psychol.* 171:105–6.

Goldberg, D. P., J. J. Steele, C. Smith, and L. Spivey. 1980. Training family doctors to recognize psychiatric illness with increased accuracy. *Lancet* ii:521–23.

Goodwin, F. K., and K. R. Jamison. 1990. *Manic Depressive Illness.* New York: Oxford University Press.

Gotlib, I. H., and S.R.H. Beach. 1995. A marital/familiy discord model of depression: Implications for therapeutic intervention. In *Clinical Handbook of Couple Therapy,* ed. Neil S. Jacobson and Alan S. Gurman, 411–36. New York: Guilford Press.

Gotlib, I. H., V. E. Whiffen, J. H. Mount, K. Milne, and N. I. Cordy. 1989. Prevalence rates and demographic characteristics associated with depression in pregnancy and the postpartum. *J. Consult. Clin. Psychol.* 57:269–74.

Gotlib, D., V. E. Whiffen, P. M. Wallace, and J. H. Mount. 1991. Prospective investigation of postpartum depression: Factors involved in onset and recovery. *J. Abnorm. Psychol.* 100:122–32.

Gould, M., and L. Davidson. 1988. Suicide contagion among adolescents. In *Advances in Adolescent Mental Health,* vol. 3, *Depression and Suicide,* ed. A. R. Stilman and R. A. Feldman, 29–59. Greenwich, Conn.: JAI Press.

Graves, J. S. 1993. Living with mania: A study of outpatient group psychotherapy for bipolar patients. *Am. J. Psychother.* 47(1):113–26.

Grumet, G. W. 1979. Telephone therapy: A review and case report. *Am. J. Orthopsychiatry* 49:574–84.

Haas, G. L., I. D. Glick, J. F. Clarkin, J. H. Spencer, A. B. Lewis, J. Peyser, N. DeMane, N. Good-Ellis, E. Harris, and V. Lestelle. 1988. Inpatient family intervention: A randomized clinical trial. II. Results at hospital discharge. *Arch. Gen. Psychiatry* 45:217–24.

Hamilton, M. 1960. A rating scale for depression. *J. Neurol. Neurosurg. Psychiatry* 25:56–62.

Hamilton, S., L. A. Mellman, G. O. Gabbard, M. E. Thase, and J. C. Markowitz. Psychotherapies in residency training. *J. Psychotherapy Practice and Research* 8:301–13.

Harrington, R., H. Fudge, M. Rutter, A. Pickles, and J. Hill. 1990. Adult outcomes of childhood and adolescent depression. *Arch. Gen. Psychiatry* 47:465–73.

Harrington, R. C., H. Fudge, M. L. Rutter, C. G. Bredenkamp, and J. Pridham. 1993. Child and adult depression: A test of continuities with family study data. *Br. J. Psychiatry* 162:627–33.

Heimberg, R. G., and D. H. Barlow. November 1991. New developments in cognitive-behavioral therapy for social phobia. *J. Clinical Psychiatry* 52 (suppl.):21–30.

Heimberg, R. G., M. R. Liebowitz, D. A. Hope, F. R. Schneier, C. S. Holt, L. A. Welkowitz, H. R. Juster, R. Campeas, M. A. Bruch, M. Cloitre, B. Fallon, and D. F. Klein. December 1998. Cognitive behavioral group therapy vs. phenelzine therapy for social phobia: 12-week outcome. *Archives of General Psychiatry* 55(12):1133–41.

Hellerstein, D., P. Yanowitch, and J. Rosenthal. 1993. A randomized double-blind study of fluoxetine versus placebo in treatment of dysthymia. *Am. J. Psychiatry* 150:1169–75.

Henderson, S. 1977. The social network, support, and neurosis: The function of attachment in adult life. *British Journal of Psychiatry* 131:185–91.

Henderson, S., P. Duncan-Jones, R. Scott, and S. Adcock. 1979. Psychiatric disorder in Canberra: A standardized study of prevalence. *Acta Psychiatrica Scandinavica* 60:355–74.

Henderson, S., P. Duncan-Jones, D. G. Byrne, R. Scott, and S. Adcock. 1980. Social relationships, adversity, and neurosis: A study of associations in a general population sample. *British Journal of Psychiatry* 136:574–83.

Hersen, M., and V. B. Van Hasselt. 1987. *Therapy with Children and Adolescents: A Clinical Approach.* New York: Wiley.

Higgins, E. S. 1994. A review of unrecognized mental illness in primary care. *Arch. Fam. Medicine* 3:908–17.

Hill, C. E., K. E. O'Grady, and I. Elkin. 1992. Applying the collaborative study psychotherapy rating scale to rate therapist adherence in cognitive-behavior therapy, interpersonal therapy, and clinical management. *J. Consult. Clin. Psychology* 60:73–79.

Hinrichsen, G. A. 1997. Interpersonal psychotherapy for depressed older adults. *J Geriatric Psychiatry* 30:239–57.

Hirschfeld, R.M.A., and C. K. Cross. 1983. Personality, life events, and social factors in depression. In *Psychiatric Update: The American Psychiatric Association Annual Review,* vol. 2, ed. Lester Grinspoon. Washington, D.C.: American Psychiatric Press.

Hirschfeld, R.M.A., M. T. Shea, and C. E. Holzer III. 1997. Personality dysfunction and depression. In *Depression: Neurobiological, Psychopathological and Therapeutic Advances,* vol. 3, ed Adriaan Honig and Herman M. van Praag, 327–41. Chichester: John Wiley & Sons.

Holland, J. C., and J. H. Rowland. 1989. *Handbook of Psychooncology.* New York: Oxford University Press.

Hollon, S. D., and R. J. DeRubeis. 1981. Placebo-psychotherapy combinations: Inappropriate representations of psychotherapy in drug-psychotherapy comparative trials. *Psychopharmacol. Bull.* 90:467–77.

Holmes, W. D., and K. D. Wagner. Fall 1992. Psychotherapy treatment for depression in children and adolescents. *Journal of Psychotherapy Practice and Research* 1(4):313–23.

Horowitz, M. J. 1976. *Stress Response Syndromes.* Northvale, N.J.: Jason Aronson.

Howard, K. I., S. M. Kopta, M. S. Krause, and D. E. Orlinsky. 1986. The dose-effect relationship in psychotherapy. *Am. Psychologist* 41:159–64.

Hsu, L. 1986. The treatment of anorexia nervosa. *Am J Psychiatry* 143:573–81.

Jacobson, E. 1929. *Progressive Relaxation.* Chicago: University of Chicago Press.

Jacobson, E. 1971. *Depression.* New York: International Universities Press, Inc.

Jacobson, G., and D. S. Jacobson. 1987. Impact of marital dissolution on adults and children: The significance of loss and continuity. In *The Psychology of Separation and Loss: Perspectives on Development, Life Transitions, and Clinical Practice,* ed. J. Bloom-Feshbach and S. Bloom-Feshbach, 316–44. San Francisco: Jossey-Bass.

Jacobson, N. S., K. Dobson, A. E. Fruzzetti, K. B. Schmaling, and S. Salusky. August 1991. Marital therapy as a treatment for depression. *Journal of Consulting & Clinical Psychology* 59(4):547–57.

Jacobson, N. S., K. Dobson, A. E. Fruzzetti, K. B. Schmaling, and S. Salusky. June 1993. Couple therapy as a treatment for depression: II. The effects of relationship quality and therapy on depressive relapse. *Journal of Consulting & Clinical Psychology* 61(3):516–19.

Jamison, K. R. 1995. *The Unquiet Mind.* New York: Alfred A. Knopf, Inc.

Jarrett, R. B., and A. J. Rush. May 1994. Short-term psychotherapy of depressive disorders: Current status and future directions. *Psychiatry: Interpersonal & Biological Preocesses* 47(2): 115–32.

Jensen, P. S., V. S. Bhatatra, B. Vitiello, K. Hoagwood, M. Feil, and L. B. Burke. 1999. Psychoactive medication prescribing practices for U.S. children: Gaps between research and clinical practice. *J. Am. Acad. Child Adolesc. Psychiatry* 38(5):557–65.

Kahn, D. A. 1993. The use of psychodynamic psychotherapy in manic-depressive illness. *J. Am. Acad. Psychoanal.* 21(3):441–55.

Kalichman, S. C. 1995. *Understanding AIDS: A Guide for Mental Health Professionals.* New York: American Psychological Association.

Kanas, N. 1993. Group psychotherapy with bipolar patients: A review and synthesis. *Int. J. Group Psychother.* 43(3):321–33.

Kandel, D. B., and M. Davies. 1982. Epidemiology of depressed mood in adolescents. *Arch. Gen. Psychiatry* 39:1205–12.

———. 1986. Adult sequelae of adolescent depressive symptoms. *Arch. Gen. Psychiatry* 43:255.

Kaplan, S., G. K. Hong, and C. Weinhold. 1984. Epidemiology of depressive symptoms in adolescents. *J. Am. Acad. Child Adolesc. Psychiatry* 23:91–98.

Karnofsky, D. A. 1949. *The Clinical Evaluation of Chemotherapeutic Agents in Cancer,* 191–205. New York: Columbia University Press.

Kashani, J. H., D. J. Burbach, and T. K. Rosenberg. 1988. Perception of family conflict resolution and depressive symptomatology in adolescents. *J. Am. Acad. Child Adolesc. Psychiatry* 27:42–48.

Kashani, J. H., G. A. Carlson, N. C. Beck, E. W. Hoeper, C. M. Corcoran, J. A. McAllister, J. A. Fallahi, T. K. Rosenberg, and J. C. Reid. 1987. Depression, depressive symptoms, and depressed mood among a community sample of adolescents. *Am. J. Psychiatry* 144:931–34.

Kashani, J. H., W. O. Shekim, and J. C. Reid. 1984. Amitriptyline in children with major depressive disorder: A double-blind crossover pilot study. *J. Am. Acad. Child Psychiatry* 23:348–51.

Kashani, J. H., and D. D. Sherman. 1988. Childhood depression: Epidemiology, etiological models and treatment applications. *Integrative Psychiatry* 6:1–21.

Keller, M. B. 1985. Chronic and recurrent affective disorders: Incidence, course, and influencing factors. In *Chronic Treatments in Neuropsychiatry*, ed. D. Kemali and F. Racagni, 111–20. New York: Raven Press.

Keller, M. B., P. W. Lavori, C. E. Lewis, and G. L. Klerman. 1983. Predictors of relapse in major depressive disorder. *JAMA* 250:3299–304.

Keller, M. B., P. W. Lavori, and T. I. Mueller. 1992. Time to recovery, chronicity, and levels of psychopathology in major depression: A five-year prospective follow-up of 431 subjects. *Arch. Gen. Psychiatry* 49:809–16.

Keller, M. B., and R. W. Shapiro. 1982. "Double depression": Superimposition of acute depressive episodes on chronic depressive disorders. *Am. J. Psychiatry* 139:438–42.

Keller, M. B., R. W. Shapiro, P. W. Lavori, and N. Wolfe. 1982a. Recovery in major depressive disorder: Analysis with the life table and regression models. *Arch. Gen. Psychiatry* 39:905–10.

———. 1982b. Relapse in major depressive disorder: Analysis with the life table. *Arch. Gen. Psychiatry* 39:911–15.

Kelly, J. A., D. A. Murphy, G. R. Bahr, S. C. Kalichman, M. G. Morgan, L. Y. Stevenson, J. J. Koob, T. L. Brasfield, and B. M. Bernstein. 1993. Outcome of cognitive-behavioral and support group brief therapies for depressed, HIV-infected persons. *Am. J. Psychiatry* 150:1679–86.

Kessler, R. C., K. A. McGonagle, C. B. Nelson, M. Hughes, M. Swartz, and D. G. Blazer. 1994a. Sex and depression in the national comorbidity survey. II: Cohort effects. *J. Affec. Disorders* (30)1:15–26.

Kessler, R. C., K. A. McGonagle, S. Zhao, C. B. Nelson, M. Hughes, S. Eshleman, H.-U. Wittchen, and K. S. Kendler. 1994b. Lifetime and 12-month prevalence of DSM-III-R psychiatric disorders in the United States: Results from the National Comorbidity study. *Arch. Gen. Psychiatry* 51:8–19.

Kestenbaum, C. J., and L. Kron. 1987. Psychoanalytic intervention with children and adolescents with affective disorders: A combined treatment approach. *J. Am. Acad. Psychoanal.* 15:153–74.

Klein, D. F., and D. C. Ross. 1993. Reanalysis of the National Institute of Mental Health treatment of depression collaborative research program general effectiveness report. *Neuropsychopharmacol* 8:241–51.

Klerman, G. L. 1990. Treatment of recurrent unipolar major depressive disorder. *Arch. Gen. Psychiatry* 47:1158–62.

———. 1991. Ideological conflicts in integrating pharmacotherapy and psychotherapy. In *Integrating Pharmacotherapy and Psychotherapy*, ed. B. D. Beitman and G. L. Klerman, 3–19. Washington, D.C.: American Psychiatric Press.

Klerman, G. L., S. Budman, D. Berwick, M. M. Weissman, J. Damico-White, A. Demby, and M. Feldstein. 1987. Efficacy of a brief psychosocial intervention for symptoms of stress and distress among patients in primary care. *Med. Care* 25(11):1078–88.

Klerman, G. L., A. DiMascio, M. M. Weissman, and E. Chevron. 1974. Treatment of depression by drugs and psychotherapy. *Am. J. Psychiatry* 131:186–91.

Klerman, G. L., and M. M. Weissman. 1992. Interpersonal psychotherapy. In *Handbook of Affective Disorders*, 2d ed., ed. E. S. Paykel, 501–10. London: Churchill Livingstone.

Klerman, G. L., and M. M. Weissman. 1993. *New Applications of Interpersonal Psychotherapy*. Washington: D.C.: American Psychiatric Press, Inc.

Klerman, G. L., M. M. Weissman, J. Markowitz, I Glick, P. J. Wilner, B. Mason, and M. K. Shear. 1994. Medication and psychotherapy. In *Handbook of Psychotherapy and Behavior Change*, 4th ed., ed. A. E. Bergin and S. L. Garfield, 734–82. New York: John Wiley.

Klerman, G. L., M. M. Weissman, B. J. Rounsaville, and E. Chevron. 1984. *Interpersonal Psychotherapy of Depression*. New York: Basic Books.

Klerman, G. L., M. M. Weissman, B. J. Rounsaville, and E. Chevron. 1997. *Interpersonal Psychotherapy of Depression*. Translated into Japanese by Hiroko Mizushima, Makoto Shimada, and Yutaka Ono. Tokyo: Iwasaki Gakujyutsa.

Klier, C., M. Muzik, and K. Rosenblum. May 1998. Interpersonal psychotherapy (IPT) adapted for the group setting in the treatment of postpartum depression: A pilot study. Presented at the American Psychiatric Association Annual Meeting, Toronto, Canada.

Kocsis, J. H., and A. J. Frances. 1987. A critical discussion of DSM-III dysthymic disorder. *Am. J. Psychiatry* 144:1534–42.

Kocsis, J. H., A. J. Frances, C. Voss, J. J. Mann, B. J. Mason, and J. Sweeney. 1988a. Imipramine and social-vocational adjustment in chronic depression. *Am. J. Psychiatry* 145:997–99.

Kocsis, J. H., A. J. Frances, C. B. Voss, J. J. Mann, B. J. Mason, and J. Sweeney. 1988b. Imipramine treatment for chronic depression. *Arch. Gen. Psychiatry* 45:253–57.

Kocsis, J. H., M. E. Thase, L. Koran, U. Halbreich, and K. Yonkers. 1994. Pharmacotherapy for "pure" dysthymia: Sertraline vs. imipramine vs. placebo. *Eur. Neuropsychopharmacol.* 4:204.

Koerner, K., S. Prince, and N. S. Jacobson. Summer 1994. Enhancing the treatment and prevention of depression in women: The role of integrative behavioral couple therapy. *Behavior Therapy* 25(3):373–90.

Koren, G., ed. 1994. *Maternal-fetal toxicology: A clinician's guide*. 2d ed. New York: Marcel Dekker.

Kovacs, M., T. L. Feinberg, M. A. Crouse-Novak, S. L. Paulauskas, and R. Finkelstein. 1984a. Depressive disorders in childhood, I: A longitudinal prospective study of characteristics and recovery. *Arch. Gen. Psychiatry* 41:229–37.

———. 1984b. Depressive disorders in childhood. II: A longitudinal study of the risk for a subsequent major depression. *Arch. Gen. Psychiatry* 41:643–49.

Kovacs, M., S. L. Paulauskas, C. Gatsonis, and C. Richards. 1988. Depressive disorders in childhood. III: A longitudinal study of comorbidity with and risk for conduct disorders. *J. Affective Disord.* 15:205–17.

Kovacs, M., A. J. Rush, A. T. Beck, and S. D. Hollon. 1981. Depressed outpatients treated with cognitive therapy or pharmacotherapy: A one-year follow-up. *Arch. Gen. Psychiatry* 38:33–39.

Kramer, E., and R. Feiguine. 1981. Clinical effects of amitriptyline in adolescent depression. *J. Am. Acad. Child Psychiatry* 20:636–44.

Kramer, R. A., V. Warner, M. Olfson, C. M. Ebanks, F. Chaput, and M. M. Weissman. 1998. General medical problems among the offspring of depressed parents: A ten-year follow-up. *J. Am. Acad. Child Adolesc. Psychiatry* 37(6):602–11.

Kroll, L., R. Harrington, D. Jayson, J. Fraser, and S. Gowers. 1996. A pilot study of continuation cognitive-behavioral therapy for major depression in adolescent psychiatric patients. *J. Am. Acad. Child Adolesc. Psychiatry* 35(9):1156–61.

Krupnick, J. 1984. Bereavement during childhood and adolescence. In *Bereavement: Reactions, Consequences, and Care*, ed. M. Osterweis, F. Solomon, and M. Green, 99–141. Washington, D.C.: National Academy Press.

Kupfer, D. J., E. Frank, and M. J. Perel. 1989. The advantage of early treatment intervention in recurrent depression. *Arch. Gen. Psychiatry* 46:771–75.

Last, C. G., D. H. Barlow, and G. T. O'Brien. 1984. Precipitants of agoraphobia: Role of streessful life events. *Psychological Reports* 54:567–70.

Lave, J. R., R. G. Frank, H. C. Schulberg, and M. S. Kamlet. 1998. Cost-effectiveness of treatments for major depression in primary care practice. *Arch. Gen. Psychiatry* 55(7):645–51.

Lebowitz, B. D., J. L. Pearson, L. S. Schneider, C. F. Reynolds III, G. S. Alexopoulos, M. L. Bruce, Y. Conwell, I. R. Katz, B. S. Meyers, M. F. Morrison, J. Mossey, G. Niederehe, and P. Parmelee. 1997. Diagnosis and treatment of depression in late life: Consensus statement update. *JAMA* 278:1186–90.

Lefkowitz, M. M., and E. P. Tesiny. 1985. Assessment of childhood depression. *J. Consult. Psychol.* 14:25–39.

Lewinsohn, P. M., G. N. Clarke, H. Hops, and J. Andrews. 1990. Cognitive-behavioral treatment for depressed adolescents. *Behavior Therapy* 21:385–401.

Liebowitz, J. H., and P. F. Kernberg. 1988. Psychodynamic psychotherapies. In *Handbook of Clinical Assessment of Children and Adolescents*, vol. 2, ed. C. J. Kestenbaum and D. T. Williams, 1045–65. New York: New York University Press.

Liebowitz, M. R., F. R. Schneier, R. Campeas, E. Hollander, J. Hatterer, A. J. Fyer, J. Gorman, L. Papp, S. Davies, R. Gully, and D. F. Klein. 1992. Phenelzine vs. atenolol in social phobia. *Archives of General Psychiatry* 49:290–300.

Lindemann, E. 1944. Symptomatology and management of acute grief. *American Journal of Psychiatry* 101:141–48.

Linehan, M. 1987. Dialectical behavior therapy for borderline personality disorder: Theory and method. *Bull. Menninger Clin.* 51:261–76.

Linehan, M. M. 1993. *Cognitive-Behavioral Treatment of Borderline Personality Disorder.* New York: Guilford.

Linehan, M. M., H. E. Armstrong, A. Suarez, D. Allman, and H. L. Heard. 1991. Cognitive-behavioral treatment of chronically parasuicidal borderline patients. *Arch. Gen. Psychiatry* 48:1060–64.

Linehan, M. M., D. A. Tutek, H. L. Heard, and H. E. Armstrong. 1994. Interpersonal outcome of cognitive behavioral treatment for chronically suicidal borderline patients. *Am. J. Psychiatry* 151:1771–76.

Lipsitz, J. D., A. J. Fyer, J. C. Markowitz, and S. Cherry. 1999. An open trial of interpersonal psychotherapy for social phobia. *American Journal of Psychiatry* 101:141–48.

Locke, H. J., and K. M. Wallace. 1959. Short marital-adjustment and prediction tests: Their reliability and validity. *Marriage & Family Living* 21:251–55.

Loranger, A. W., M. F. Lenzenweger, A. F. Gartner, et al. 1991. Trait-state artifacts and the diagnosis of personality disorders. *Arch. Gen. Psychiatry* 48:720–28.

Lorentzen, S. 1993. Referat fra Nordisk Psykoterapi-symposium i Reykjavik, Island, 5–8 August 1993. *Felles Nytt.* 3:10–12.

Luborsky, L. 1984. *Principles of Psychoanalytic Psychotherapy: A Manual for Support-ive/Expressive Treatment.* New York: Basic Books.

Maddison, D. 1968. The relevance of conjugal bereavement for preventive psychiatry. *British Journal of Medical Psychology* 41:223–33.

Maddison, D., and W. Walker. 1967. Factors affecting the outcome of conjugal bereavement. *British Journal of Psychiatry* 113:1057–67.

Malan, D. H. 1963. A Study of Brief Psychotherapy. London: Tavistock Publications.

Markowitz, J. C. Manual for Interpersonal Psychotherapy for Patients with Primary Dysthymic Disorder and Secondary Alcohol Abuse. Cornell University Medical College. Unpublished.

_____. 1993a. Comorbidity of dysthymia. *Psychiatric Annals* 23(11):617–24.

———. 1993b. Psychotherapy of the post-dysthymic patient. *Journal of Psychotherapy Practice and Research* 2:157–63.

———. 1994. Psychotherapy of dysthymia. *Am. J. Psychiatry* 151:1114–21.

_____. 1995. Teaching interpersonal psychotherapy to psychiatric residents. *Academic Psychiatry* 19:167–73.

———. 1998. *Interpersonal Psychotherapy for Dysthymic Disorder.* Washington, D.C.: American Psychiatric Press.

———. 2000. Learning the new psychotherapies. In *Treatment of Depression: Bridging the 21st Century,* ed. M. M. Weissman. Washington, D.C.: American Psychiatric Press.

Markowitz, J. C., G. L. Klerman, K. F. Clougherty, L. A. Spielman, L. B. Jacobsberg, B. Fishman, A. J. Frances, J. H. Kocsis, and S. W. Perry. 1995. Individual psychotherapies for depressed HIV-positive patients. *Am. J. Psychiatry* 152:1504–9.

Markowitz, J. C., G. L. Klerman, and S. Perry. 1992b. Interpersonal psychotherapy of depressed HIV-seropositive outpatients. *Hospital and Community Psychiatry* 43:885–90.

Markowitz, J. C., G. L. Klerman, S. W. Perry, K. F. Clougherty, and L. S. Josephs. 1993. Interpersonal therapy for depressed HIV-seropositive patients. In *New Applications of Interpersonal Therapy,* ed. G. L. Klerman and M. M. Weissman, 199–224. Washington, D.C.: American Psychiatric Press.

Markowitz, J. C., J. H. Kocsis, B. Fishman, L. A. Spielman, L. B. Jacobsberg, A. J. Frances, G. L. Klerman, and S. W. Perry. 1998. Treatment of HIV-positive patients with depressive symptoms. *Arch. Gen. Psychiatry* 55:452–57.

Markowitz, J. C., M. E. Moran, J. H. Kocsis, and A. J. Frances. 1992a. Prevalence and comorbidity of dysthymic disorder among psychiatric outpatients. *J. Affective Disord.* 24:63–71.

Markowitz, J. C., and S. W. Perry. 1990. AIDS: A medical overview for psychiatrists. In *Annual Review of Psychiatry,* vol. 9, ed. A. Tasman, S. Goldfinger, and C. A. Kaufmann, 574–92. Washington, D.C.: American Psychiatric Press.

Markowitz, J. C., J. G. Rabkin, and S. W. Perry. 1994a. Treating depression in HIV-positive patients. *AIDS* 8:403–12.

Markowitz, J. C., P. A. Scarvalone, L. A. Spielman, and S. W. Perry. 1994b. Adherence in psychotherapy for depressed HIV-positive patients. Presented at the meeting of the Society for Psychotherapy Research, York, England, July 1994.

Markowitz, J. C., M. Svartberg, and H. A. Swartz. 1998. Is IPT time-limited psychodynamic psychotherapy? *Journal of Psychotherapy Practice and Research* 7:185–95.

Markowitz, J. C., and H. A. Swartz. 1997. Case formulation in interpersonal psychotherapy of depression. In *Handbook of psychotherapy case formulation*, ed. T. D. Eels, 192–222. New York: Guilford.

Markowitz, J. C., and M. M. Weissman. 1999. Interpersonal psychotherapy. In *Therapies for Suicidal Behavior*, ed. D. Clark, J. Fawcett, and S. Hollon. Washington, D.C.: American Psychiatric Press.

Marks, I., and J. Michan. 1988. Dysmorphophobia avoidance with disturbed bodily perception: A pilot study of exposure therapy. *Br. J. Psychiatry* 152:674–78.

Marziali, E., and H. Munroe-Blum. 1994. *Interpersonal Group Psychotherapy for Borderline Personality Disorder.* New York: Basic Books.

Mason, B. J., J. Markowitz, and G. L. Klerman. 1993. IPT for dysthymic disorder. In *New Applications of Interpersonal Therapy*, ed. G. L. Klerman and M. M. Weissman, 225–64. Washington, D.C.: American Psychiatric Press.

McCullough, J. P. 1992. *The Manual for Therapists Treating the Chronic Depressions and Using the Cognitive-Behavioral Analysis System of Psychotherapy.* Virginia Commonwealth University. Unpublished manuscript.

McGee, R., M. Feehan, S. Williams, F. Partridge, P. A. Silva, and J. Kelly. 1990. DSM-III disorders in a large sample of adolescents. *J. Am. Acad. Child Adolesc. Psychiatry* 29:611–19.

McKenry, P. C., D. H. Browne, J. B. Kotch, and M. J. Symons. August 1990. Mediators of depression among low-income, adolescent mothers of infants: A longitudinal perspective. *Journal of Youth & Adolescence* 19(4):327–47.

Mechanic, D., and S. Hansell. 1989. Divorce, family conflict, and adolescents' well-being. *J. Health Soc. Behav.* 30:105–16.

Menninger, K. A., and P. S. Holzman. 1973. *Theory of Psychoanalytic Technique.* New York: Basic Books.

Merikangas, K., C. Ranelli, and D. Kupfer. 1979. Marital interaction in hospitalized depressed patients. *Journal of Nervous and Mental Disease* 167:689–95.

Merikangas, K. R., and D. G. Spiker. 1982. Assortative mating among in-patients with primary affective disorder. *Psychological Medicine* 12(4):753–64.Merikangas, K., and M. M. Weissman. 1986. Epidemiology of DSM-III Axis II personality disorders in psychiatry update. In *American Psychiatric Association annual review*, vol. 5, ed. A. Frances and R. Hales. Washington, D.C.: American Psychiatric Association.

Merikangas, K. R., W. Wich, and J. Angst. 1994. Heterogeneity of depression: Classification of depressive subtypes by longitudinal course. *Br. J. Psychiatry* 164:342–48.

Mermelstein, H. T., and J. C. Holland. 1991. Psychotherapy by telephone: A therapeutic tool for cancer patients. *Psychosomatics* 32(4):407–12.

Meyer, A. 1957. *Psychobiology: A Science of Man.* Springfield, Ill.: Charles C. Thomas.

Miklowitz, D. J. 1996. Psychotherapy in combination with drug treatment for bipolar disorder. *J. Clin. Psychopharmacol.* 16(2) Suppl. 1:56S–66S.

Miklowitz, D. J., E. Frank, and E. L. George. 1996. New psychosocial treatments for the outpatient management of bipolar disorder. *Psychopharmacol. Bull.* 32:613–21.

Miklowitz, D. J., and M. J. Goldstein. 1990. Behavioral family treatment for patients with bipolar affective disorder. *Behav. Modification* 14(4):457–89.

Miklowitz, D. J., M. J. Goldstein, and K. H. Nuechterlein. 1995. Verbal interactions in the families of schizophrenic and bipolar affective patients. *J. Abnorm. Psychol.* 104(2):268–76.

Miklowitz, D. J., M. J. Goldstein, K. H. Nuechterlein, K. S. Snyder, and J. Mintz. 1988. Family factors and the course of bipolar affective disorder. *Arch. Gen. Psychiatry* 45:225–31.

Miller, D. 1974. *Adolescence: Psychology, Psychopathology, Psychotherapy*. New York: Jason Aronson.

Miller, I. W., G. I. Keitner, N. B. Epstein, D. S. Bishop, and C. E. Ryan. 1991. Families of bipolar inpatients: Dysfunction, course of illness, and pilot treatment study. In *Proceedings of the 22nd meeting of the Society for Psychotherapy Research*, Pittsburgh, Society for Psychotherapy Research.

Miller, M. D., E. Frank, C. Cornes, S. D. Imber, B. Anderson, L. Ehrenpreis, J. Malloy, R. Silberman, L. Wolfson, J. Zaltman, and C. F. Reynolds III. 1994. Applying interpersonal psychotherapy to bereavement-related depression following loss of a spouse in late life. *J. Psychotherapy Practice and Research* 3:149–62.

Miller, M. D., and R. L. Silberman. 1996. Using interpersonal psychotherapy with depressed elders. In *A guide to Psychotherapy and Aging: Effective Clinical Interventions in a Life-Stage Context*, ed. S. H. Zarit and B. G. Knight, 83–99. Washington, D.C.: American Psychological Association.

Miller, M. D., L. Wolfson, E. Frank, C. Cornes, R. Silberman, L. Ehrenpreis, J. Zaltman, J. Malloy, and C. F. Reynolds III. 1998. Using interpersonal psychotherapy (IPT) in a combined psychotherapy/medication research protocol with depressed elders. *J. Psychotherapy Practice and Research* 7:47–55.

Miller, P., and J. G. Ingham. 1976. Friends, confidants and symptoms. *Social Psychiatry* 11:51–58.

Mintz, J., L. I. Mintz, M. J. Arruda, and S. S. Hwang. 1992. Treatments of depression and the functional capacity to work. *Arch. Gen. Psychiatry* 49:761–68.

Minuchin, S., B. L. Rosman, and L. Baker. 1978. *Psychosomatic Families: Anorexia Nervosa in Context*. Cambridge: Harvard University Press.

Moreau, D., L. Mufson, M. M. Weissman, and G. L. Klerman. 1991. Interpersonal psychotherapy for adolescent depression: Description of modification and preliminary application. *J. Am. Acad. Child Adolesc. Psychiatry* 30(4):642–51.

Mossey, J. M., K. Knott, and R. Craik. 1990. The effects of persistent depressive symptoms on hip fracture recovery. *J. Gerontol.* 45(5):M163–68.

Mossey, J. M., K. A. Knott, M. Higgins, and K. Talerico. 1996. Effectiveness of a psychosocial intervention, interpersonal counseling for subdysthymic depression in medically ill elderly. *J. Gerontol.* 51A(4):M172–78.

Mufson, L., and J. Fairbanks. 1996. Interpersonal psychotherapy for depressed adolescents: A one-year naturalistic follow-up study. *J. Am. Acad. Child Adolesc. Psychiatry* 35(9):1145–55.

Mufson, L., D. Moreau, M. M. Weissman, and G. L. Klerman. 1993. *Interpersonal Therapy for Depressed Adolescents*. New York: Guilford.

Mufson, L., D. Moreau, M. M. Weissman, P. Wickramaratne, J. Martin, and A. Samoilov. 1994. Modifications of interpersonal psychotherapy with depressed adolescents (IPT-A): Phase I and II studies. *J. Am. Acad. Child Adolesc. Psychiatry* 33(5):695–705.

Mufson, L., M. M. Weissman, D. Moreau, and R. Garfinkel. 1999. Efficacy of interpersonal psychotherapy for depressed adolescents. *Arch. Gen. Psychiatry* 56:573–79.

Müller-Popkens, K., and G. Hajak. 1996. Interpersonelle Psychotherapie zur Behandling von Patienten mit primärer Insomnie—Vorlaufige Daten zur polysomnographischen Makroanalyse. *Wien Med. Wochenschrift* 153:303–5.

Murray, C. L., and A. D. Lopez, eds. 1996. *The Global Burden of Disease*. World Health Organization. Distributed by Harvard University Press.

Murray, L., and P. J. Cooper. 1997. Editorial: Postpartum depression and child development. *Psychological Medicine* 27:253–60.

Murray, L., C. Stanley, R. Hooper, F. King, and A. Fiori-Cowley. 1996. The role of infant factors in postnatal depression and mother-infant interactions. *Developmental Medicine and Child Neurology* 38:109–19.

Musselman, D. L., D. L. Evans, and C. B. Nemeroff. 1998. The relationship of depression to cardiovascular disease: Epidemiology, biology, and treatment. *Arch. Gen. Psychiatry* 55:580–92.

Nissen, G. 1986. Treatment for depression in children and adolescents. *Psychopathology* 19:156–61.

Nulman, I., J. Rovet, D. E. Stewart, and J. Wolpin. 1997. Neurodevelopment of children exposed in utero to antidepressant drugs. *New England Journal of Medicine* 336:258–62.

Offer, D. 1969. *The psychological world of the teenager: A study of normal adolescent boys.* New York: Basic Books.

Offer, D., E. Ostrov, and K. I. Howard. 1981. The mental health professionals' concept of the normal adolescent. *Arch. Gen. Psychiatry* 38:149–52.

Offord, D. R., M. H. Boyle, and P. Szatmari. 1987. Ontario Child Health Study. II: Six-month prevalence of disorder and rates of service utilization. *Arch. Gen. Psychiatry* 44:832–36.

O'Hara, M. W., D. J. Neunobaer, and G. H. Zekoski. 1984. Prospective study of postpartum depression: Prevalence and predictive factors. *J. Abnorm. Psychol.* 93:158–71.

O'Hara, M. W., and S. Stuart. In press. Pregnancy and postpartum. In *Psychiatric Treatment of the Medically Ill*, ed. R. G. Robinson and W. R. Yates. New York: Marcel Dekker.

O'Leary, K. D., and S. R. Beach. February 1990. Marital therapy: A viable treatment for depression and marital discord. *American Journal of Psychiatry* 147(2):183–86.

O'Leary, K. D., J. L. Christian, and N R. Mendell. Spring 1994. A closer look at the link between marital discord and depressive symptomatology. *Journal of Social and Cilnical Psychology* 13(1):33–41.

Opdyke, K. S., C. F. Reynolds III, E. Frank, A. E. Begley, D. J. Buysse, M. A. Dew, B. H. Mulsant, M. K. Shear, S. Mazumdar, and D. J. Kupfer. 1996/1997. Effect of continuation treatment on residual symptoms in late-life depression: How well is "well"? *Depression and Anxiety* 4:312–19.

Orvaschel, H., M. M. Weissman, and K. K. Kidd. 1981. Children and depression: The children of depressed parents; The childhood of depressed patients; Depression in children. *J. Affective Disord.* 2:1–16.

Overholser, J. C., and D. M. Adams. 1997. Stressful life events and social support in depressed psychiatric inpatients. In *Clinical Disorders and Stressful Life Events*, ed. T. W. Miller et al. Madison, Conn.: International Universities Press.

Parker, G. 1979. Parental characteristics in relation to depressive disorders. *British Journal of Psychiatry* 134:138–47.

Parkes, C. M., and R. S. Weiss. 1983. *Recovery from Bereavement.* New York: Basic Books.

Parsons, T. 1951. Illness and the role of the physician: A sociological perspective. *American Journal of Orthopsychiatry* 21:452–60.

Pastuszak, A., B. Schick-Boschetto, C. Zuber, M. Feldkamp, M. Pinelli, S. Sihn, A. Donnenfield, M. McCormack, M. Leen-Mitchell, and C. Woodland. 1993. Pregnancy outcome following first-trimester exposure to fluoxetine (Prozac). *JAMA* 269:2246–48.

Paykel, E. S., J. K. Myers, M. N. Dienelt, G. L. Klerman, J. J. Lindenthal, and M. P. Pepper. 1969. Life events and depression: A controlled study. *Archives of General Psychiatry* 21:753–60.

Paykel, E. S., A. DiMascio, G. L. Klerman, B. A. Prusoff, and M. M. Weissman. 1976. Maintenance therapy of depression. *Pharmakopsychiatrie Neuropsychopharmakologie* 9:127–36.

Pearlin, L. I., and M. A. Lieberman. 1977. Social sources of emotional distress. In *Research in Community and Mental Health,* ed. R. Simmons. Greenwich, Conn.: JAI Press.

Peet, M., and N. S. Harvey. 1991a. Lithium maintenance: 1. A standard education programme for patients. *Br. J. Psychiatry* 158:197–200.

_____. 1991b. Lithium maintenance: 2. Effects of personality and attitude on health information acquisition and compliance. *Br. J. Psychiatry.* 158:200–204.

Phillips, K. A. 1991. Body dysmorphic disorder: The distress of imagined ugliness. *Am. J. Psychiatry* 148:1138–49.

Phillips, K. A., S. L. McElroy, P. E. Keck, J. I. Hudson, and H. G. Pope. 1994. A comparison of delusional and nondelusional body dysmorphic disorder in one hundred cases. *Pharmacol. Bull.* 30(2):179–86.

Polinsky, M. L., C. Fred, and P. A. Ganz. 1991. Quantitative and qualitative assessment of a case management program for cancer patients. *Health and Social Work* 16(3):176–83.

Post, R. M., D. R. Rubinow, and J. C. Ballenger. 1986. Conditioning and sensitization in the longitudinal course of affective illness. *Br. J. Psychiatry* 149:191–201.

Pratt, L. A., D. E. Ford, R. M. Crum, H. K. Armenian, J. J. Gallo, and W. W. Eaton. 1996. Depression, psychotropic medication, and risk of myocardial infarction: Prospective data from the Baltimore ECA follow-up. *Circulation* 94:3123–29.

Prigerson, H. G., A. J. Bierhals, S. V. Kasl, C. F. Reynolds III, M. K. Shear, J. T. Newsom, and S. Jacobs. 1996. Complicated grief as a disorder distinct from bereavement-related depression and anxiety: A replication study. *Am. J. Psychiatry* 153:1484–86.

Prigerson, H. G., E. Frank, S. V. Kasl, C. F. Reynolds, B. Anderson, G. Zubenko, M. S. Houch, C. J. George, and D. J. Kupfer. 1995. Complicated grief and bereavement-related depression as distinct disorders: Preliminary empirical validation in elderly bereaved spouses. *Am. J. Psychiatry* 152:22–30.

Prigerson, H. G., E. Frank, C. F. Reynolds, and C. J. George. 1993. Protective psychosocial factors in depression among spousally bereaved elders. *Am. J. Geriatric Psychiatry* 1:296–309.

Puig, J. S. 1995. Psicoterapia interpersonal (I). *Rev. Psiquiatría Fac. Med. Barna.* 22(4):91–99.

————. 1997. The European launch of interpersonal psychotherapy in the Tenth World Congress of Psychiatry. *Eur. Psychiatry* 12:46–48.

Puig-Antich, J., E. Lukens, M. Davies, D. Goetz, J. Brennan-Quattrock, and G. Todak. 1985. Psychosocial functioning in prepubertal major depression disorders, II: Interpersonal relationships after sustained recovery from the depressive episode. *Arch. Gen. Psychiatry* 42:511–17.

Puig-Antich, J., J. M. Perel, W. Luptakin, W. J. Chambers, M. A. Tabrize, J. King, R. Goetz, M. Davies, and R. L. Stiller. 1987. Imipramine in prepubertal major depressive disorders. *Arch. Gen. Psychiatry* 44:81–89.

Puig-Antich, J., and B. Weston. 1983. The diagnosis and treatment of major depressive disorder in childhood. *Annu. Rev. Med.* 34:231–45.

Rao, U., N. D. Ryan, B. Birmaher, R. F. Dahl, D. E. Williamson, J. Kaufman, R. Rao, and B. Nelson 1995. Unipolar depression in adolescents: Clinical outcome in adulthood. *J. Am. Acad. Child Adolesc. Psychiatry* 34(5):566–77.

Regier, D. A., W. E. Narrow, D. S. Rae, R. W. Manderscheld, B. Z. Locke, and F. K. Goodwin. 1993. The de facto U.S. mental and addictive disorders service system: Epidemiologic catchment area prospective one-year prevalence rates and services. *Arch. Gen. Psychiatry* 50:85–94.

Reinherz, H. Z., G. Stewart-Berghauer, B. Pakiz, A. K. Frost, B. A. Moeykens, and W. M. Holmes. 1989. The relationship of early risks and current mediators to depressive symptomatology in adolescence. *J. Am. Acad. Child Adolesc. Psychiatry* 28:942–47.

Reynolds, C. F., III, E. Frank, P. R. Houck, S. Mazumdar, M. A. Dew, C. Cornes, D. J. Buysse, A. Begley, and D. J. Kupfer. 1997. Which elderly patients with remitted depression remain well with continued interpersonal psychotherapy after discontinuation of antidepressant medication? *Am. J. Psychiatry* 154:958–62.

Reynolds, C. F., III, E. Frank, D. J. Kupfer, M. E. Thase, J. M. Perel, S. Mazumdar, and P. R. Houck. 1996a. Treatment outcome in recurrent major depression: A post-hoc comparison of elderly and midlife patients. *Am. J. Psychiatry* 1288–92.

Reynolds, C. F., III, E. Frank, J. M. Perel, S. D. Imber, C. Cornes, M. D. Miller, S. Mazumdar, P. R. Houck, M. A. Dew, J. A. Stack, B. G. Pollock, and D. J. Kupfer. 1999. Nortriptyline and interpersonal psychotherapy as maintenance therapies for recurrent major depression: A randomized controlled trial in patients older than fifty-nine years. *JAMA* 281:39–45.

Reynolds, C. F., III, E. Frank, J. M. Perel, S. D. Imber, C. Cornes, R. K. Morycz, S. Mazumdar, M. D. Miller, B. G. Pollock, A. H. Rifai, J. A. Stack, C. J. George, P. R. Houck, and D. J. Kupfer. 1992. Combined pharmacotherapy and psychotherapy in the acute and continuation treatment of elderly patients with recurrent major depression: A preliminary report. *Am. J. Psychiatry* 149:1687–92.

Reynolds, C. F., III, E. Frank, J. M. Perel, S. Mazumdar, M. A. Dew, A. Begley, P. R. Houck, M. Hall, B. Mulsant, M. K. Shear, M. D. Miller, C. Cornes, and D. J. Kupfer. 1996b. High relapse rates after discontinuation of adjunctive medication in elderly patients with recurrent major depression. *Am. J. Psychiatry* 153:1418–22.

Reynolds, C. F., III, E. Frank, J. M. Perel, M. D. Miller, C. Cornes, A. H. Rifai, B. G. Pollock, S. Mazumdar, C. J. George, P. R. Houck, and D. J. Kupfer. 1994. Treatment of consecutive episodes of major depression in the elderly. *Am. J. Psychiatry* 151:1740–43.

Reynolds, W. M., and K. I. Coats. 1986. A comparison of cognitive-behavioral therapy and relaxation training for the treatment of depression in adolescents. *J. Consult. Clin. Psychol.* 44:653–60.

Rhodes, J. E., and M. Woods. 1995. Comfort and conflict in the relationships of pregnant, minority adolescents: Social support as a moderator of social strain. *Journal of Community Psychology* 23(1):74–84.

Richman, N., J. E. Stevenson, and P. J. Graham. 1975. Prevalence of behavior problems in three-year-old children: An epidemiological study in a London borough. *J. Child Psychol. Psychiatry* 16:277–87.

Robbins, D. R., N. E. Allesi, and M. V. Colfer. 1989a. Treatment of adolescents with major depression: Implications of the DST and the melancholic clinical subtype. *J. Affective Disord.* 17:99–104.

———. 1989b. The use of the Research Diagnostic Criteria (RDC) for depression in adolescent psychiatric inpatients. *J. Am. Acad. Child Adolesc. Psychiatry* 21:215–55.

Rogers, C. R. 1951. *Client-centered therapy.* Boston: Houghton Mifflin.

Rohde, P., P. M. Lewinsohn, and J. R. Seeley. 1994. Response of depressed adolescents to cognitive-behavioral treatment: Do differences in initial severity clarify the comparison of treatments? *J. Consult. Clin. Psychol.* 62(4):851–54.

Rossello, J., and G. Bernal. 1996. Adapting cognitive-behavioral and interpersonal treatment for depressed Puerto Rican adolescents. In *Psychosocial Treatments for Child and Adolescent Disorders: Empirically Based Strategies for Clinical Practice,* ed. E. D. Hibbs and P. S. Jensen, 157–85. Washington, D.C.: American Psychological Association.

Rossello, J., and G. Bernal. 1999. The efficacy of cognitive-behavioral and interpersonal treatments for depression in Puerto Rican adolescents. *Journal of Consulting & Cinical Psychology* 67(5):734–45.Roth, A. D., and P. Fonagy. 1996. *What Works for Whom?* New York: Guilford.

Rothblum, E. D., A. J. Sholomskas, C. Berry, and B. A. Prusoff. 1982. Issues in clinical trials with the depressed elderly. *J. Am. Geriatrics Society* 30:694–99.

Rounsaville, B., and K. Carroll. 1993. Interpersonal psychotherapy for patients who abuse drugs. In *New Applications of Interpersonal Psychotherapy,* ed. G. L. Klerman and M. M. Weissman, 319–53. Washington, D.C.: American Psychiatric Press.

Rounsaville, B. J., W. Glazer, C. H. Wilber, M. M. Weissman, and H. D. Kleber. 1983. Short-term interpersonal psychotherapy in methadone-maintained opiate addicts. *Arch. Gen. Psychiatry* 40:629–36.

Rounsaville, B. J., T. R. Kosten, M. M. Weissman, and H. D. Kleber. 1986. A 2.5 year follow-up of short-term interpersonal psychotherapy in methadone-maintained opiate addicts. *Compr Psychiatry* 27:201–10.

Rounsaville, B. J., S. O'Malley, S. Foley, and M. M. Weissman. 1988. Role of manual-guided training in the conduct and efficacy of interpersonal psychotherapy for depression. *J. Consult. Clin. Psychology* 56:681–88.

Roy-Byrne, P. P., M. Geraci, and T. W. Uhde. 1986. Life events and the onset of panic disorder. *Am. J. Psychiatry* 143:1424–27.

Rutter, M., P. Graham, O. F.. Chadwick, and W. Yule. 1976. Adolescent turmoil: Fact or fiction. *J. Child. Psychol. Psychiatry* 17:35–56.

Ryan, N. D. 1990. Pharmacotherapy of adolescent major depression: Beyond TCA's. *Psychopharmacol. Bull.* 26:75–79.

Ryan, N. D., V. S. Bhatara, and J. M. Perel. 1999. Mood stabilizers in children and adolescents. *J. Am. Acad. Child Adolesc. Psychiatry* 38(5):529–38.

Ryan, N. D., V. Meyer, S. Dachille, D. Mazzie, and J. Puig-Antich. 1988a. Lithium antidepressant augmentation in TCA-refractory depression in adolescents. *J. Am. Acad. Child Adolesc. Psychiatry* 27:371–76.

———. 1988b. MAOIs in adolescent major depression unresponsive to tricyclic antidepressants. *J. Am. Acad. Child Adolesc. Psychiatry* 27:755–58.

Ryan, N. D., and J. Puig-Antich. 1986. Affective illness in adolescence. In *Psychiatry Update: The American Psychiatric Association Annual Review*, vol. 5, ed. A. J. Frances and R. E. Hales, 420–50. Washington, D.C.: American Psychiatric Press.

Ryan, N. D., J. Puig-Antich, P. Ambrosini, H. Rabinovich, D. Robinson, B. Nelson, S. Iyengar, and J. Twomey. 1987. The clinical picture of major depression in children and adolescents. *Arch. Gen. Psychiatry* 44:854–61.

Ryan, N. D., J. Puig-Antich, T. B. Cooper, H. Rabinovich, P. Ambrosini, M. Davies, J. King, D. Torres, and J. Fried. 1986. Imipramine in adolescent major depression: Plasma level and clinical response. *Acta Psychiatr. Scand.* 73:275–88.

Sargent, J. K., M. L. Bruce, L. P. Florio, and M. M. Weissman. 1990. Factors associated with one-year outcome of major depression in the community. *Arch. Gen. Psychiatry* 47:519–26.

Schneider, L. S., R. B. Sloane, F. R. Staples, and M. Bender. 1986. Pretreatment orthostatic hypotension as a predictor of response to nortriptyline in geriatric depression. *J. Clin. Psychpharmacol.* 6:172–76.

Schneier, F. R., J. Johnson, C. D. Hornig, M. R. Liebowitz, and M. M. Weissman. 1992. Social phobia: Comorbidity and morbidity in an epidemiologic sample. *Archives of General Psychiatry* 49:282–88.

Schou, M. 1997. Forty years of lithium treatment. *Arch Gen Psychiatry* 54:9–13.

Schulberg, H., M. Madonia, M. Block, J. Coulehan, C. Scott, E. Rodriguez, and A. Black. 1995. Major depression in primary care practice: Clinical characteristics and treatment implications. *Psychosomatics* 36:129–37.

Schulberg, H. C., M. R. Block, M. J. Madonia, P. Scott, E. Rodriguez, S. D. Imber, J. Perel, J. Lave, P. R. Houck, and J. L. Coulehan. 1996. Treating major depression in primary care practice. *Arch. Gen. Psychiatry* 53(10):913–19.

Schulberg, H. C., C. P. Scott, M. J. Madonia, and S. D. Imber. 1993. Applications of interpersonal psychotherapy to depression in primary care practice. In *New Applications of Interpersonal Psychotherapy*, ed. G. L. Klerman and M. M. Weissman. Washington, D.C.: American Psychiatric Press.

Schwartz, R. S., and J. Olds. 1997. Loneliness. *Harvard Rev. Psychiatry* 5:94–98.

Scott, J. 1995. Psychotherapy for bipolar disorder. *Br J Psychiatry.* 167:581–88.

Scott, J., and G. Ikkos. 1996. A pilot study of interpersonal psychotherapy for the treatment of chronic somatization in primary care. Presented at First Congress of the World Council of Psychotherapy, June 30–July 4, 1996, Vienna, Austria.

Shaffer, D., A. Garland, M. Gould, P. Fisher, and P. Trautman. 1988. Preventing teenage suicide: A critical review. *J. Am. Acad. Child Adolesc. Psychiatry* 27:675–87.

Shaila, M. 1995. *Shouldn't I Be Happy? Emotional Problems of Pregnant and Postpartum Women.* New York: Free Press.

Shain, B. N., M. Naylor, and N. Alessi. 1990. Comparison of self-rated and clinician-rated measures of depression in adolescents. *Am. J. Psychiatry* 147:793–95.

Shea, M. T., I. Elkin, S. D. Imber, S. M. Sotsky, J. T. Watkins, J. F. Collins, P. A. Pilkonis, E. Beckham, D. R. Glass, R. T. Dolan, and M. B. Parloff. 1992. Course of depressive symptoms over follow-up: Findings from the National Institute of Mental Health Treatment of Depression Collaborative Research Program. *Arch. Gen. Psychiatry* 49:782–87.

Shea, M. T., D. Glass, P. A. Pilkonis, J. Watkins, and J. Docherty. 1987. Frequency and implications of personality disorders in a sample of depressed outpatients. *J. Personality Disorders* 1:27–42.

Shea, M. T., P. A. Pilkonis, E. Beckham, J. F. Collins, I. Elkin, S. M. Sotsky, and J. P. Docherty. 1990. Personality disorders and treatment outcome in the National Institute of Mental Health Treatment of Depression Collaborative Research Program. *Am. J. Psychiatry* 147:711–18.

Shear, M. K., A. M. Cooper, G. L. Klerman, F. N. Busch, and T. Shapiro. 1993. A psychodynamic model of panic disorder. *Am. J. Psychiatry* 150:859–66.

Sholomskas, A. J., E. S. Chevron, B. A. Prusoff, and C. Berry. 1983. Short-term interpersonal therapy (IPT) with the depressed elderly: Case reports and discussion. *Am. J. Psychotherapy* 37:552–66.

Sifneos, P. E. 1979. *Short-Term Dynamic Psychotherapy*. New York: Plenum.

Simeon, J. E., V. F. Dinicola, H. B. Ferguson, and W. Copping. 1990. Adolescent depression: A placebo control fluoxetine study and follow-up. *Prog. Neuropsychopharm. Biol. Psy.* 14:791–95.

Sloane, R. B., F. R. Stapes, and L. S. Schneider. 1985. Interpersonal therapy versus nortriptyline for depression in the elderly. In *Clinical and Pharmacological Studies in Psychiatric Disorders*, ed. G. D. Burrow, T. R. Norman, and L. Dennerstein, 344–46. London: John Libbey.

Smucker, M. R., W. E. Craighead, L. W. Craighead, and B. J. Green. 1986. Normative and reliability data for the Children's Depression Inventory. *J. Abnormal Child Psychol.* 14:25–39.

Solé-Puig, J. 1995a. Psicoterapia interpersonal (I). *Rev. Psiquiatria Fac. Med. Barna* 22(4):91–99.

———. 1995b. Psicoterapia interpersonal (II). *Rev. Psiquiatria Fac. Med. Barna* 22(5):120–31.

Solé-Puig, J. 1997. The European launch of interpersonal psychotherapy in the Tenth World Congress of Psychiatry. *Eur. Psychiatry* 12:46–48.

Solé-Puig, J. 1998. *Psicoterapia interpersonal*. Barcelona: Masson.

Sotsky, S. M. May 1997a. Pharmacotherapy and psychotherapy response in atypical depression: Findings from the NIMH Treatment of Depression Collaborative Research Program. Presented as part of Symposium 73 at the American Psychiatric Association 150th Annual Meeting, San Diego, California.

———. 1997b. Therapeutic alliance in treatment outcome for depression. Presented as part of Symposium 13 at the American Psychiatric Association 150th Annual Meeting, San Diego, California.

Sotsky, S. M., D. R. Glass, M. T. Shea, P. A. Pilkonis, J. F. Collins, I. Elkin, J. T. Watkins, S. D. Imber, W. R. Leber, J. Moyer, and M. E. Oliveri. 1991. Patient predictors of response to psychotherapy and pharmacotherapy: Findings in the NIMH treatment of depression collaborative research program. *Am. J. Psychiatry* 148:997–1008.

Spanier, G. B. February 1976. Measuring dyadic adjustment: New scales for assessing the quality of marriage and similar dyads. *Journal of Marriage & the Family* 38(1):15–28.

Spinelli, M. G. 1997a. Interpersonal psychotherapy for depressed pregnant HIV-positive women: A pilot study. *Am. J. Psychiatry* 154:1028–30.

———. 1997b. Manual of interpersonal psychotherapy for antepartum depressed women (IPT-P). Available through Dr. Spinelli, Maternal Mental Health Program, Columbia University College of Physicians and Surgeons and New York State Psychiatric Institute, 722 West 168 St., Unit 14, New York, N.Y. 10032.

———. 1997c. Interpersonal psychotherapy for depressed antepartum women: A pilot study. *American Journal of Psychiatry* 154(7):1028–30.

Spinelli, M. G., and M. M. Weissman. 1997. The clinical application of interpersonal psychotherapy for depression during pregnancy. *Primary Psychiatry* 10:50–57.

Spitzer, R. L., J.B.W. Williams, M. Gibbon, and M. B. First. 1992. The Structured Clinical Interview for DSM-III-R (SCID): History, rationale and description. *Arch. Gen. Psychiatry* 49:624–29.

Spitzer, R. L., and J. Endicott. 1979. *Schedule for Affective Disorders and Schizophrenia— Lifetime Version*, 3d ed. New York: New York State Psychiatric Institute, Biometrics Research.

Spitzer, R. L., J. Endicott, and E. Robins. 1978. *Research Diagnostic Criteria (RDC) for a Selected Group of Functional Disorders*, 3d ed. New York: New York State Psychiatric Institute, Biometrics Research.

Steiner, M., G. Browne, J. Roberts, A. Gafni, C. Byrne, B. Bell, and E. Dunn. 1998. Sertraline and IPT in dysthymia: One-year follow-up. Poster presented at the Thirty-eighth Annual Meeting of the NIMH New Clinical Drug Evaluation Unit (NCDEU), Boca Raton, Florida, June 1998.

Stewart, J. W., F. M. Quitkin, P. J. McGrath, J. G. Rabkin, J. S. Markowitz, E. Tricamo, and D. F. Klein. 1988. Social functioning in chronic depression: Effect of six weeks of antidepressant treatment. *Psychiatr. Res.* 25:213–22.

Stone, M. 1989. The course of borderline personality disorder. In *Review of Psychiatry*, vol. 8, ed. A. Tasman, R. Hales, and A. Frances, 103–22. Washington, D.C.: American Psychiatric Press.

Strober, M. 1985. Depression in adolescents. *Psychiatric Annals* 16:375–78.

Strober, M., and G Carlson. 1982. Bipolar illness in adolescents with major depressive disorder: Clinical, genetic, and psychopharmacological predictors. *Arch. Gen. Psychiatry* 39:549–55.

Strober, M., M. De Antonio, C. Lampert, and J. Diamond. 1998. Intensity and predictors of treatment received by adolescents with unipolar major depression prior to hospital admission. *Depression* 7:40–46.

Strober, M., R. Freeman, and J. Rigali. 1990. The pharmacotherapy of depressive illness in adolescence, I: An open label trial of imipramine. *Psychopharmacol. Bull.* 26:80–84.

Strober, M., J. Green, and G. Carlson. 1981. Phenomenology and subtypes of major depressive disorder in adolescence. *J. Affective Disord.* 3:281–90.

———. 1997. Use of interpersonal psychotherapy for depression. *Directions in Psychiatry* 17:263–274.

Stuart, S. 1999. Interpersonal psychotherapy for postpartum depression. In *Postpartum Psychiatric Disorders*, ed. L. Miller, 143–62. Washington, D.C.: American Psychiatric Press.

Stuart, S., and V. Cole. 1996. Treatment of depression following myocardial infarction with interpersonal psychotherapy. *Annals Clin. Psychiatry* 8(4):203–6.

Stuart, S., and M. W. O'Hara. 1995a. Interpersonal psychotherapy for postpartum depression. *Journal of Psychotherapy Practice and Research* 4:18–29.

————. 1995b. Treatment of postpartum depression with interpersonal psychotherapy. *Arch. Gen. Psychiatry* 52:75–76.

Stuart, S., M. W. O'Hara, and M. C. Blehar. 1998. Mental disorders associated with childbearing: Report of the biennial meeting of the Marce Society. *Psychopharmacol. Bull.* 34:333–38.

Sullivan, H. S. 1953. *The Interpersonal Theory of Psychiatry*. New York: W. W. Norton.

Swartz, H. A., J. C. Markowitz, and M. G. Spinelli. 1997. Interpersonal psychotherapy of a dysthymic, pregnant, HIV-positive woman. *Journal of Psychotherapy Practice and Research* 6:165–78.

Targ, E. F., D. H. Karasic, P. N. Diefenbach, D. A. Anderson, A. Bystritsky, and F. I. Fawzy. 1994. Structured group therapy and fluoxetine to treat depression in HIV-positive persons. *Psychosomatics* 35:132–37.

Tennant, C., P. Bebbington, and J. Hurry. 1980. Parental death in childhood and risk of adult depressive disorders: A review. *Psychol. Medicine* 10(2):289–99.

Thase, M. E., D. J. Buysse, E. Frank, C. R. Cherry, C. L. Cornes, A. G. Mallinger, and D. J. Kupfer. 1997. Which depressed patients will respond to interpersonal psychotherapy? The role of abnormal EEG profiles. *Am. J. Psychiatry* 154:502–9.

Thompson, L. W., D. E. Gallagher, and J. S. Breckenridge. Comparative effectiveness of psychotherapies for depressed elders. *J. Consult. Clin. Psychol.* 55:385–90.

Van Hermert, A. M., M. W. Hengeveld, J. H. Bolk, H. G. Rooijmans, and J. P. Vanderbroucke. 1993. Psychiatric disorders in relation to medical illness among patients of a general medical outpatient clinic. *Psychol. Med.* 23(1):167–73.

Veale, D., A. Boocock, K. Gournay, W. Dryden, F. Shah, R. Willson, and J. Walburn. 1996a. Body dysmorphic disorder: A survey of fifty cases. *Br. J. Psychiatry* 169:1962.

————. 1996b. Body dysmorphic disorder: A cognitive behavior model and pilot randomized controlled trial. *Behav. Res. Ther.* 34(9):717–29.

Versiani, M. 1994. Pharmacotherapy of dysthymia: A controlled study of imipramine, moclobemide or placebo. *Neuropsychopharmacology* 10:298.

Viederman, M. 1995. Grief: Normal and pathological variants. *Am. J. Psychiatry* 152:1–4.

Walker, K., A. MacBride, and M. Vachon. 1977. Social support networks and the crisis of bereavement. *Soc. Sci. Med.* 11:35–41.

Waring, E. M., C. H. Chamberlaine, E. W. McCrank, C. A. Stalker, C. Carver, R. Fry, and S. Barnes. 1988. Dysthymia: A randomized study of cognitive marital therapy and antidepressants. *Can. J. Psychiatry* 33:96–99.

Warner, V., M. M. Weissman, M. Fendrich, P. Wickramaratne, and D. Moreau. 1992. The course of major depression in the offspring of depressed parents: Incidence, recurrence, and recovery. *Arch. Gen. Psychiatry* 49:795–801.

Warner, V., M. M. Weissman, L. Mufson, and P. J. Wickramaratne. 1999. Grandparents, parents, and grandchildren at high risk for depression: A three-generation study. *J. Am. Acad. Child Adolesc. Psychiatry* 38:289–296.

Wasson, J., C. Gaudette, F. Whaley, A. Sauvigne, P. Baribeau, and H. G. Welch. 1992. Telephone care as a substitute for routine clinic follow-up. *JAMA* 267:1788–93.

Weissman, M. M. 1993. The epidemiology of personality disorders. *Psychiatry Update*, vol. 3, ed. L. Grinspoon. Washington, D.C.: American Psychiatric Press.

Weissman, M. M., B. J. Rounsaville, and E. S. Chevron. 1982. Training psychotherapists to participate in psychotherapy outcome studies: Identifying and dealing with the research requirement. *American Journal of Psychiatry* 139:1442–46.

Weissman, A. N., and A. T. Beck. 1979. *The Dysfunctional Attitudes Scale*. University of Pennsylvania. Unpublished manuscript.

Weissman, M. M., R. B. Jarrett, and A. J. Rush. 1987. Psychotherapy and its relevance to the pharmacotherapy of major depression: A decade later(1976–1985). In *Psychopharmacology: The Third Generation of Pregress*, ed. H. Meltzer, 1059–69. New York: Raven Press.

Weissman, M. M., and J. C. Markowitz. 1994. Interpersonal psychotherapy: Current status. *Archives of General Psychiatry* 51:599–606.

Weissman, M. M., and E. S. Paykel. 1974. *The Depressed Woman: A Study of Social Relationships*. Chicago: University of Chicago Press.Weissman, M. M. 1995. *Mastering Depression Through Interpersonal Psychotherapy*. Available through the Psychological Corporation, Order Service Center, P.O. Box 839954, San Antonio, Tex. 78283–3954.

Weissman, M. M., and H. S. Akiskal. 1984. The role of psychotherapy in chronic depressions: A proposal. *Compr. Psychiatry* 25:23–31.

Weissman, M. M., and S. Bothwell. 1976. Assessment of social adjustment by patient self-report. *Arch. Gen. Psychiatry* 33:1111–15.

Weissman, M. M., and G. L. Klerman. 1993. Interpersonal counseling for stress and distress in primary care settings. In *New Applications of Interpersonal Psychotherapy*, ed. G. L. Klerman and M. M. Weissman. Washington, D.C.: American Psychiatric Press.

Weissman, M. M., and G. L. Klerman. 1977. The chronic depressive in the community: Underrecognized and poorly treated. *Compr. Psychiatry* 18:523–31.

———.1993. Interpersonal counseling for stress and distress in primary care settings. In *New Applications of Interpersonal Psychotherapy*, ed. G. L. Klerman and M. M. Weissman, 295–318. Washington, D.C.: American Psychiatric Press.

Weissman, M. M., R. G. Bland, G. Canino, C. Faravelli, S. Greenwald, H. G. Hwu, P. R. Joyce, E. G. Karem, C. K. Lee, J. Lellouch, J. P. Lepine, S. C. Newman, M. Rubio-Stipec, J. E. Wells, P. J. Wickramaratne, H. U. Wittchen, and E. K. Yeh. 1996. Cross-national epidemiology of major depression and bipolar disorder. *JAMA* 276: 293–99.

Weissman, M. M., G. D. Gammon, K. John, K. R. Merikangas, V. Warner, B. A. Prusoff, and D. Sholomskas. 1987a. Children of depressed parents: Increased psychopathology and early-onset major depression. *Arch. Gen. Psychiatry* 44:847–53.

———. 1987b. Psychotherapy and its relevance to the pharmacotherapy of major depression: A decade later (1976–1985). In *Psychopharmacology: The Third Generation of Progress*, ed. H. Y. Meltzer, 1059–69. New York: Raven.

Weissman, M. M., G. L. Klerman, B. A. Prusoff et al. 1981. Depressed outpatients: Results one year after treatment with drugs and/or interpersonal psychotherapy. *Arch. Gen. Psychiatry* 38:51–55.

Weissman, M. M., G. L. Klerman, B. A. Prusoff, D. Sholomskas, and N. Padian. 1981. Depressed outpatients: Results one year after treatment with drugs and/or interpersonal psychotherapy. *Arch. Gen. Psychiatry* 38:52–55.

Weissman, M. M., P. J. Leaf, M. L. Bruce et al. 1988. The epidemiology of dysthymia in five communities: Rates, risks, comorbidity, and treatment. *Am. J. Psychiatry* 145:815–19.

Weissman, M. M., and M. Olfson. 1995. Depression in women: Implications for health care research. *Science* 269:799–801.

Weissman, M. M., B. A. Prusoff, A. DiMascio, C. Neu, M. Goklaney, and G. L. Klerman. 1979. The efficacy of drugs and psychotherapy in the treatment of acute depressive episodes. *Am. J. Psychiatry* 136:555–58.

Weissman, M. M., V. Warner, P. Wickramaratne, D. Moreau, and M. Olfson. 1997. Offspring of depressed parents: 10 years later. *Arch. Gen. Psychiatry* 54:932–40.

Weissman, M. M., B. J. Rounsaville, and E. S. Chevron. 1982. Training psychotherapists to participate in psychotherapy outcome studies. *American Journal of Psychiatry* 139:1442–46.

Weissman, M. M., V. Warner, P. J. Wickramaratne, D. Moreau, and M. Olfson. 1997. Offspring of depressed parents: Ten years later. *Arch. Gen. Psychiatry* 54(10):932–40.

Wells, K. B., M. A. Burnam, W. Rogers, R. Hays, and P. Camp. 1992. The course of depression in adult outpatients: Results from the medical outcomes study. *Arch. Gen. Psychiatry* 49:788–94.

Wells, K. B., A. Stewart, R. D. Hayes, M. A. Burnam, W. Rogers, M. Daniels, S. Berry, S. Greenfield, and J. Ware. 1989. The functioning and well-being of depressed patients: Results of the medical outcomes study. *JAMA* 262:914–19.

Wells, V. E., E. Y. Deykin, and G. L. Klerman. 1985. Risk factors for depression in adolescents. *Psychiatr. Dev.* 3:85–108.

Whiffen, V. 1988. Vulnerability to postpartum depression: A prospective multivariate study. *J. Abnorm. Psychol.* 97:647–674.

Wickramaratne, P. J., and M. M. Weissman. 1998. Onset of psychopathology in offspring by development phase and parental depression. *J. Am. Acad. Child Adolesc. Psychiatry* 37(9):933–42.

Wilfley, D. E., W. S. Agras, C. F. Telch, E. M. Rossiter, J. A. Schneider, A. G. Cole, L. A. Sifford, and S. D. Raeburn. 1993. Group cognitive-behavioral therapy and group interpersonal psychotherapy for the nonpurging bulimic individual: A controlled comparison. *J. Consult. Clin. Psychol.* 61(2):296–305.

Wilkes, T.C.R., G. Belscher, A. J. Rush, and E. Frank. 1994. *Cognitive Therapy for Depressed Adolescents.* New York: Guilford.

Wittchen, U. 1994. Reliability and validity studies of the WHO-Compositive International Diagnostic Interview (CIDI): A critical review. *J. Psychiatr. Res.* 28:57–84.

Wolfson, L., M. Miller, P. Houch, L. Ehrenpreis, J. A. Stack, E. Frank, C. Cornes, S. Mazumdar, D. J. Kupfer, and C. F. Reynolds III. 1997. Foci of interpersonal psychotherapy (IPT) in depressed elders: Clinical and outcome correlates in a combined IPT/nortriptyline protocol. *Psychotherapy Research* 7:45–55.

Wolk, S. I., and M. M. Weissman. 1996. Psychiatric problems of women. In *Current Practice in Medicine,* ed. R. C. Bone, 12.1–12.8. New York: Churchill Livingstone.

Woody, G. E., L. Luborsky, A. T. McLellan, C. P. O'Brien, A. Beck, J. Blaine, I Herman, and A. Hole. 1983. Psychotherapy for opiate addicts: Does it help? *Arch. Gen. Psychiatry* 40:639–45.

Woody, G. E., A. T. McLellan, L. Luborsky, and C. P. O'Brien. 1985. Sociopathy and psychotherapy outcome. *Arch. Gen. Psychiatry* 42:1081–86.

Zaretsky, A. E., and Z. V. Segal. 1994/1995. Psychosocial interventions in bipolar disorder. *Depression* 2:179–88.

Zuckerman, D. M., B. A. Prusoff, M. M. Weissman, and N. S. Padian. 1980. Personality as a predictor of psychotherapy and pharmacotherapy outcome for depressed outpatients. *Journal of Consulting and Clinical Psychology* 48:730–35.

Index

Abraham, 269
Activities, diminished interest or
    pleasure in, 30
Affect, encouragement of, 67, 125–128,
    240–241, 422–426
Age, and depression, 2, 6
Agency for Health Care Policy and
    Research, Depression Guideline
    Panel, 36
Agras, W. S., 322
Alcohol, abuse of, 38, 161. *See also*
    Substance abuse and dependence
Allesi, N. E., 197–198
American Psychiatric Association (APA)
    diagnostic criteria, 36
    treatment guidelines for bipolar
        disorder, 268, 270
AMI. *See* Amitriptyline
Amitriptyline (AMI), 163–164, 178–179.
    See also Pharmacotherapy
Anorexia, 326–327
Antepartum depression, 300–302
Antidepressants, 7, 41–43, 196. *See also*
    Pharmacotherapy
Anxiety
    affects and interpersonal
        relationships, 127
    examples, 337–338
    panic disorder, 336–338
    posttraumatic stress disorder, 338–339
    social phobia. *See* Social phobia
    symptoms, 33, 37–38
APA. *See* American Psychiatric
    Association
Appetite, change in, 30–31

Appointments, patient misses or is late
    for, 145–147
Arieti, S., 7
Armstrong, H. E., 351
Arzt, 336, 372
Australia, 370
Austria, 370

Barber, J. P., 168
Basco, 272
Bauer, 371
Baugher, M., 197
BDD. *See* Body dysmorphic disorder
Beach, 263
Becker, 7
Behavioral family management, 271
Behavior change techniques
    decision analysis, 135–136
    directive, 133–135
    in integrative case example, 430–434
    role playing, 136–137
Bell, B., 192
Bemporad, J., 7
Bereavement. *See* Grief
Berg, Roland, 373
Bernal, G., 209
Berwick, D., 283
Bibring, 123
Bipolar disorder, 267–268, 278
    adaptation for treatment of, 272–276
    efficacy for treatment of, 277
    examples, 276–277
    as a mood disorder, 5
    in pregnant women, 277–278
    psychotherapies for, 270–272

rationale for treatment of, 268–270
symptoms, assessing in initial
    sessions, 37
Birmaher, B., 197
Blame, 142–143
Blatt, S. J., 168
Block, M. R., 280
Blom, M. B. J., 166, 372
Body dysmorphic disorder (BDD),
    341–344
Boocock, A., 342, 344
Borderline personality disorder (BPD),
    350–351
    adaptation for treatment of, 352–354
    efficacy for treatment of, 357–358
    examples, 354–357
Boston-New Haven study, 163–164
BPD. *See* Borderline personality
    disorder
Brazil, 370
Brent, D. A., 197
Browne, G., 192, 280, 282, 370–371
Budman, S., 283
Bulimia, 317
    adaptation for treatment of, 318–320
    efficacy for treatment of, 321–322, 326
    examples, 320–326
    group therapy for, 322
    rationale for treatment, 317–318
Byrne, C., 192

Canada, 370, 383
Cancer, therapy over the phone for
    patients with, 363–364
Carroll, 312
Casework in training, 380–383
Catharsis, 67, 127
CBT. *See* Cognitive behavioral therapy
Centers for Disease Control, 289
Ceroni, Giuseppe Berti, 371
Certification, 384, 397–399
Cherry, S., 332
Chevron, E. S., xi, 178–179, 371–372
Childbirth and pregnancy, 299, 306–307
    antepartum depression, adaptation
        for treatment of, 300–302
    antepartum depression, efficacy for
        treatment of, 302

examples, 301–302, 304–305
    postpartum depression, adaptation
        for treatment of, 303–306
    postpartum depression, efficacy for
        treatment of, 305
    rationale for treatment, 300
Chodoff, 7
Clarification techniques, 128–130, 246,
    426–430
Clarke, G. N., 196–197
Clarke Institute, 210
Clougherty, Kathleen, 289
Coats, K. I., 197
Cochran, 272
Cognitive behavioral therapy (CBT)
    bipolar disorder, 272
    bulimia, 321–322
    certification and quality control,
        397–399
    compared to Interpersonal
        Psychotherapy, 12, 164–168, 209,
        295–297, 318
    depressed adolescents, treatment of,
        197–198
    depression, treatment of, 3–4, 188
    extension to treatment of disorders
        beyond depression, 173
    social phobia, 330
Cohen, 7
Cole, A. G., 322
Cole, V., 347–348
Colfer, M. V., 197–198
Communication analysis techniques,
    130–131, 239–241, 434
Compulsive symptoms, 35–36
Concentrate, diminished ability to, 32
Conjoint treatment (IPT-CM), 223
    adaptation for, 224–225
    efficacy for, 263–266
    examples, 234, 252–262
    initial sessions, 225–232
    intermediate sessions, 232–238
    problems arising during therapy,
        246–252
    rationale for, 223–224
    techniques, 238–246
    termination sessions, 238
Conte, 21

Continuation treatment, 177
Control, loss of, 141
Cornell University Medical College,
    186, 188–190, 192–193, 289
Cornes, C., 175, 179, 182–183, 215,
    217–220
Costs
    of depression, 279
    finances and/or coverage of patient,
        158–159
    future of psychotherapy, 395–396
    primary-care patients, 279–282
Coulehan, J. L., 280
Couples, treatment of. *See* Conjoint
    treatment
Crisis management, depressed
    adolescents, 207–208

Davanloo, 416
DBT. *See* Dialectical behavior therapy
Death, recurrent thoughts of, 32
Decision analysis, 135–136, 241–242
Decisions, diminished ability to make,
    32
Demby, A., 283
De Mello, Marcelo Feijo, 370
Depersonalization, 35
Depressed adolescents
    adaptation for treatment of, 195,
        198–208
    efficacy for treatment of, 209–211
    examples, 208–209
    learning disabilities, 206–207
    medication, 203–204
    pregnant, 210–211
    protective service agencies, 206
    rationale for treatment of,
        195–196
    school, 205–206
    sexual abuse, 206
    sexual identity problems, 207
    substance abuse, 205
    suicide, 204
    treatments of, 196–198
    violent behavior, 204–205
Depressed HIV-positive patients,
    289–290
    adaptation for treatment of, 291–294

efficacy for treatment of, 295–297
    examples, 294–295
    rationale for treatment, 291
Depression
    adolescents. *See* Depressed
        adolescents
    biological v. psychological, 160
    childbirth and pregnancy, associated
        with. *See* Childbirth and
        pregnancy
    costs of, 279
    feelings of, 36
    genetic transmission of, 161
    HIV-positive patients. *See* Depressed
        HIV-positive patients
    and interpersonal deficits. *See*
        Interpersonal deficits
    and interpersonal role disputes. *See*
        Interpersonal role disputes
    manifested in therapy by patients,
        139–145
    and role transitions. *See* Role
        transitions
Depression, chronic. *See* Dysthmic
    disorder
Depression, clinical, 8
Depression, major
    and disability, 6
    and grief. *See* Grief
    incidence of, 6
    late-life. *See* Late-life depression
    manic. *See* Bipolar disorder
    medical causes of, 37
    recurring. *See* Recurrent major
        depression
    symptoms, 1–2, 5–6. *See also*
        Symptoms
    treatment, advances in, 7
    treatment, different approaches to,
        3–4, 10
Derealization, 35
DeRubeis, R. J., 179
Dew, M. A., 182–183, 217–220
Diagnosis
    conditions related to depression,
        36–38
    criteria for major depressive episode,
        29

dysthmic disorder, 186
grief, 62–64
initial sessions, 27
interpersonal deficits, 104
interpersonal role disputes, 75–76
role transition problems, 91–92
See also Symptoms
Dialectical behavior therapy (DBT), 351
Dickens, Charles, 73n
DiMascio, A., 178–179
Diminished abilities to think,
concentrate, or make decisions, 32
Directive techniques, 133–135
Disability, depression as cause of, 6
Diurnal variation, 35
Donnelly, 362
Dreams, 11
Drug abuse, 38, 198, 205. *See also*
Substance abuse and dependence
Dryden, W., 342, 344
Dunn, E., 192
Dysthmic disorder, 185–187
adaptation for treatment of, 188–190
distinguished from major depression,
5
efficacy for treatment of, 192–193
example, 191
as problem for therapy, 139–140
rationale for treatment of, 187–188

Eating disorders. *See* Anorexia; Bulimia
Education as part of therapy. *See*
Psychoeducation
Efficacy. *See* Research
Ehrenpreis, L., 215
Electroconvulsive therapy, 42
Elkin, I., 165
Energy, loss of, 32
Examples
antepartum depression, 301–302
appointments, patient misses, 147
bipolar disorder, 276–277
body dysmorphic disorder, 342–344
borderline personality disorder,
354–357
bulimia, 320–326
complaining patient, 150
conjoint treatment, 234, 252–262

delayed emergence of issues, 58–59
depressed adolescents, 208–209
depressed HIV-positive patients,
294–295
dysthmic disorder, treatment of, 191
early termination of therapy, patient's
desire for, 156
excessive dependence of patient, 151
exercises, 244
feelings of therapist toward patient,
153
financial concerns for the patient, 159
grief, 66, 68–72, 215–216
integrative case example, 403–434
interpersonal deficits, 105–106,
108–116
interpersonal role disputes, 80–88, 285
late-life depression, 215–216
myocardial infarction, depression
following, 347–348
panic disorder, 337–338
patient guide to Interpersonal
Psychotherapy, 368
postpartum depression, 304–305
recurrent depression, 180–181
role transitions, 95–101
social phobia, 331, 334–335
somatization disorder, 345–346
substance abuse, 313–314
telephone, therapy over the, 364–367
treatment contract, setting up the, 54
Exercises, 242–246
Exploratory techniques, 124–125,
420–422

Fairburn, Christopher, 123, 317–319, 321,
374
Families
and depression, 2
participation of significant other in
therapy, 154–155
single-parent and depressed
adolescents, 202–203
termination sessions with depressed
adolescents, 203
Family therapy
bipolar disorder, 271
depression, treatment of, 3

Fatigue, 32
Feldstein, M., 283
Foley, 169
Fonagy, P., 10, 374, 395
Foreign languages, Interpersonal
      Psychotherapy in, 369–374
Formats for therapy
   foreign languages, 369–374
   group. *See* Group therapy
   patient guide, 367–369
   telephone, 362–367
France, 371
Frank, E.
   bipolar disorder, 269, 272, 274–278
   focus on interpersonal themes, 169
   late-life depression, 215, 217–220
   psychotherapy, foundations of,
      8, 10
   recurrent major depression, 175, 179,
      181–183
Fraser, J., 198
Fromm-Reichmann, 7, 269
Future of Interpersonal Psychotherapy
   certification and quality control,
      397–399
   decline of psychotherapy, fighting
      the, 395–396
   psychotherapists of the future,
      396–397
   range of, 399–401
Fyer, A. J., 332

Gastrointestinal symptoms, 33
Gender, and depression, 2, 6, 185
Genetic transmission of depression,
   161
Germany, 371
Gillies, L., 210, 349, 352, 357–358, 362,
   369–370
Glick, 271
Goldstein, 271
Gorman, 362
Gournay, K., 342, 344
Gowers, S., 198
Grief
   abnormal, 62–63
   bereavement late in life, 220–221
   and bipolar disorder, 275

depressed adolescents, treatment of,
   200
diagnosis of, 62–64
examples, 66, 68–72, 403–416
initial sessions, 37, 48
normal, 61
overgrieving, 70–71
therapeutic relationship as therapy
   technique, 133
treatment, goals and strategies, 64–68
Grochocinski, V. J., 175, 179
Group therapy
   adaptation for, 361–362
   bulimia, 322–326
   postpartum depression, 305–306
   social phobia, 335
Guilt, feelings of inappropriate, 32

Hajak, G., 349
Handbook of Psychiatric Measures, 36
Harrington, R., 198
Harvard Community Health Plan,
   285–286
Harvey, 271
Health, attitudes regarding, 34
Heard, H. L., 351
Higgins, M., 286–287
Hinrichsen, 215, 217
HIV. *See* Human immunodeficiency
   virus
Hoencamp, E., 166, 372
Holder, D., 197
Holland, 362
Hollon, S. D., 179
Holzman, 123
Hopelessness, 140
Hops, H., 197
Houch, P., 215
Houck, P. R., 182–183, 217–220, 280
Hovaguimian, Theodore, 374
Human immunodeficiency virus (HIV)
   and depressed patients. *See*
      Depressed HIV-positive patients
   incidence of, 289
Hypersomnia, 31

Iceland, 371
Ikkos, G., 346

Imber, S. D., 165, 182–183, 217–220, 280
IMI. *See* Imipramine
Imipramine (IMI), 164–166, 179–181,
    183. *See also* Pharmacotherapy
Initial sessions, 27–28
    bipolar disorder, 274–275
    borderline personality disorder, 352
    bulimia, 319
    communication of diagnosis, 39
    conjoint treatment, 225–232, 252–257
    depressed adolescents, treatment of,
        198–200
    explaining depression and its
        treatment, 39–41
    explaining interpersonal factors and
        techniques of treatment, 51–53
    grief, examples of, 69
    integrative case example, 403–410
    interpersonal deficits, examples of,
        109–110, 114–116
    interpersonal inventory, 45–51
    interpersonal role disputes, examples
        of, 81, 84, 86–87
    medication, determining need for,
        41–43
    related diagnoses, consideration of,
        36–38
    role transitions, examples of, 95–97,
        99–100
    "sick role", giving the patient the,
        43–45
    symptoms, review of, 28–36
    teaching patients their role, 56
    therapy over the phone, 365
    treatment contract, setting the, 53–56
Insomnia, 31, 349–350
Intermediate sessions
    beginning the, 57–60
    bipolar disorder, 275–276
    borderline personality disorder,
        352–354
    conjoint treatment, 232–238, 257–261
    depressed adolescents, treatment of,
        200–203
    grief. *See* Grief
    integrative case example, 410–413
    interpersonal deficits. *See*
        Interpersonal deficits

interpersonal role disputes. *See*
    Interpersonal role disputes
    role transitions. *See* Role transitions
    therapy over the phone, 365–366
Interpersonal counseling (IPC), 280
    adaptation of, 283–285
    efficacy of, 285–287
Interpersonal deficits, 103–104
    bipolar disorder, 276
    depressed adolescents, treatment of,
        201–202
    diagnosis of, 104
    examples, 105–106, 108–116
    initial sessions, 48
    postpartum depression, 304
    treatment, goals and strategies of,
        104–108
    use of therapeutic relationship as
        therapy technique, 133
Interpersonal factors
    explaining to the patient, 51–53
    inventory of, 45–51, 230–231, 256
Interpersonal Psychotherapy of Depression,
    xi, 387
Interpersonal Psychotherapy (IPT)
    conjoint for depressed patients with
        marital disputes. *See* Conjoint
        treatment
    contrasted with other
        psychotherapies, 10–13, 164–168,
        209, 295–297, 318, 416–419
    development and design, xi, 4–5
    examples of. *See* Examples
    in foreign languages, 369–374
    formats for. *See* Formats for
        therapy
    future of. *See* Future of Interpersonal
        Psychotherapy
    initial sessions. *See* Initial sessions
    intermediate sessions. *See*
        Intermediate sessions
    maintenance form of. *See* Recurrent
        major depression
    and mood disorders. *See* Mood
        disorders
    outline, 22–25
    primary-care patients, treatment of.
        See Primary-care patients

problems commonly encountered in.
See Problems
research on. *See* Research
strategies, 19–21
techniques of. *See* Techniques
termination sessions. *See* Termination
sessions
theoretical and empirical
foundations, 7–10
therapist, role of in, 13–16
training in. *See* Training
Interpersonal role disputes, 75
bipolar disorder, 275–276
depressed adolescents, treatment of,
200–201
diagnosis of, 75–76
examples, 80–88, 285
initial sessions, 48
treatment, goals and strategies of,
76–79
use of therapeutic relationship as
therapy technique, 132–133
Interpersonal and Social Rhythm
Therapy (IPSRT), 274–278
IPC. *See* Interpersonal Counseling
IPSRT. *See* Interpersonal and Social
Rhythm Therapy
IPT-CM. *See* Conjoint treatment
Italy, 371
ITP. *See* Interpersonal Psychotherapy

Jacobson, 263, 335
Japan, 372
Jarrett, R. B., 21, 169, 175, 179
Jayson, D., 198
Johnson, B., 197
Jonker, Kosse, 372
Joyce, Peter, 373
Judd, Fiona, 369–370

Kalichman, S. C., 292
Kingsley Communications, 383
Klein, 165
Klerman, G. L.
depressed adolescents, 195, 198,
203
depressed HIV-positive patients, 289,
295

development of Interpersonal
Psychotherapy, xi, 21
interpersonal counseling, 283
maintenance therapy, 178–179
research and treatment, 400
training and quality control, 397–398
translation into foreign languages,
371–372
Klier, C., 305–306, 362, 370
Knott, K. A., 286–287
Kolko, D., 197
Kölling, Pieternel, 373
Kornbluth, 362
Kraan, Herro, 372–373
Kroll, L., 198
Krupnick, J., 338, 362
Kupfer, D. J., 175, 179, 181–183, 215,
217–220

Late-life depression, 213
adaptation for treatment of, 214–215
bereavement, 220–221
efficacy for treatment of, 217–220
example, 215–216
rationale for treatment, 214
Lave, J., 280
Learning disabilities, and depressed
adolescents, 206–207
Levels of intervention, 419–420
Lewinsohn, P. M., 196–197
Linehan, M. M., 351
Lipsitz, J. D., 330, 332, 335
Luborsky, L., 193
Lundbeck International Psychiatric
Institute, 383

McAnanama, 349
McEachran, A. B., 175, 179
McKenzie, Janice, 327
Madonia, M. J., 280
Maintenance therapy, 177–178. *See also*
Recurrent major depression
Malan, 416
Mallinger, A. G., 175, 179
Manic depression. *See* Bipolar disorder
Marital disputes
assessing relation to depression,
226–230

conjoint treatment for depressed patients with. *See* Conjoint treatment

examples, 80–86, 95–99, 180–181, 234, 252–262, 337–338

extramarital affairs, 247, 259

as focus of therapy, 48

grievances to renegotiation, moving from, 231–232

marital role contract, renegotiating, 237–238

transgressions, dealing with, 251–252

Markowitz, J. C., 21, 289, 295, 302, 311, 332, 369

Marks, I., 342

Martin, Elizabeth, 374

Martin, S., 166, 374

Mastering Depression: A Patient's Guide to Interpersonal Psychotherapy, 49, 138, 367–369

Mayers, Aviva, 373

Mazumdar, S., 182–183, 215, 217–220

Medical conditions, and depression. *See* Primary-care patients

Melancholic features specifier, 42

Memorial Sloan-Kettering Cancer Center, 362

Menninger, 123

Meyer, Adolf, 7

MI. *See* Myocardial infarction

Miklowitz, 271

Miller, M. D., 182–183, 215, 217–220, 271

Mood, 29–30

Mood disorders

adaptation for treatment of, 173–174

bipolar disorder. *See* Bipolar disorder

childbirth and pregnancy, depression associated with. *See* Childbirth and pregnancy

chronic depression. *See* Dysthmic disorder

defined, 5

depressed adolescents. *See* Depressed adolescents

depressed HIV-positive patients. *See* Depressed HIV-positive patients

late-life depression. *See* Late-life depression

recurrent major depression. *See* Recurrent major depression

Moreau, D., 195, 198, 203, 210

Mossey, J. M., 286–287

Muenz, L. R., 168

Mufson, L., 21, 195, 198, 203, 209–210, 362

Müller-Popkes, K., 349, 371

Myocardial infarction (MI), depression following, 346–348

Nancy Pritzker Network, 192

National Alliance of the Mentally Ill, 272

National Depressive and Manic Depressive Association, 272

National Institute of Mental Health (NIMH)

funding of research, 192

Treatment of Depression Collaborative Research Program (TDCRP), 164–168, 295, 297

Netherlands, the, 166, 372, 383

Neuroimaging, 166–167

New Zealand, 373

NIMH. *See* National Institute of Mental Health

Nortriptyline, 182, 215, 217–218, 280–281. *See also* Pharmacotherapy

Norway, 373

Obsessional symptoms, 35–36

O'Hara, M. W., 303–306, 307n, 330, 333, 335, 362

O'Leary, 263

Ono, Yutaka, 372

Opdyke, 220

Oskarsson, H., 371

Paranoid symptoms, 35

Parents, and depressed adolescents, 199–201

Parsons, Talcott, 43

Patients

and alcohol abuse, 161

appointments, missing or late for, 145–147

biological depression, concern regarding, 160

complaining or uncooperative, 150
depressed adolescents. *See* Depressed
    adolescents
with dysthmic disorder, 185–186
early termination of therapy desired
    by, 155–156
elderly. *See* Late-life depression
excessively dependent, 150–151
finances or limited insurance
    coverage, 158–159
genetic transmission of depression to
    children, concern regarding, 161
guide to Interpersonal
    Psychotherapy, 367–369
HIV-positive and depressed. *See*
    Depressed HIV-positive patients
insight into condition, 34
interpersonal problem areas. *See*
    Problem areas
with physical disabilities, 348–349
primary-care and medically ill. *See*
    Primary-care patients
problems of depression manifested in
    therapy, 139–145
role in Interpersonal Psychotherapy,
    56
self-disclosure, problems with, 157
"sick role," 43–45
silent in therapy sessions, 147–149
subject, changes or avoids, 149–150
suicidal, 144–145
symptoms. *See* Symptoms
therapist, relationship with. *See*
    Patient-therapist relations
Patient-therapist relations
interpersonal deficits, 106–107
in Interpersonal Psychotherapy, 13–16
powerful feelings of therapist toward
    the patient, 152–153
sabotaging of treatment by the
    patient, 151–152
substituting of therapist for family or
    friends, 145
therapeutic relationship, use of as
    therapy technique, 131–133
Peet, 271
Perel, J. M., 175, 179, 181–183, 217–220,
    280

Pergami, Andrea, 372
Perry, Samuel, 289, 295
Personality, 12–13
Pessimism, of one or both spouses in
    conjoint treatment, 246–249
Pharmacotherapy, 7, 41–43
amitriptyline, 163–164, 178–179
bipolar disorder, 173, 268
borderline personality disorder,
    350–351
bulimia, 317
depressed adolescents, 196, 203–204
dysthmic disorder, 187
imipramine, 164–166, 179–181, 183
late-life depression, 213–214, 217–220
nortriptyline, 182, 215, 217–218,
    280–281
pregnant women, 300
recurring depression, 176
social phobia, 330
Phillips, K. A., 341
Physical disabilities, depressed patients
    with, 348–349
Physical examination, 28
Pilokonis, P. A., 168
Pollock, B. G., 182–183, 217–220
Postpartum depression, 303–306
Posttraumatic stress disorder (PTSD),
    338–339
Pregnancy, depression associated with.
    See Childbirth and pregnancy
Prien, R. F., 169, 175
Primary-care patients, 279–280
adaptation for treatment of, 280
cost-effectiveness for treatment of,
    282
efficacy for treatment of, 280–281
See also Interpersonal counseling
    (IPC)
Problem areas, 20–21
commonly encountered by patients,
    47–50
grief. *See* Grief
interpersonal deficits. *See*
    Interpersonal deficits
interpersonal role disputes. *See*
    Interpersonal role disputes
loss of health, 348

role transitions. *See* Role transitions
syndromes other than depression,
   application to, 174
Problems
  alternative treatment sought by
   patient, 158
  appointments, patient misses or is
   late for, 145–147
  common patient concerns, 159–161
  complaining or uncooperative
   patient, 150
  early termination of therapy desired
   by patient, 155–156
  excessively dependent patient,
   150–151
  finances or insurance coverage of
   patient, 158–159
  patient's manifestations of
   depression, 139–145
  pessimism in conjoint treatment,
   246–249
  relations between partners in conjoint
   therapy, 249–250
  sabotaging of treatment by patient,
   151–152
  self-disclosure, patient problems
   with, 157
  significant other, participation of,
   154–155
  silence, 147–149
  stalled, therapy is, 250–251
  subjects, patient changes or avoids,
   149–150
  substitution of therapist for family or
   friends, 145
  therapist's feelings towards the
   patient, 152–153
  transgressions, dealing with in
   conjoint treatment, 251–252
Prophylactic therapy, 177
Psychoeducation
  bipolar disorder, 271
  conjoint treatment, 254
  in initial sessions, 39–41, 51–53, 56
  techniques, 137–138
Psychomotor agitation or retardation,
  31–32
Psychotic symptoms, 42

PTSD. *See* Posttraumatic stress
  disorder
Pull, Charles, 371

Rand Medical Outcomes Study, 185
Recurrent major depression, 175–176,
  182–183
  adaptation for treatment of,
   179–180
  efficacy for treatment of, 181–182
  rationale for maintenance therapy,
   176–179
Relationship Management Therapy
  (RPT), 357
Research, 9–10
  antepartum depression, 302
  bipolar disorder, 277
  Boston-New Haven study, 163–164
  bulimia, 321–322, 326
  Columbia study, 363–364
  conjoint treatment, 263–266
  depressed adolescents, treatment of,
   209–211
  depressed HIV-positive patients,
   295–297
  Dutch studies, 166
  dysthmic disorder, treatment of, 188,
   192–193
  future directions, 399–401
  interpersonal counseling, 285–287
  late-life depression, 213, 215,
   217–220
  Memorial Sloan-Kettering Study,
   362–363
  National Institute of Mental Health
   Treatment of Depression
   Collaborative Research Program,
   164–168
  neuroimaging, 166–167
  primary-care patients, 280–282
  recurrent major depression,
   maintenance treatment of,
   178–183
  response, predictors of, 167–169
  substance abuse, 314–315
Reynolds, C. F., III, 182–183, 215
Reynolds, W. M., 197, 217–220
Rivera, 209

RMT. *See* Relationship Management
Therapy
Robbins, D. R., 197–198
Roberts, J., 192
Rodriguez, E., 280
Role disputes. *See* Interpersonal role
disputes
Role playing, 136–137
Role transitions, 89–91
and bipolar disorder, 276
depressed adolescents, treatment of,
201
diagnosis of, 91–92
examples, 95–101
initial sessions, 48
postpartum depression, 304
treatment, planning for,
92–95
Rosello, J., 209
Ross, 165
Rossiter, E. M., 322
Roth, A. D., 10, 374, 395
Rothblum, 213, 217
Roth, C., 197
Rounsaville, B. J., xi, 21, 312, 314,
371–372, 387
Rush, 21, 272

Schools, and depressed adolescents,
199, 205–206
Schramm, E., 349, 371
Schulberg, H. C., 280
Scott, J., 346
Scott, P., 280
Self-help, for bipolar disorder, 272
Seminars on Interpersonal
Psychotherapy, 377–380
Sexual abuse, and depressed
adolescents, 206
Sexual identity, and depressed
adolescents, 207
Sexual symptoms, 34
Shah, F., 342, 344
Shea, M. T., 165, 168
Sholomskas, 214
Sick role, 43–45
Sifford, L. A., 322
Sifneos, 416

Significant others, participation in
therapy, 154–155
Sloane, 213, 217
Social phobia, 329–330
adaptation for treatment of,
330–331
efficacy for treatment of, 335
examples, 331, 334–335
group therapy, 335
rationale for treatment, 330
treatment of compared to treatment
for depression, 331–334
Solé-Puig, Jose, 373
Somatic symptoms, general, 33
Somatization disorder, 344–346
Sophocles, 70
Sotsky, 167, 169
Spain, 373
Spinelli, M. G., 300, 302, 307n
Stack, J. A., 182–183, 215, 217–220
Steiner, M., 192, 280–282
Stuart, S.
myocardial infarction, depression
following, 347–348
postpartum depression, 303–306,
307n
social phobia, 330, 333, 335
somatization disorder, 344–346
Substance abuse and dependence,
311–312
adaptation for treatment of, 312–314
assessing in initial sessions, 38
depressed adolescents, 205
efficacy for treatment of, 314–315
examples, 313–314
rationale for treatment, 312
Sughondhabirom, 374
Suicide, 144–145
bipolar disorder, 268
depressed adolescents, 204
pharmacotherapy, 42
thoughts about as symptom,
32
Sullivan, Harry Stack, 7
Svartberg, Martin, 373
Swartz, H. A., 302
Sweden, 373
Switzerland, 374

Symptoms
  of grief, 62–63
  psychotic, 42
  review of, 28–36
  See also Depression, major, symptoms;
    Diagnosis

TDCRP. *See* National Institute of Mental
  Health, Treatment of Depression
  Collaboration Research Program
Techniques, 123, 238
  adjunctive, 137
  behavior change, 133–137, 430–434
  clarification, 128–130, 246, 426–430
  communication analysis, 130–131,
    239–241, 434
  decision analysis, 135–136, 241–242
  directive, 133–135
  encouragement of affect, 125–128,
    240–241, 422–426
  exercises, 242–246
  explaining to patient, 137–138
  exploratory, 124–125, 420–422
  role playing, 136–137
  therapeutic relationship, use of the,
    131–133, 434
Telch, C. F., 322
Telephone, as vehicle for therapy,
  362–367
Termination sessions, 117–120
  bipolar disorder, 276
  borderline personality disorder,
    354
  conjoint treatment, 261–262
  depressed adolescents, treatment of,
    203
  difficulties with termination, 120–121
  grief, examples of, 70
  integrative case example, 414–415
  interpersonal deficits, examples of,
    112–113, 116
  interpersonal role disputes, examples
    of, 83, 85–86, 88
  long-term treatment, indications for,
    121
  role transitions, examples of, 98–99,
    101
  therapy over the phone, 366

Termination of therapy, premature,
    155–156
Thailand, 374
Thase, M. E., 169, 175, 179, 219
Therapeutic relationship, use of as
    therapy technique, 131–133
Therapies
  behavioral family management,
    271
  biological psychiatry, 3
  cognitive behavioral. *See* Cognitive
    behavioral therapy (CBT)
  dialectical behavior, 351
  electroconvulsive, 42
  family. *See* Family therapy
  group. *See* Group therapy
  Interpersonal Psychotherapy. *See*
    Interpersonal Psychotherapy (IPT)
  Interpersonal and Social Rhythm
    Therapy (IPSRT), 274–278
  psychoanalysis, 3
  radical feminist, 3–4
  Relationship Management Therapy
    (RPT), 357
Therapists
  of the future, 396–397
  patients, relationship with. *See*
    Patient-therapist relations
  termination of treatment, difficulties
    with, 121
Think, diminished ability to, 32
Training, 375–377
  casework, 380–383
  certification, 384
  evaluation methods, 381–382
  informal, 385
  seminars, 377–380
  tapes, 383
  training centers, 385–386
  written material, 377, 383–384
Transference, 14
Treatment contract, 53–56, 137
Treatment manuals, 386–387
  developing, 390–393
  for particular populations, 387–389
Tutek, D. A., 351

United Kingdom, 374

van Bemmel, Alex, 373
van Rijsoort, M., 336, 372–373
Veale, D., 342, 344
Violent behavior, depressed
    adolescents, 204–205

Weight, change in, 30–31
Weissman, M. M.
    depressed adolescents, 195, 198, 203,
        210
    depressed mothers, 306
    development of Interpersonal
        Psychotherapy, xi, 21
    patient guide to Interpersonal
        Psychotherapy, 367, 369
    social phobia, 335
    training and quality control, 398
    translation into foreign languages,
        371–372
Wilfley, D. E., 322, 361

Willson, R., 342, 344
Wolfson, L., 215
Women
    bipolar disorder in, 277–278
    childbirth and pregnancy, depression
        associated with. *See* Childbirth and
        pregnancy
    depressed HIV-positive patients and
        desire to have a child, 297–298n
    depression in, 2, 6, 185, 300
    eating disorders. *See* Anorexia;
        Bulimia
    treatment during pregnancy and
        nursing, 282
Woody, 315
World Bank, depression and disability,
    6
World Health Organization, depression
    and disability, 6
Worthlessness, feelings of, 32